Pet-Based Novel Imaging Techniques with Recently Introduced Radiotracers

Editors

MONA-ELISABETH REVHEIM
ABASS ALAVI

PET CLINICS

www.pet.theclinics.com

Consulting Editor
ABASS ALAVI

April 2021 • Volume 16 • Number 2

ELSEVIER

1600 John F. Kennedy Boulevard • Suite 1800 • Philadelphia, Pennsylvania, 19103-2899

http://www.pet.theclinics.com

PET CLINICS Volume 16, Number 2
April 2021 ISSN 1556-8598, ISBN-13: 978-0-323-78957-8

Editor: John Vassallo (j.vassallo@elsevier.com)
Developmental Editor: Karen Solomon

PET Clinics (ISSN 1556-8598) is published quarterly by Elsevier Inc., 360 Park Avenue South, New York, NY 10010-1710. Months of issue are January, April, July, and October. Periodicals postage paid at New York, NY, and additional mailing offices. Subscription prices per year are $254.00 (US individuals), $501.00 (US institutions), $100.00 (US students), $282.00 (Canadian individuals), $514.00 (Canadian institutions), $100.00 (Canadian students), $275.00 (foreign individuals), $514.00 (foreign institutions), and $140.00 (foreign students). To receive student and resident rate, orders must be accompanied by name of affiliated institution, date of term, and the signature of program/residency coordinator on institution letterhead. Orders will be billed at individual rate until proof of status is received. Foreign air speed delivery is included in all Clinics subscription prices. All prices are subject to change without notice. POSTMASTER: Send address changes to PET Clinics, Elsevier Health Sciences Division, Subscription Customer Service, 3251 Riverport Lane, Maryland Heights, MO 63043. **Customer Service: 1-800-654-2452 (U.S. and Canada); 314-447-8871 (outside U.S. and Canada). Fax: 314-447-8029. E-mail: journalscustomerservice-usa@elsevier.com (for print support); journalsonlinesupport-usa@elsevier.com (for online support).**

Reprints. For copies of 100 or more of articles in this publication, please contact the Commercial Reprints Department, Elsevier Inc., 360 Park Avenue South, New York, NY 10010-1710. Tel.: 212-633-3874; Fax: 212-633-3820; E-mail: reprints@elsevier.com.

Printed in the United States of America.

PET Clinics is covered in MEDLINE/PubMed (Index Medicus).

Contributors

CONSULTING EDITOR

ABASS ALAVI, MD, MD (Hon), PhD (Hon), DSc (Hon)
Professor of Radiology, Division of Nuclear Medicine, Department of Radiology, Hospital of the University of Pennsylvania, University of Pennsylvania Perelman School of Medicine, Philadelphia, Pennsylvania, USA

EDITORS

MONA-ELISABETH REVHEIM, MD, PhD, MHA
Associate Professor, Division of Radiology and Nuclear Medicine, Oslo University Hospital, Institute of Clinical Medicine, Faculty of Medicine, University of Oslo, Oslo, Norway

ABASS ALAVI, MD, MD (Hon), PhD (Hon), DSc (Hon)
Professor of Radiology, Division of Nuclear Medicine, Department of Radiology, Hospital of the University of Pennsylvania, University of Pennsylvania Perelman School of Medicine, Philadelphia, Pennsylvania, USA

AUTHORS

ABASS ALAVI, MD, MD (Hon), PhD (Hon), DSc (Hon)
Professor of Radiology, Division of Nuclear Medicine, Department of Radiology, Hospital of the University of Pennsylvania, University of Pennsylvania Perelman School of Medicine, Philadelphia, Pennsylvania, USA

CYRUS AYUBCHA, MSc
Department of Radiology, Hospital of the University of Pennsylvania, Philadelphia, Pennsylvania, USA; Harvard Medical School, Boston, Massachusetts, USA

PETER M. BLOOMFIELD, MSc
Head of Imaging Methodology, Brain Health Imaging Centre, Centre for Addiction and Mental Health, Toronto, Ontario, Canada

NICOLAAS I.L.J. BOHNEN, MD, PhD
Professor of Radiology (Nuclear Medicine and Molecular Imaging) and Neurology, University of Michigan, Ann Arbor Veterans Administration Medical Center, Ann Arbor, Michigan, USA

AUSTIN J. BORJA, BA
Department of Radiology, Hospital of the University of Pennsylvania, Perelman School of Medicine, University of Pennsylvania, Philadelphia, Pennsylvania, USA

PACO E. BRAVO, MD
Division of Cardiovascular Medicine, Department of Medicine, Division of Nuclear Medicine and Clinical Molecular Imaging, Department of Radiology, Division of Cardiothoracic Imaging, Department of Radiology, Perelman School of Medicine, University of Pennsylvania, Philadelphia, Pennsylvania, USA

XIAOYUAN CHEN, PhD
Yong Loo Lin School of Medicine and Faculty of Engineering, National University of Singapore, Singapore, Singapore

KENNETH DAHL, PhD
Independent Scientist, Azrieli Centre for Neuro-Radiochemistry, Brain Health Imaging Centre, Centre for Addiction and Mental Health, Toronto, Ontario, Canada

DONALD K. DETCHOU, BA
Department of Radiology, Hospital of the University of Pennsylvania, Perelman School of Medicine, University of Pennsylvania, Philadelphia, Pennsylvania, USA

KIRK A. FREY, MD, PhD
David E. Kuhl Collegiate Professor of Radiology (Nuclear Medicine and Molecular imaging), Professor of Neurology, University of Michigan, Ann Arbor, Michigan, USA

EMILY C. HANCIN, MS, BA
Department of Radiology, Hospital of the University of Pennsylvania, Lewis Katz School of Medicine, Temple University, Philadelphia, Pennsylvania, USA

EIVOR HERNES, MD, PhD
Department of Nuclear Medicine, Division of Radiology and Nuclear Medicine, Oslo University Hospital, Oslo, Norway

KNUT HÅKON HOLE, MD, PhD
Division of Radiology and Nuclear Medicine, Oslo University Hospital, Institute of Clinical Medicine, University of Oslo, Oslo, Norway

CAMILLA BARDRAM JOHNBECK, MD, PhD
Staff Specialist, Department of Clinical Physiology, Nuclear Medicine and PET, Rigshospitalet, European Neuroendocrine Tumor Society Center of Excellence, Rigshospitalet, Copenhagen, Denmark

VLADIMIR JOSEPH, MD
Division of Cardiovascular Medicine, Department of Medicine, Perelman School of Medicine, University of Pennsylvania, Philadelphia, Pennsylvania, USA

HOWARD M. JULIEN, MD, MPH
Division of Cardiovascular Medicine, Department of Medicine, Perelman School of Medicine, University of Pennsylvania, Philadelphia, Pennsylvania, USA

RAKESH KUMAR, MD, PhD
Professor and Head, Division of Diagnostic Nuclear Medicine, Department of Nuclear Medicine, All India Institute of Medical Sciences, New Delhi, India

WOLFGANG LILLEBY, MD, PhD
Department of Oncology, Oslo University Hospital, Oslo, Norway

YAPING LUO, MD
Department of Nuclear Medicine, Chinese Academy of Medical Sciences and Peking Union Medical College Hospital, Beijing, P. R. China; Beijing Key Laboratory of Molecular Targeted Diagnosis and Therapy in Nuclear Medicine

MATEEN MOGHBEL, MD
Department of Radiology, Massachusetts General Hospital, Boston, Massachusetts, USA

JANN MORTENSEN, MD, DMSc
Clinical Professor, Chief Physician, Department of Clinical Physiology, Nuclear Medicine and PET, Rigshospitalet, European Neuroendocrine Tumor Society Center of Excellence, Rigshospitalet, Copenhagen, Medical Faculty, University of Copenhagen, Denmark

VIDYA NARAYANASWAMI, PhD
Postdoctoral Fellow, Azrieli Centre for Neuro-Radiochemistry, Brain Health Imaging Centre, Centre for Addiction and Mental Health, Toronto, Ontario, Canada

ANDREW NEWBERG, MD
Department of Integrative Medicine and Nutritional Sciences, Marcus Institute of Integrative Health, Thomas Jefferson University, Department of Radiology, Thomas Jefferson University, Philadelphia, Pennsylvania, USA

WILLIAM Y. RAYNOR, BS
Department of Radiology, Hospital of the University of Pennsylvania, Drexel University College of Medicine, Philadelphia, Pennsylvania, USA

MONA-ELISABETH REVHEIM, MD, PhD, MHA
Associate Professor, Division of Radiology and Nuclear Medicine, Oslo University Hospital, Institute of Clinical Medicine, Faculty of Medicine, University of Oslo, Oslo, Norway

CHRISTIN SCHIFANI, PhD
Project Scientist, Brain Health Imaging Centre, Centre for Addiction and Mental Health, Toronto, Ontario, Canada

THERESE SEIERSTAD, MSc, PhD, MHA
Department of Research and Development, Division of Radiology and Nuclear Medicine, Oslo University Hospital, Oslo, Norway

HILDE STRØMME, MSc
Library of Medicine and Science, University of Oslo, Norway

JUNCHAO TONG, PhD
Head of Preclinical Imaging, Brain Health Imaging Centre, Centre for Addiction and Mental Health, Toronto, Ontario, Canada

ANDREAS JULIUS TULIPAN, MD
Department of Nuclear Medicine, Oslo University Hospital, Institute of Clinical Medicine, University of Oslo, Oslo, Norway

NEIL VASDEV, PhD
Azrieli Chair of Brain and Behaviour, Department of Psychiatry, Director, Brain Health Imaging Centre, Director, Azrieli Centre for Neuro-Radiochemistry, Centre for Addiction and Mental Health, University of Toronto, Toronto, Ontario, Canada

THOMAS J. WERNER, MSc
Department of Radiology, Hospital of the University of Pennsylvania, Philadelphia, Pennsylvania, USA

DIVYA YADAV, MD
Department of Nuclear Medicine, All India Institute of Medical Sciences, New Delhi, India

Contents

Prostate-specific membrane antigen PET is a promising diagnostic tool in prostate cancer. The gold standard for the detection of prostate tumor and lymph node metastases is histopathology. The aim of the present review was to investigate accuracy measures of ^{68}Ga/^{18}F-labeled prostate-specific membrane antigen PET tracers in primary and recurrent prostate cancer with systematic sector-based histopathology as the reference standard. A systematic literature search was performed and 34 studies were included. Overall, prostate-specific membrane antigen PET showed high specificity, but variable sensitivity to localize known prostate cancer and detect pelvic lymph node metastases.

The PET tracer ^{18}F-fluciclovine (Axumin) was recently approved in the United States and Europe for men with suspected prostate cancer recurrence following prior treatment. This article summarizes studies where systematic sector-based histopathology was used as reference standard to assess the diagnostic accuracy of the tracer ^{18}F-fluciclovine PET in patients with prostate cancer.

2-[18F]-fluoro-2-deoxyglucose (FDG) is the most commonly used radiotracer and provides valuable information about glucose metabolism. With the advent of newer receptor-based tracers in the management of hormonally active malignancies, the focus has been shifted from FDG. These tracers might be more specific than FDG because they target specific hormone receptors. But because FDG is widely available, this review discusses what information still can be harnessed from this workhorse of molecular imaging. The personalized implementation of FDG imaging in undifferentiated malignancies will help in characterization of tumor and may aid in patient management.

PET/computed tomography (CT) imaging increasingly is used in neuroendocrine neoplasms (NENs) for diagnosis, staging, monitoring, prognostication, and choosing treatment. Somatostatin PET analog tracers have added to the specificity by obtaining higher affinity to somatostatin receptors with ^{68}Ga-labeled or ^{64}Cu-labeled DOTA peptides compared with single-photon emission CT imaging isotopes. PET uptake correlates to tumor grade and is an essential part of theranostics with peptide receptor radionuclide treatment. This article focuses on the literature on head-to-head studies and meta-analyses of different combinations of peptide agonists and a few antagonists. Overall, the published data support the diagnostic capability of PET/CT imaging in NENs.

Glucagonlike peptide-1 (GLP-1) receptor imaging, using radiolabeled exendin-4, was recently established for detecting insulinoma in patients with hyperinsulinemic hypoglycemia. It has proven to be a sensitive and specific method for preoperative localization of insulinoma. This review introduces the development, clinical research, and perspective of GLP-1 receptor imaging mainly in insulinoma.

The brain is a common site for metastases as well as primary tumors. Although evaluation of these malignancies with contrast-enhanced MR imaging defines current clinical practice, ^{18}F-fluorodeoxyglucose (FDG)-PET has shown considerable utility in this area. In addition, many other tracers targeting various aspects of tumor biology have been developed and tested. This article discusses recent developments in PET imaging and the anticipated role of FDG and other tracers in the assessment of brain tumors.

Discovery of novel PET radiotracers targeting neuroinflammation (microglia and astrocytes) is actively pursued. Employing a lipopolysaccharide (LPS) rat model, this longitudinal study evaluated the translocator protein 18-kDa radiotracer [^{18}F] FEPPA (primarily microglia) and monoamine oxidase B radiotracers [^{11}C]L-deprenyl and [^{11}C]SL25.1188 (astrocytes preferred). Increased [^{18}F]FEPPA binding peaked at 1 week in LPS-injected striatum whereas increased lazabemide-sensitive [^{11}C]L-deprenyl binding developed later. No increase in radiotracer uptake was observed for [^{11}C]SL25.1188. The unilateral intrastriatal LPS rat model may serve as a useful tool for benchmarking PET tracers targeted toward distinct phases of neuroinflammatory reactions involving both microglia and astrocytes.

William Y. Raynor, Austin J. Borja, Emily C. Hancin, Thomas J. Werner, Abass Alavi, and Mona-Elisabeth Revheim

PET imaging with ^{18}F-sodium fluoride (NaF), combined with computed tomography or magnetic resonance, is a sensitive method of assessing bone turnover. Although NaF-PET is gaining popularity in detecting prostate cancer metastases to bone marrow, osseous changes represent secondary effects of cancer cell growth. PET tracers more appropriate for assessing prostate cancer metastases directly portray malignant activity and include ^{18}F-fluciclovine and prostatic specific membrane antigen ligands. Recent studies investigating NaF-PET suggest utility in the assessment of benign musculoskeletal disorders. Emerging applications in assessing traumatic injuries, joint disease, back pain, orthopedic complications, and metabolic bone disease are discussed.

PET CLINICS

SERIES OF RELATED INTEREST

Advances in Clinical Radiology
Available at: Advancesinclinicalradiology.com
MRI Clinics of North America
Available at: MRI.theclinics.com
Neuroimaging Clinics of North America
Available at: Neuroimaging.theclinics.com
Radiologic Clinics of North America
Available at: Radiologic.theclinics.com

THE CLINICS ARE AVAILABLE ONLINE!
Access your subscription at:
www.theclinics.com

PROGRAM OBJECTIVE

The goal of the PET Clinics is to keep practicing radiologists and radiology residents up to date with current clinical practice in positron emission tomography by providing timely articles reviewing the state of the art in patient care.

TARGET AUDIENCE

Practicing radiologists, radiology residents, and other health care professionals who provide patient care utilizing radiologic findings.

LEARNING OBJECTIVES

Upon completion of this activity, participants will be able to:
1. Review the clinical role of PET imaging in detecting breast, thyroid, neuroendocrine and prostate malignancies.
2. Discuss clinical and research applications for positron emitting radioisotopes.
3. Recognize the role of NaF PET/CT in detecting and characterizing musculoskeletal disorders with emphasis on traumatic injuries, joint diseases, back pain, orthopedic complications, and metabolic bone disorders.

ACCREDITATION

The Elsevier Office of Continuing Medical Education (EOCME) is accredited by the Accreditation Council for Continuing Medical Education (ACCME) to provide continuing medical education for physicians.

The EOCME designates this journal-based CME activity for a maximum of 12 *AMA PRA Category 1 Credit*(s)™. Physicians should claim only the credit commensurate with the extent of their participation in the activity.

All other health care professionals requesting continuing education credit for this enduring material will be issued a certificate of participation.

DISCLOSURE OF CONFLICTS OF INTEREST

The EOCME assesses conflict of interest with its instructors, faculty, planners, and other individuals who are in a position to control the content of CME activities. All relevant conflicts of interest that are identified are thoroughly vetted by EOCME for fair balance, scientific objectivity, and patient care recommendations. EOCME is committed to providing its learners with CME activities that promote improvements or quality in healthcare and not a specific proprietary business or a commercial interest.

The planning committee, staff, authors, and editors listed below have identified no financial relationships or relationships to products or devices they or their spouse/life partner have with commercial interest related to the content of this CME activity:

Abass Alavi, MD, MD (Hon), PhD (Hon), DSc (Hon); Cyrus Ayubcha, MSc; Peter M. Bloomfield, MSc; Nicolaas I.L.J. Bohnen, MD, PhD; Austin J. Borja, BA; Paco E. Bravo, MD; Regina Chavous-Gibson, MSN, RN; Xiaoyuan Chen, PhD; Kenneth Dahl, PhD; Donald K. Detchou, BA; Kirk A. Frey, MD, PhD; Emily C. Hancin, MS, BA; Eivor Hernes, MD, PhD; Knut Håkon Hole, MD, PhD; Camilla Bardram Johnbeck, MD, PhD; Vladimir Joseph, MD; Howard M. Julien, MD, MPH; Rakesh Kumar, MD, PhD; Wolfgang Lilleby, MD, PhD; Yaping Luo, MD; Mateen Moghbel, MD; Jann Mortensen, MD, DMSc; Vidya Narayanaswami, PhD; Andrew Newberg, MD; William Y. Raynor, BS; Mona-Elisabeth Revheim, MD, PhD, MHA; Christin Schifani, PhD; Therese Seierstad, MSc, PhD, MHA; Hilde Strømme, MSc; Junchao Tong, PhD; Andreas Julius Tulipan, MD; Neil Vasdev, PhD; John Vassallo; Vignesh Viswanathan; Thomas J. Werner, MSc; Divya Yadav, MD

UNAPPROVED/OFF-LABEL USE DISCLOSURE

The EOCME requires CME faculty to disclose to the participants:
1. When products or procedures being discussed are off-label, unlabelled, experimental, and/or investigational (not US Food and Drug Administration [FDA] approved); and
2. Any limitations on the information presented, such as data that are preliminary or that represent ongoing research, interim analyses, and/or unsupported opinions. Faculty may discuss information about pharmaceutical agents that is outside of FDA-approved labelling. This information is intended solely for CME and is not intended to promote off-label use of these medications. If you have any questions, contact the medical affairs department of the manufacturer for the most recent prescribing information.

TO ENROLL

To enroll in the PET Clinics Continuing Medical Education program, call customer service at 1-800-654-2452 or sign up online at http://www.theclinics.com/home/cme. The CME program is available to subscribers for an additional annual fee of USD 254.00

METHOD OF PARTICIPATION

In order to claim credit, participants must complete the following:
1. Complete enrolment as indicated above.
2. Read the activity.

3. Complete the CME Test and Evaluation. Participants must achieve a score of 70% on the test. All CME Tests and Evaluations must be completed online.

CME INQUIRIES/SPECIAL NEEDS
For all CME inquiries or special needs, please contact elsevierCME@elsevier.com.

Preface

PET-based Novel Imaging Techniques with Recently Introduced Radiotracers

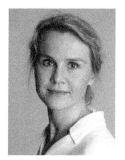
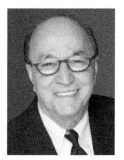

Mona-Elisabeth Revheim, MD, PhD, MHA   Abass Alavi, MD, MD (Hon), PhD (Hon), DSc (Hon)

Editors

Today, imaging research is an integral component of basic and clinical investigation in medicine. With the introduction of novel interventions, which are complex and systemic in nature, sophisticated imaging techniques along with new blood biomarkers, molecular histology, and advanced data analysis schemes have become a necessity in modern practice of medicine. These advances are allowing assessment of response at a molecular level with high precision and accuracy. In particular, molecular imaging modalities provide noninvasive and quantitative measures of the in vivo disease activity at the focal and global levels, which are well suited for longitudinal studies. These approaches are based on targeting the intended sites by well-characterized mechanisms that have been identified and characterized over the past decades. These exciting developments have been well illustrated by the articles in the current issue of PET Clinics, which includes 12 reviews covering a broad spectrum of relevant topics in the field of molecular imaging. We have made an effort to include scientific communications that describe clinical and research applications of novel PET tracers that are currently of great interest to the medical community.

Oncology still is one of the most active domains for applications of PET tracers, and therefore, 6 reviews in this issue have been dedicated to cancer-related molecular imaging techniques. Hernes and colleagues and Seierstad and colleagues present systematic reviews of the clinical role of PET imaging with prostate-specific membrane antigen and fluciclovine (Axumin) in this cancer, respectively. With the advent of new receptor-based tracers in the assessment of hormonally active malignancies, the focus has now been shifted to some extent from fluorodeoxyglucose (FDG), since these compounds are more specific in nature. However, since the availability of such receptor-based tracers is limited worldwide, Yadav and colleagues discuss the strengths and limitations of various imaging techniques and point out that, despite recent development, we can still harness useful information from FDG imaging by focusing on breast, thyroid, neuroendocrine, and prostate malignancies. FDG-PET is particularly very sensitive in detecting undifferentiated cancer cells, which frequently occur in such malignancies and cannot be visualized by the specific tracers.

In recent years, new PET compounds have been synthesized by employing ^{68}Ga instead of ^{18}F or ^{11}C, and many of these tracers have been tested successfully and validated for examining several serious diseases and disorders. Positron emitting radioisotopes with long half-lives, such as ^{64}Cu, have also gained recognition for certain applications for clinical and research purposes. In this issue, Johnbeck and colleagues describe the potential role of somatostatin-binding compounds that are labeled by both ^{68}Ga and ^{64}Cu for imaging neuroendocrine neoplasms. Insulinomas, neuroendocrine tumors with insufficient expression of somatostatin receptors (<60%), are poor

PET Clin 16 (2021) xv–xvi
https://doi.org/10.1016/j.cpet.2021.01.001
1556-8598/21/© 2021 Published by Elsevier Inc.

candidates for this approach. Therefore, a glucagon-like peptide-1 (GLP-1) receptor-based PET imaging agent, like radiolabeled exendin-4, has been introduced for targeting pancreatic β cells in patients with hyperinsulinism. An article by Luo and colleagues provides an introduction to the development, clinical research, and perspective of GLP-1 receptor imaging and its high sensitivity and specificity in localizing insulinomas.

The introduction of novel PET tracers to image and assess central nervous system disorders has met serious challenges due to the PET tracers' ability to cross the blood-brain barrier and their specificity for the intended targets. Because of the nonspecificity of structural imaging techniques, there is a dire need for imaging brain tumors with tracers that allow assessing tumor response and the course of the disease. The role of PET tracers that are currently used to characterize brain tumors is discussed in a critical review by Borja and colleagues.

There has also been an emerging interest in understanding the role of the neuroimmune system in the pathophysiology of neurodegenerative and psychiatric diseases, and several PET tracers have been investigated with somewhat divergent and confusing results. Narayanaswami and colleagues summarize the findings from imaging with different generations of translocator protein 18-kDa tracers (primarily microglia) and monoamine oxidase-B radiotracers (astrocytes preferred). They also present results from a preclinical study in a lipopolysaccharide rat model of neuroinflammation. Another focus of investigation in molecular neuroimaging dealt with the protein depositions in head injuries and movement disorders. In the review by Ayubcha and colleagues, the state of tau radiotracer developments and the potential clinical role of tau-PET imaging are described in this domain. Furthermore, Bohnen and Frey evaluate possible targeting of protein depositions that are specific to neurodegenerative parkinsonism disorders. These include aggregates of misfolded tau proteins characteristic of progressive supranuclear palsy and α-synuclein in Parkinson disease and multiple system atrophy.

Two articles are devoted to PET imaging of the cardiovascular system with different perspectives.

Hancin and colleagues describe a summary of non-FDG/NaF radiotracers that have been proposed for the diagnosis and management of cardiovascular disorders. The review by Joseph and colleagues deals with imaging of cardiac amyloidosis by both planar/single-photon emission computed tomography and PET/computed tomography (CT) and describes the current state of these modalities as they relate to this serious disease. The final article is a review of the role of NaF PET/CT in detecting and characterizing musculoskeletal disorders with an emphasis on traumatic injuries, joint diseases, back pain, orthopedic complications, and metabolic bone disorders.

By now, it has become quite clear that among the existing modalities, molecular imaging with PET has the greatest prospects for becoming the examination of choice for personalized medicine in the foreseeable future. During the past 4 decades, many novel radiotracers have been introduced for PET imaging and have been shown to be of great value in certain settings. However, we must emphasize that FDG as a single tracer has brought about a revolution to medical imaging, and without its substantial impact, PET could not have survived as a sustainable discipline. As such, we salute our distinguished colleague, Henry Wagner, for labeling FDG as the "Molecule of the 20th Century."

Mona-Elisabeth Revheim, MD, PhD, MHA
Division of Radiology and
Nuclear Medicine
Oslo University Hospital
Sognsvannsveien 20
0372 Oslo, Norway

Abass Alavi, MD, MD (Hon), PhD (Hon), DSc
(Hon)
Division of Nuclear Medicine
Department of Radiology
University of Pennsylvania
School of Medicine, Hospital of the
University of Pennsylvania
3400 Spruce Street
Philadelphia, PA 19104, USA

E-mail addresses:
monar@ous-hf.no (M.-E. Revheim)
Abass.Alavi@pennmedicine.upenn.edu (A. Alavi)

Prostate-Specific Membrane Antigen PET for Assessment of Primary and Recurrent Prostate Cancer with Histopathology as Reference Standard
A Systematic Review and Meta-Analysis

Eivor Hernes, MD, PhD[a],*, Mona-Elisabeth Revheim, MD, PhD, MHA[a,b],
Knut Håkon Hole, MD, PhD[a,b], Andreas Julius Tulipan, MD[a,b],
Hilde Strømme, MSc[c], Wolfgang Lilleby, MD, PhD[d],
Therese Seierstad, MSc, PhD, MHA[a]

KEYWORDS

- Prostate cancer • PSMA PET • Histopathology • Primary tumor location • Lymph node metastases
- Personalized medicine

KEY POINTS

- A total of 34 studies of prostate-specific membrane antigen PET in prostate cancer had systematic-sector based histopathology and data for diagnostic accuracy measures.
- Prostate-specific membrane antigen PET showed overall high specificity, but variable sensitivity, to localize known prostate cancer and detect pelvic lymph node metastases.
- Sensitivity for the detection of pelvic lymph node metastases is better in the recurrent than in the primary setting.

BACKGROUND

Prostate cancer is a major health problem. It is one of the most common cancers in males, and worldwide a substantial number of men die from prostate cancer each year.[1,2] Radical prostatectomy and external radiotherapy and/or brachytherapy are standard curative treatment options. However, more than 30% experience disease recurrence with an increasing prostate-specific antigen (PSA) level.[3,4]

A key factor for treatment planning is knowledge of extent of spread and location of disease, thus selecting patients for local treatment options and/or combination with systemic therapy. Conventional imaging with computed tomography (CT) and bone scans is of limited value, particularly in primary and early biochemically recurrent prostate cancer. Multiparametric MR imaging is increasingly used, yet another promising option

[a] Division of Radiology and Nuclear Medicine, Oslo University Hospital, P.O. Box 4956 Nydalen, 0424 Oslo, Norway; [b] Institute of Clinical Medicine, University of Oslo, P.O. Box 1171 Blindern, 0318 Oslo, Norway; [c] Library of Medicine and Science, University of Oslo, Sognsvannsveien 20, 0372 Oslo, Norway; [d] Department of Oncology, Oslo University Hospital, P.O. Box 4953 Nydalen, 0424 Oslo, Norway
* Corresponding author. Department of Nuclear Medicine, Division of Radiology and Nuclear Medicine, Oslo University Hospital, P.O. Box 4956 Nydalen, 0424 Oslo, Norway.
E-mail address: ehh@ous-hf.no

PET Clin 16 (2021) 147–165
https://doi.org/10.1016/j.cpet.2020.12.001
1556-8598/21/© 2020 Elsevier Inc. All rights reserved.

of molecular imaging is PET with prostate-specific membrane antigen (PSMA)-based tracers. The diagnostic principle has been further developed by theranostic medicine into PSMA-based targeted radiotherapy.[5–7]

PSMA is a transmembrane glycoprotein with catalytic properties, named glutamate carboxypeptidase II. It is not specific for prostate cancer, but has proven useful because it is highly overexpressed in prostate cancer cells in about 95% of these patients.[8–11] When the ligand binds to the extracellular domain, it is internalized. Hence, the PET tracer accumulates in the cancer cells providing, a high tumor-to-background ratio

(Fig. 1).[12] In biochemical recurrence, PSMA PET is included in the European guidelines,[13] and ^{68}Ga-PSMA-11 is currently under review by the US Food and Drug Administration.[14]

The present review aims to investigate accuracy measures of [68]Ga- and ^{18}F-labeled PSMA PET tracers for the assessment of primary and recurrent prostate cancers with systematic sector-based histopathology as the reference standard.

EVIDENCE ACQUISITION
Search Strategy

The systematic review followed the PRISMA guidelines.[15] An information specialist (H.S.) planned and

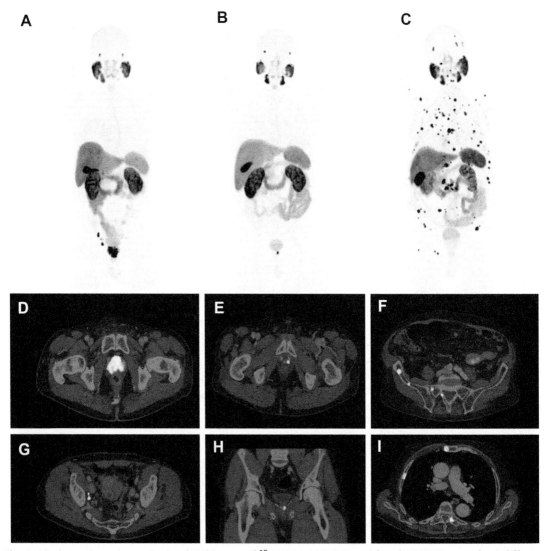

Fig. 1. Maximum intensity projection (MIP) image of ^{18}F-PSMA-1007 PET and fused PET/CT images for 3 different patients. One patient had a large primary prostate cancer and pelvic lymph node metastases (*A, D, G*). Another patient with biochemically recurrent prostate cancer (PSA of 2.3) and disease located to the prostate bed only (*B, E, H*). A third patient, also with biochemically recurrent disease (PSA of 21), but with extensive bone metastases (*C, F, I*).

performed the systematic literature search in MEDLINE (Ovid), Embase (Ovid), Cochrane Database of Systematic Reviews (Wiley), Cochrane Central Register of Controlled Trials, including references from ClinicalTrials.gov, The World Health Organization International Clinical Trials Registry Platform (Wiley), and Scopus (Elsevier). Search terms were discussed in detail with 2 reviewers (E.H., T.S.) and we searched for a combination of subject headings, where applicable, and text words, including synonyms for PSMA and PSMA PET tracers. In addition, we did a search for various terms for prostate cancer combined with PSMA. The following strategy was used in MEDLINE (Ovid) and adapted to the other databases: ((("glutamate carboxypeptidase II" or "PSMA antigen" or "PSM antigen" or (("folate hydrolase 1" or "FOLH1 protein") adj1 human) or "prostate specific membrane antigen" or "68Ga-PSMA-11" or "68Ga-HBED-CC" or "68Ga-PSMA-HBED-CC" or "Glu-NH-CO-NH-Lys-(Ahx)-((68)Ga(HBED-CC))" or "68Ga-PSMA-617" or "PSMA-617" or "68 Ga-PSMA-I-T" or "68 Ga-PSMA-I and T" or "68 Ga-PSMA-I &T" or "18F-PSMA-1007" or "PSMA-1007" or "18F-DCFPyL" or "2-(3-(1-carboxy-5-((6-fluoropyridine-3-carbonyl)amino)pentyl)ureido)pentanedioic acid" or "18F-DCFBC" or "N-(N-((S)-1,3-Dicarboxypropyl)carbamoyl)-4-(18F)fluorobenzyl-L-cysteine" or "18F-JK-PSMA-7" or "18F-PSMA-11" or CTT1057 or BAY1075553 or 68Ga-THP-PSMA or CTT-54 or "(2RS,4S)-2-[(18)F]Fluoro-4-phosphonomethyl-pentanedioic acid" or "18F-rhPSMA-7").mp.) OR (exp Prostatic Neoplasms/or (prostat* adj3 (neoplasm* or cancer* or tumo?r* or carcinom*)).mp.) and (FOLH1 protein, human.rn. or Glutamate Carboxypeptidase II/or PSMA.mp.)). Filters to exclude animal studies were applied in MEDLINE and Embase. Publication types such as editorials, conference abstracts, reviews, surveys, and letters were excluded. All searches were performed on July 13, 2020. The complete search strategies for all databases can be obtained from the corresponding author. The results from all searches were imported into EndNote and duplicates were removed.

Eligibility Criteria

The PICO framework (patient, intervention, comparator, outcome) was used to define the eligibility criteria: The study must consist of patients with prostate cancer (P), the patients must have had [68]Ga- or ^{18}F-labeled PSMA PET (I), the reference standard (comparator) must be systematic sector-based histopathology (C) and the outcome must be diagnostic performance given as sensitivity and specificity (O). Furthermore, the study must report the sector-based data either as individual 2 × 2 data or as summary diagnostic accuracy measurements for more than 15 patients fulfilling all these criteria. In case of studies with mixed clinical settings (primary/recurrence) and anatomic location (prostate tumor location/lymph nodes), each subgroup must fulfill all criteria. Only original articles in English were eligible. Brief communications with substantial data were accepted. Editorials, letters, review articles, comments, conference proceedings, and case reports were excluded.

Screening and Study Selection

Two reviewers independently screened the titles and abstracts (E.H., T.S.) using the Rayyan software,[16] and conflicts were resolved by consensus. The remaining articles assessed for inclusion eligibility were read in full text and excluded with reasons when appropriate.

Quality Assessment

Two reviewers (E.H., T.S.) in consensus used the Quality Assessment of Diagnostic Accuracy Studies-2 tool to assess the risk of bias in 4 domains: patient selection, index test, reference standard and reference test timing.[17] For the first 3 domains applicability concerns were also assessed.

Data Extraction

For each selected study the following information was collected:

- Basic study characteristics: authors, year of publication, country, PSMA tracer, study design (prospective/retrospective), clinical setting (primary/recurrence), and anatomy (prostate/lymph nodes).
- Clinicopathologic data: number of patients, age, PSA at time of PSMA PET, Gleason score of primary prostate cancer and pathologic T category (pT).
- Diagnostic accuracy data: number of true positives, true negatives, false positives, and false negatives were recorded when available to obtain 2 × 2 contingency tables. Authors of studies that only reported summary diagnostics were contacted by email and asked for additional data.

Data Synthesis and Analysis

Sensitivity and specificity with 95% confidence intervals were calculated from the 2 × 2 contingency tables for each study using the MedCalc diagnostic test evaluator calculator,[18] or extracted from studies where 2 × 2 data were not available. Forest plots were drawn to show the variation and explore heterogeneity for sensitivity and specificity. Studies were assessed for inclusion in the quantitative analyses, performed separately for different subgroups with respect to clinical setting (primary/recurrent disease) and disease location (prostate gland/ lymph nodes). Summarized receiver operating characteristic curves were estimated using the Python software (www.python.org/), and area under the curve was calculated.[19,20]

EVIDENCE SYNTHESIS
Literature Search and Study Selection

A total of 9053 records were retrieved; after removing duplicate publications, 3843 articles remained (**Fig. 2**).[15] After screening of titles and abstracts, 3762 records were excluded. The remaining 81 studies were read in full text and 47 studies were excluded. The reasons for exclusion were most often a reference standard inappropriate for the review question or patient-based data only.[21–43] Other reasons for exclusion were insufficient data to extract the required accuracy measures,[44–47] too few patients,[48–54] or study objective and design outside scope of the review.[55–67] Finally, a total of 34 studies were included.[68–101]

Study and Patient Characteristics

The included studies were published between 2016 and 2020 (**Table 1**). Patient populations originated worldwide, the majority from Germany. All but 2 studies used ^{68}Ga-labeled PSMA PET tracers. The imaging modality was PET/CT scans in all but 5 studies, which used either PET/MR imaging[75,82,91] or mixed PET/CT scan and PET/MR imaging.[86,89] There were 26 studies in primary prostate cancer (1083 patients) and 8 studies (256 patients) in biochemically recurrent prostate cancer. Patient and tumor characteristics are outlined in **Tables 2–4**. The median PSA was 6.1 to 55.9 ng/mL in the primary setting, and the median was 0.8 to 2.4 ng/mL in biochemically recurrent prostate cancer (mean PSA of 3.9 ng/mL in 1 study).

Quality Assessment

Table 5 outlines the results of assessment according to the Quality Assessment of Diagnostic Accuracy Studies-2 tool. Most studies had low risk of bias and low applicability concerns with regard to patient selection, index test and reference standard. A substantial number of studies did not report time from PET to surgery; thus, the flow and timing remained unclear.

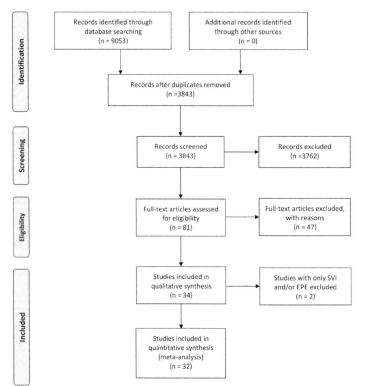

Fig. 2. PRISMA flow diagram showing the selection of studies.

Table 1
Study characteristics

Author, Year	Journal	Country	PET Tracer	Design	Setting	Anatomy
Abufaraj et al,[68] 2019	EJNMMI	Austria	68Ga-PSMA-11	Prospective	Recurrence	Nodes
Berger et al,[69] 2018	Prostate Cancer Prostatic Dis	Australia	68Ga-PSMA-HBED-CC	Retrospective	Primary	Prostate
Bettermann et al,[70] 2019	Radiat Oncol	Germany	68Ga-PSMA-11	Prospective	Primary	Prostate
Budäus et al,[71] 2016	Eur Urol	Germany	68Ga-PSMA	Retrospective	Primary	Nodes
Cytawa et al,[72] 2020	EJNMMI	Germany	68Ga-PSMA I&T	Retrospective	Primary	Nodes
Dekalo et al,[73] 2019	Urol Oncol-Semin Ori	Israel	68Ga-PSMA-HBED-CC	Retrospective	Primary	Prostate
Dundee et al,[74] 2018	Urology	Australia	68Ga-PSMA-HBED-CC	Prospective	Recurrence	Nodes
Eiber et al,[75] 2016[a]	Eur Urol	Germany	68Ga-PSMA-HBED-CC	Retrospective	Primary	Prostate
El Hajj et al,[76] 2019	Medicine	Lebanon	68Ga-PSMA-11	Retrospective	Primary	Prostate
Fendler et al,[77] 2016	JNM	Germany	68Ga-PSMA-HBED-CC	Retrospective	Primary	Prostate
Gorin et al,[78] 2018	J Urol	USA	18F-DCFPyL	Prospective	Primary	Nodes
Gupta et al,[79] 2018	World J Nucl Med	India	68Ga-PSMA-11	Retrospective	Primary	Prostate + nodes
Hanske et al,[80] 2019	Urol Oncol-Semin Ori	Germany	68Ga-PSMA	Retrospective	Recurrence	Nodes
Herlemann et al,[81] 2016[c]	Eur Urol	Germany	68Ga-PSMA-HBED-CC	Retrospective	Primary	Nodes
Hicks et al,[82] 2018[a]	Radiology	USA	68Ga-PSMA-11	Retrospective	Primary	Prostate
Jilg et al,[83] 2017	Theranostics	Germany	68Ga-PSMA-HBED-CC	Retrospective	Recurrence	Nodes
Jilg et al,[84] 2020	EJNMMI Research	Germany	68Ga-PSMA-HBED-CC	Retrospective	Recurrence	Nodes
Kopp et al,[85] 2020	World J Urol	Germany	68Ga-PSMA	Retrospective	Primary	Nodes
Kroenke et al,[86] 2020[b]	JNM	Germany	18F-rhPSMA-7	Retrospective	Primary	Nodes
Liu et al,[87] 2020	JNM	China	68Ga-PSMA-617	Prospective	Prediagnostic	Prostate
Mandel et al,[88] 2020	Eur Urol Focus	Germany	68Ga-PSMA	Retrospective	Recurrence	Nodes
Maurer et al,[89] 2016[b]	J Urol	Germany	68Ga-PSMA-HBED-CC	Retrospective	Primary	Nodes
Muehlematter et al,[90] 2019	Radiology	Switzerland	68Ga-PSMA-11	Retrospective	Primary	Prostate
Park et al,[91] 2018[a]	Radiology	USA	68Ga-PSMA-11	Prospective	Primary	Prostate + nodes
Petersen et al,[92] 2020	World J Urol	Denmark	68Ga-PSMA-11	Prospective	Primary	Nodes
Pfister et al,[93] 2016	EJNMMI	Germany	68Ga-PSMA-HBED-CC	Retrospective	Recurrence	Nodes

(continued on next page)

Table 1
(continued)

Author, Year	Journal	Country	PET Tracer	Design	Setting	Anatomy
Rauscher et al,[94] 2016	JNM	Germany	68Ga-PSMA-HBED-CC	Retrospective	Recurrence	Nodes
Rhee et al,[95] 2016	J Urol	Australia	68Ga-PSMA-HBED-CC	Prospective	Primary	Prostate
Scheltema et al,[96] 2019	BJUI	The Netherlands	68Ga-PSMA-11	Retrospective	Primary	Prostate
van Kalmthout et al,[97] 2020	J Urol	The Netherlands	68Ga-PSMA-11	Prospective	Primary	Nodes
van Leuween et al,[98] 2017	BJUI	Australia	68Ga-PSMA-HBED-CC	Prospective	Primary	Nodes
von Klot et al,[99] 2017	Nucl Med Mol Imaging	Germany	68Ga-PSMA I&T	Retrospective	Primary	Prostate
Yilmaz et al,[100] 2019	The Prostate	Turkey	68Ga-PSMA-11	Retrospective	Primary	Prostate
Zhang et al,[101] 2017	J Transl Med	China	68Ga-PSMA-11	Retrospective	Primary	Nodes

PET/CT scan was used unless otherwise notified.

[a] PET/MR imaging.

[b] Mixed PET/CT scan and PET/MR imaging.

[c] Patients with recurrent disease were excluded owing to the number of patients being less than 15.

Table 2
Patient characteristics: primary prostate tumor

Author, Year	Patients	Age (years) Median	Age (years) Range	PSA (ng/mL) Median	PSA (ng/mL) Range	Gleason Score (%)	pT Category (%)
Berger et al,[69] 2018	50[a]	65	5.6[c]	10.6	8.1[c]	6 (2), 7a (36), 7b (30), 8 (12), 9 (20)	T2 (46), T3a (36) T3b (18)
Bettermann et al,[70] 2019	17	67	48–76	17.4	6.1–218	7a (35), 7b (29), 8 (18), 9 (18)	T2 (41), T3a (29), T3b (29)
Dekalo et al,[73] 2019	59/61[b]	65	7.0[c]	13.0	11.9[c]	7a (37), 7b (36), 8 (17), 9 (10)	T2 (51), T3a (29), T3b (20)
Eiber et al,[75] 2016	53/66[b]	66	62–72[d]	12.0	6.9–18.8[d]	6 (6), 7 (66), 8 (19), 9 (8), 10 (2)	T2 (43), T3a (34), T3b (21) T4 (2)
El Hajj et al,[76] 2019	23	69	8.7[c]	10.8	7.5[c]	7a (26), 7b (48), 8 (13), 9 (9), 10 (4)	T2 (70), T3a (4), T3b (26)
Fendler et al,[77] 2016	21	71	59–80	31.0	3–363	6 (14), 7a (10), 7b (29), 8 (14), 9 (33)	T2 (24), T3a (24), T3b (48), T4 (5)
Gupta et al,[79] 2018	23	66	50–77	36.1	5.5–200	6 (4), 7a (13), 7b (22), 8 (39), 9 (22)	T2 (17), T3a (22), T3b (61)
Hicks et al,[82] 2018	32	68	62–71[d]	13.4	8.4–19.7[d]	7a (6), 7b (56), 8 (3), 9 (28), 10 (6)	T2 (31), T3a (41), T3b (22), T4 (6)
Liu et al,[87] 2020	31	65	53–81	18.0	5.5–49.8	no cancer (52), 6 (10), ≥7a (39)	NR
Muehlematter et al,[90] 2019	40	63	6[c]	8.1	7–56[d]	7a (5), 7b (15), 8 (53), 9 (28)	T2 (68), T3a (20), T3b (13)
Park et al,[91] 2018	33	66	55–74	9.6	3.7–34.5	7 (55), 8 (24), 9 (21)	T1c (45), T2 (48), T3a (6)[e]
Rhee et al,[95] 2016	20	62	41–71	6.1	3.5–45	7a (60), 7b (20), 9 (20)	T2 (65), T3a (20), T3b (15)
Scheltema et al,[96] 2019	54	64	59–6[d]	7.7	4.4–11[d]	7a (41), 7b (59)	T1c (46), T2 (50), T3 (4)[e]
von Klot et al,[99] 2017	21	68	56–77	11.9	1.8–58	6 (10), 7a (48), 7b (19), 8 (14), 9 (10)	T2 (52), T3a (29), T3b (19)
Yilmaz et al,[100] 2019	24	63	49–73	12.0	2.4–32	6 (13), 7a (25), 7b (42), 8 (8), 9 (13)	NR

Abbreviation: NR, not reported.
[a] Two patients with recurrent disease after definite radiotherapy included.
[b] Patients with histology/total number of patients.
[c] Standard deviation.
[d] Interquartile range.
[e] Clinical T category.

Table 3
Patient characteristics: primary lymph nodes

Author, Year	Patients	Age (Years) Median	Range	PSA (ng/mL) Median	Range	Gleason Score (%)c	pT Category (%)c
Budäus et al,[71] 2016	30	63	44–75	8.8	1.4–376	7a (30), 7b (33), ≥8 (37)	T2 (37), T3a (13), T3b (40) T4 (10)
Cytawa et al,[72] 2020	40/82a	67	53–83	11.0	0.7–872	median 7, range 6–10	NR
Gorin et al,[78] 2018	25	61	49–75	9.3	3.6–125.5	7b (20), 8 (8), 9 (72)	T2 (20), T3a (52), T3b (28)
Gupta et al,[79] 2018	23	66	50–77	36.1	5.5–200	6 (4), 7a (13), 7b (22), 8 (39), 9 (22)	T2 (17), T3a (22), T3b (61)
Herlemann et al,[81] 2016	20	71	59–80	55.9	3.3–363	6 (10), 7 (40), 8 (15), 9 (35)	T2 (15), T3a (25), T3b (60)
Kopp et al,[85] 2020	90	65	60–71b	7.4	5.5–12.5b	6 (1), 7a (43), 7b (33), ≥8 (24)	T2 (55), T3a (27), T3b (18)
Kroenke et al,[86] 2020	58	68	48–80	12.2	1.2–81.6	7a (19), 7b (43), 8 (7), 9 (31)	≤T2 (45), T3a (21), ≥T3b (35)
Maurer et al,[89] 2016	130	67	45–84	11.6	0.6–244	median 7, 7–8,b range 6–10	≤T2 (43), T3a (23), ≥T3b (34)
Park et al,[91] 2018	33	66	55–74	9.6	3.7–34.5	7 (55), 8 (24), 9 (21)	T1c (45), T2 (48), T3a (6)d
Petersen et al,[92] 2020	20	71	58–76	12.5	2.8–66.0	7a (10), 7b (30), 8 (15), 9 (45)	T1c (10), T2 (40), T3 (50)d
van Kalmthout et al,[97] 2020	97/103a	69	53–82	21.8	1.7–298	6 (4), 7a (16), 7b (30), 8 (34), 9 (15), 10(2)	T2 (32), T3a (42), T3b (26)
van Leuween et al,[98] 2017	30	65	60–71b	8.1	5.2–10.1	7b (17), 8 (17), 9 (67)	T2 (30), T3a (43), T3b (27)
Zhang et al,[101] 2017	42	69	55–82	52.3	7.2–348	7a (21), 7b (21), ≥8 (57)	T2 (26), T3a (19), T3b (55)

Abbreviation: NR, not reported.
a Patients with histology/total number of patients.
b Interquartile range.
c Gleason score and pT category from the primary tumor.
d Clinical T category.

Table 4
Patient characteristics: recurrent lymph nodes

Author, Year	Patients	Age (Years)		PSA (ng/mL)		Gleason Score (%)[e]	pT Category (%)[e]
		Median	Range	Median	Range		
Abufaraj et al,[68] 2019	65	65	63–69[c]	1.4	0.8–2.9[c]	6 (2), 7a (22), 7b (31), ≥8 (46)	T2 (19), T3a (47), T3b (31)
Dundee et al,[74] 2018	17	66	60–70[c]	1.6	0.8–2.7[c]	7a (6), 7b (35), 8 (35), 9 (24)	T2 (24), T3a (41), T3b (35)
Hanske et al,[80] 2019	22/43[a]	62	55–66[c]	0.8	0.4–1.7[c]	≤6 (7), 7a (23), 7b (26), 8 (19), 9 (25)	T2 (30), T3a (28), T3b (42)
Jilg et al,[83] 2017	30	66	52.4–70	1.7	0.1–12.2	7 (40), ≥8 (60)	NR
Jilg et al,[84] 2020	23[b]	67	52–78	1.8	0.03–56.2	7a (17), 7b (31), 8 (22), 9 (30)	NR
Mandel et al,[88] 2020	23	64[d]	NR	3.9[d]	NR	NR	NR
Pfister et al,[93] 2016	28	67	46–79	2.4	0.04–8.0	≤7 (57), >7 (32), NR (11)	NR
Rauscher et al,[94] 2016	48	71	66–74[c]	1.3	0.75–2.6[c]	Median 7, 7–9[c]	NR

Abbreviation: NR, not reported.
[a] Patients with histology/total number of patients.
[b] Two patients with primary prostate cancer included.
[c] Interquartile range.
[d] Mean.
[e] Gleason score and pT category from the primary tumor.

Table 5
Quality of the included studies using Quality Assessment of Diagnostic Accuracy Studies-2

	Risk of Bias				Applicability Concerns		
Author, Year	Patient Selection	Index Test	Reference Standard	Flow and Timing	Patient Selection	Index Test	Reference Standard
Abufaraj et al,[68] 2019	Low	Low	Low	Unclear	Low	Low	Low
Berger et al,[69] 2018	Low	Low	Low	Low	Low	Low	Low
Bettermann et al,[70] 2019	Low	Low	Low	Unclear	Low	Low	Low
Budäus et al,[71] 2016	High	Unclear	Unclear	Unclear	Low	Low	Low
Cytawa et al,[72] 2020	Low	Low	Low	Unclear	Low	Low	Low
Dekalo et al,[73] 2019	Low	Low	Unclear	Unclear	Low	Low	Low
Dundee et al,[74] 2018	Low	Low	Low	Unclear	Low	Low	Low
Eiber et al,[75] 2016	Low	Low	Low	Low	Low	Low	Low
El Hajj et al,[76] 2019	Low	Low	Low	Low	Low	Low	Low
Fendler et al,[77] 2016	Low	Low	Low	Low	Low	Low	Low
Gorin et al,[78] 2018	Low	Low	Low	Unclear	Low	Low	Low
Gupta et al,[79] 2018	Low	Low	Unclear	Low	Low	Low	Low
Hanske et al,[80] 2019	High	Unclear	Low	Unclear	Unclear	Low	Low
Herlemann et al,[81] 2016	Low	Low	Unclear	Low	Low	Low	Low
Hicks et al,[82] 2018	Low	Low	Low	Low	Low	Low	Low
Jilg et al,[83] 2017	Low	Low	Low	Low	Low	Low	Low
Jilg et al,[84] 2020	Low	Low	Unclear	Unclear	Low	Low	Unclear
Kopp et al,[85] 2020	Low	Low	Low	Unclear	Low	Low	Low
Kroenke et al,[86] 2020	Low	Unclear	Low	Unclear	Low	Unclear	Low
Liu et al,[87] 2020	High	Low	Low	Low	Low	Low	Low
Mandel et al,[88] 2020	Unclear	Unclear	Low	Unclear	Unclear	Low	Low
Maurer et al,[89] 2016	Low	Unclear	Low	Low	Low	Low	Low
Muehlematter et al,[90] 2019	Low	Low	Low	Unclear	Low	Low	Low
Park et al,[91] 2018	Low	Low	Low	Low	Low	Low	Low
Petersen et al,[92] 2020	Low	Low	Low	Low	Low	Low	Low
Pfister et al,[93] 2016	Low	Low	Low	Unclear	Low	Low	Low
Rauscher et al,[94] 2016	Low	Unclear	Low	Low	Low	Low	Low
Rhee et al,[95] 2016	Low	Low	Low	Low	Low	Low	Low
Scheltema et al,[96] 2019	Low	Low	Low	Low	Low	Low	Low
van Kalmthout et al,[97] 2020	Low	Low	Low	Low	Low	Low	Low
van Leuween et al,[98] 2017	Low	Low	Low	Low	Low	Low	Low
von Klot et al,[99] 2017	Low	Low	Unclear	Unclear	Low	Low	Low
Yilmaz et al,[100] 2019	Low	Low	Low	Low	Unclear	Low	Low
Zhang et al,[101] 2017	Low	Low	Low	Unclear	Low	Low	Low

Prostate Tumor Location

A total of 12 included studies assessed tumor location within the prostate gland. The 2 × 2 contingency data are outlined in **Table 6**. Most studies used multiple sectors of whole mount prostatectomy specimens, whereas 3 studies used lobe-based data.[73,91,99] One study was prediagnostic in men with suspected prostate cancer and previous negative biopsies.[87] Sensitivity ranged from 42% to 98%, and specificity from 71% to 99% (**Fig. 3**A).

The presence of extraprostatic extension (EPE) was reported in one study using merged data from 4 different PET readers.[90] The sensitivity was limited (47%), but the specificity was high (90%). Four studies reported data on seminal vesicle infiltration (SVI). The sensitivity for SVI

Table 6
2× 2 contingency data for PSMA PET/CT scan assessment of primary prostate tumor

Author, year	Patients	TP	FN	FP	TN	Total
Berger et al,[69] 2018	50	79	2	2	317	400
Bettermann et al,[70] 2019	17	356	58	46	312	772
Dekalo et al,[73] 2019	59	90	18	0	10	118
Eiber et al,[75] 2016[a]	53	153	49	3	113	318
El Hajj et al,[76] 2019	23	150	204	54	420	828
Fendler et al,[77] 2016	21	67	33	2	24	126
Gupta et al,[79] 2018[b]	23	17	7	4	18	46
Hicks et al,[82] 2018[a]	32	275	137	159	389	960
Liu et al,[87] 2020[d]	31	88	17	38	297	440
Muehlematter et al,[90] 2019[c]	40	10	10	18	282	320
Muehlematter et al,[90] 2019[e]	40	36	40	55	509	640
Park et al,[91] 2018[a]	33	52	8	1	5	66
Rhee et al,[95] 2016	20	92	97	16	335	540
Scheltema et al,[96] 2019	54	NR	NR	NR	NR	648
von Klot et al,[99] 2017	21	36	2	1	3	42
von Klot et al,[99] 2017[b]	21	3	1	0	38	42
Yilmaz et al,[100] 2019[b]	24	NR	NR	NR	NR	48

Abbreviations: FN, false negatives; FP, false positives; NR, not reported; TN, true negatives; TP, true positives.
[a] PET/MR imaging.
[b] Seminal vesicle infiltration.
[c] Seminal vesicle infiltration pooled data for 4 different readers.
[d] Prediagnostic data with template and targeted biopsies.
[e] Extraprostatic extension pooled data for 4 different readers.

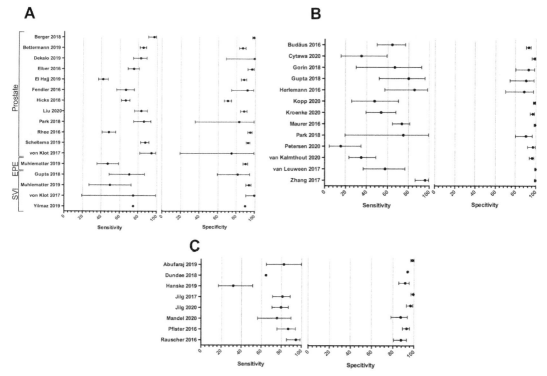

Fig. 3. (*A–C*) Forest plots of sensitivity and specificity (mean values, 95% confidence interval) for localization of primary prostate cancer tumor, EPE and SVI (*A*), primary lymph node metastases (*B*) and recurrent lymph node metastases (*C*).

Table 7
The 2 × 2 contingency data for PSMA PET/CT scan assessment of primary lymph node metastases

Author, Year	Patients	TP	FN	FP	TN	Total
Budäus et al,[71] 2016	30	34	19	40	515	608
Cytawa et al,[72] 2020	40	7	13	4	246	270
Gorin et al,[78] 2018	25	NR	NR	NR	NR	50
Gupta et al,[79] 2018	23	12	3	3	28	46
Herlemann et al,[81] 2016	20	12	2	3	23	40
Kopp et al,[85] 2020	90	10	11	5	432	458
Kroenke et al,[86] 2020[a]	58	28	24	10	313	375
Maurer et al,[89] 2016[a]	130	86	31	5	612	734
Park et al,[91] 2018[b]	33	3	1	6	56	66
Petersen et al,[92] 2020	20	4	22	3	102	131
van Kalmthout et al,[97] 2020	97	NR	NR	NR	NR	NR
van Leuween et al,[98] 2017	30	15	11	1	509	536
Zhang et al,[101] 2017	42	49	2	2	568	621

Abbreviations: FN, false negatives; FP, false positives; NR, not reported; TN, true negatives; TP, true positives.
[a] Mixed PET/CT scan and PET/MR imaging.
[b] PET/MR imaging.

detection was variable (47%–75%), and the specificity was high (81%–100%).[79,90,99,100]

Primary Lymph Node Metastases

A total of 13 included studies assessed regional lymph node metastases in primary prostate cancer. The 2 × 2 contingency data are outlined in **Table 7**. Data were reported either per side,[78,79,81,91] for multiple sectors,[72,85,86,89,92,97] or per node (many).[71,98,99] The sensitivity ranged from 15% to 96%, and the specificity from 88% to 100% (**Fig. 3B**). Studies reported the size of true PET-positive lymph node metastases to be larger (median, 4.0–13.6 mm) than false PET-negative lymph node metastases (median, 2.5–5.0 mm).[71,72,86,92,97,98]

Recurrent Lymph Nodes Metastases

A total of 8 included studies assessed regional lymph node metastases in biochemically recurrent prostate cancer after curative intent therapy. The 2 × 2 contingency data are outlined in **Table 8**. The sensitivity ranged from 32% to 95% and the specificity from 88% to 100% (**Fig. 3**C). Studies reported size of true PET-positive lymph node metastases to be larger (median, 5.8–10.0 mm) than false PET-negative lymph node metastases (median, 3.8–4.0 mm).[68,74,83]

Meta-Analysis

A total of 32 studies were included in the quantitative synthesis (meta-analysis). Two studies with

EPE and/or SVI data only were excluded.[90,100] In 1 study, the mean values for the sensitivity and specificity of the subregions were used.[68] The summarized receiver operating characteristic curves and area under the curve for localization

Table 8
The 2 × 2 contingency data for PSMA PET/CT assessment of recurrent lymph node metastases

Author, Year	Patients	TP	FN	FP	TN	Total
Abufaraj et al,[68] 2019[a]	65	NR	NR	NR	NR	NR
Dundee et al,[74] 2018	17	NR	NR	NR	NR	NR
Hanske et al,[80] 2019	22	NR	NR	NR	NR	NR
Jilg et al,[83] 2017	30	69	16	1	203	289
Jilg et al,[84] 2020[b]	23	83	21	5	158	267
Mandel et al,[88] 2020	23	22	7	10	70	109
Pfister et al,[93] 2016	28	53	8	17	230	308
Rauscher et al,[94] 2016	48	53	3	15	108	179

Abbreviations: FN, false negatives; FP, false positives; NR, not reported; TN, true negatives; TP, true positives.
[a] The 2 × 2 data for subregions.
[b] Radioguided surgery (RGS) used for ex situ measurement of surgically removed lymph nodes.

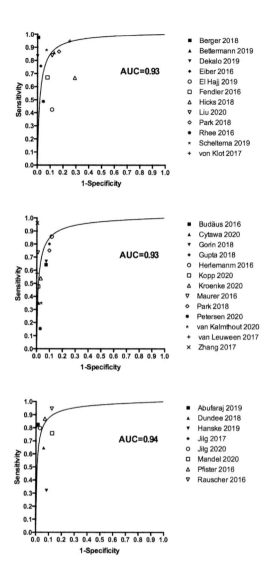

Fig. 4. Summarized receiver operating characteristic (SROC) curves for localization of primary tumor within the prostate (*top*), primary lymph node metastases (*middle*), and recurrent lymph node metastases (*bottom*).

of primary tumor within the prostate,[69,70,73,75–77,87,91,95,96,99] primary lymph node metastases,[71,72,78,79,81,85,86,89,91,92,97,98,101] and recurrent lymph node metastases[68,74,80,83,84,88,93,94] are shown in **Fig. 4.**

DISCUSSION

This systematic review of PSMA PET in prostate cancer identified 34 studies with systematic sector-based histopathology as the reference standard. Fourteen of the studies were in primary prostate cancer, 13 in primary lymph nodes, and 8 in recurrent lymph nodes.

Overall, the sensitivity was variable and the specificity was high.

This review revealed 2 main trends. First, the specificity was consistently higher than the sensitivity. Second, the sensitivity for the detection of lymph node metastases was better in the recurrent than in the primary setting. The overall high specificity probably reflects a high tumor-to-background ratio from a high accumulation of tracer in prostate tumors and pelvic lymph node metastases compared with surrounding normal tissue. The PSMA protein is not specific for prostate cancer cells, but the combination of high overexpression in tumor cells and internalization after ligand binding yields high tumor specificity. This notion is supported by the findings from Calais and colleagues,[102] who reported better interreader agreement for PSMA than for fluciclovine PET. The uptake value threshold for positive versus negative PET findings remains a challenge for all tracers.

A small amount of tumor cells is challenging to detect by imaging and many of the included studies reported detection rate to be linked to size.[68,71,72,74,83,86,89,92,97,98] Furthermore, Perera and colleagues[103] found in a large meta-analysis that likelihood of PSMA PET findings increased with PSA level, possibly reflecting larger tumor amounts. Hanske and colleagues[80] reported that the least sensitivity for the detection of recurrent lymph node metastases also had the lowest PSA level.

In a study of 4846 pelvic lymph nodes, Thoeny and colleagues[104] found that the majority of metastases were 3 mm or smaller at histopathology. With the limited spatial resolution of PET, false negatives are unavoidable. Another source of false negatives is tumors with low PSMA expression (5%–10% of patients with prostate cancer).[8,9] Clinical parameters that may contribute to the variable sensitivity of PSMA PET within the prostate gland are T category that often reflects tumor size, and Gleason grade (aggressiveness). The 2 studies with lowest sensitivity, El Hajj and colleagues[76] and Rhee and colleagues,[95] had the highest percentage of T2 stage tumors, at 65% or more. Rhee and colleagues also had a high percentage of low-grade cancers. Information regarding EPE and SVI is important in personalized treatment planning. We found 1 study investigating SVI and EPE and 3 studies investigating SVI. These studies also showed limited sensitivity and high specificity. The potential of EPE and SVI detection by PSMA PET is probably limited by spatial resolution of PET and short extent of tumor growth beyond the prostate gland. In addition, tracer excretion in the urine may out-signal discrete uptake in the seminal vesicles.

The review revealed that there was consistently greater sensitivity for recurrent lymph node metastases than for primary lymph node metastases. We can only speculate why. Based on our findings as discussed elsewhere in this article, the amount of tumor and the aggressiveness of the tumor seem to influence the sensitivity and specificity of PSMA PET. In terms of tumor biology, it is possibly the more aggressive tumors that recur as lymph node metastases. This factor could contribute to the higher PSMA PET tracer uptake and better sensitivity. Furthermore, it might be that recurrent lymph node metastases are larger than the primary lymph nodes. However, this finding is not supported by the studies in this review that revealed similar wide and largely overlapping range for both settings (see Results primary and recurrent lymph nodes).

Distant metastases (M+) and local relapse in biochemically recurrent prostate cancer are not assessed by the present review, because systematic sector-based histopathology is not feasible and targeted biopsies cannot provide false negatives. The clinical usefulness of PSMA PET in these clinical settings therefore cannot be assessed by sensitivity or specificity. Clinical outcome measured as time to progression, time to systemic treatment and/or survival is needed. There is a concern among clinicians to use new diagnostic tools when the impact on patient outcomes is unknown.[105] The increasing use of PSMA-based radionuclide therapy must also be evaluated in controlled studies with clinical end points, such as, the ongoing VISION study.[6,14]

In many centers PSMA PET/CT scanning has replaced choline PET/CT scanning, as is reflected by the literature.[106] Also, ^{18}F-fluciclovine PET/CT scanning has demonstrated superiority compared with choline PET/CT scans.[107] In comparison with PSMA PET, there is limited evidence for ^{18}F-fluciclovine PET/CT scans.[108] All but 2 of the included studies used ^{68}Ga-PSMA. Owing to its physical properties with a longer half-life and shorter positron traveling distance, ^{18}F-labeled PSMA may improve the detection of smaller lesions compared with ^{68}Ga-labeled PSMA. Within the criteria for our literature search there were no studies comparing [68]Ga- and ^{18}F-PSMA. Future ^{18}F-PSMA studies are awaited.

In conclusion, PSMA PET in prostate cancer has overall high specificity, but variable sensitivity, to localize known prostate cancer and detect pelvic lymph node metastases. Sensitivity seems to depend on tumor size and aggressiveness.

ACKNOWLEDGMENTS

The authors thank the corresponding authors Snir Dekalo (Dekalo and colleagues 2019) and Handoo Rhee (Rhee and colleagues 2016) for providing additional data for a 2 × 2 contingency table (true positives, false negatives, false positives, and true negatives). The authors thank Torgeir Mo for constructing the summarized receiver operating characteristic curves.

DISCLOSURE

The authors declare that they have no conflicts of interest that relates to the subject matter of the present review.

REFERENCES

1. Culp MB, Soerjomataram I, Efstathiou JA, et al. Recent global patterns in prostate cancer incidence and mortality rates. Eur Urol 2020;77:38–52.
2. SEER cancer Stat Facts: prostate cancer. National cancer Institute. Bethesda, MD. Available at: https://seer.cancer.gov/statfacts/html/prost.html. Accessed September 15, 2020.
3. Kishan AU, Chu FI, King CR, et al. Local failure and survival after definitive radiotherapy for aggressive prostate cancer: an individual patient-level meta-analysis of six randomized trials. Eur Urol 2020;77:201–8.
4. Vatne K, Stensvold A, Myklebust TÅ, et al. Pre- and post-prostatectomy variables associated with pelvic post-operative radiotherapy in prostate cancer patients: a national registry-based study. Acta Oncol 2017;56:1295–301.
5. Kratochwil C, Haberkorn U, Giesel FL. Radionuclide therapy of metastatic prostate cancer. Semin Nucl Med 2019;49:313–25.
6. Rahbar K, Bodei L, Morris MJ. Is the Vision of radioligand therapy for prostate cancer becoming a reality? an overview of the phase III VISION trial and its importance for the future of theranostics. J Nucl Med 2019;60:1504–6.
7. Giesel FL, Cardinale J, Schäfer M, et al. 18F-Labelled PSMA-1007 shows similarity in structure, biodistribution and tumour uptake to the theragnostic compound PSMA-617. Eur J Nucl Med Mol Imaging 2016;43:1929–30.
8. Mannweiler S, Amersdorfer P, Trajanoski S, et al. Heterogeneity of prostate-specific membrane antigen (PSMA) expression in prostate carcinoma with distant metastasis. Pathol Oncol Res 2009;15:167–72.
9. Minner S, Wittmer C, Graefen M, et al. High level PSMA expression is associated with early PSA recurrence in surgically treated prostate cancer. Prostate 2011;71:281–8.

10. Sheikhbahaei S, Afshar-Oromieh A, Eiber M, et al. Pearls and pitfalls in clinical interpretation of prostate-specific membrane antigen (PSMA)-targeted PET imaging. Eur J Nucl Med Mol Imaging 2017;44:2117–36.

11. Sheikhbahaei S, Werner RA, Solnes LB, et al. Prostate-Specific Membrane Antigen (PSMA)-targeted PET imaging of prostate cancer: an update on important pitfalls. Semin Nucl Med 2019;49:255–70.

12. Giesel FL, Hadaschik B, Cardinale J, et al. F-18 labelled PSMA-1007: biodistribution, radiation dosimetry and histopathological validation of tumor lesions in prostate cancer patients. Eur J Nucl Med Mol Imaging 2017;44:678–88.

13. Mottet N, Cornford P, van den Bergh RCN, et al. EAU guidelines prostate cancer. Available at: https://uroweb.org/guideline/prostate-cancer/. Accessed September 14, 2020.

14. Miyahira AK, Pienta KJ, Babich JW, et al. Meeting report from the Prostate Cancer Foundation PSMA theranostics state of the science meeting. Prostate 2020;80(15):1273–96.

15. Moher D, Liberati A, Tetzlaff J, et al, PRISMA Group. Preferred reporting items for systematic reviews and meta-analyses: the PRISMA statement. PLoS Med 2009;6:e1000097.

16. Ouzzani M, Hammady H, Fedorowicz Z, et al. Rayyan – a web and mobile app for systematic reviews. Syst Rev 2016;5:210.

17. Whiting PF, Rutjes AWS, Westwood ME, et al. QUADAS-2: a revised tool for the quality assessment of diagnostic accuracy studies. Ann Intern Med 2011; 155:529–36.

18. MedCalc Diagnostic test evaluation calculator. Available at: https://www.medcalc.org/calc/diagnostic_test.php. Accessed September 10, 2020.

19. Jones CM, Athanasiou T. Summary receiver operating characteristic curve analysis techniques in the evaluation of diagnostic tests. Ann Thorac Surg 2005;79:16–20.

20. Littenberg B, Moses LE. Estimating diagnostic accuracy from multiple conflicting reports: a new meta-analytic method. Med Decis Making 1993; 13:313–21.

21. Afshar-Oromieh A, Avtzi E, Giesel FL, et al. The diagnostic value of PET/CT imaging with the (68)Ga-labelled PSMA ligand HBED-CC in the diagnosis of recurrent prostate cancer. Eur J Nucl Med Mol Imaging 2015;42(2):197–209.

22. Al-Bayati M, Grueneisen J, Lütje S, et al. Integrated 68Gallium labelled prostate-specific membrane antigen-11 positron emission tomography/magnetic resonance imaging enhances discriminatory power of multi-parametric prostate magnetic resonance imaging. Urol Int 2018;100(2):164–71.

23. Basha MAA, Hamed MAG, Hussein O, et al. 68Ga-PSMA-11 PET/CT in newly diagnosed prostate cancer: diagnostic sensitivity and interobserver agreement. Abdom Radiol 2019;44:2545–56.

24. Chen M, Zhang Q, Zhang C, et al. Combination of 68Ga-PSMA PET/CT and multiparametric MRI improves the detection of clinically significant prostate cancer: a lesion-by-lesion analysis. J Nucl Med 2019;60(7):944–9.

25. Chen M, Zhang Q, Zhang C, et al. Comparison of 68Ga-prostate-specific membrane antigen (PSMA) positron emission tomography/computed tomography (PET/CT) and multi-parametric magnetic resonance imaging (MRI) in the evaluation of tumor extension of primary prostate cancer. Transl Androl Urol 2020;9(2):382–90.

26. Damjanovic J, Janssen JC, Furth C, et al. 68 Ga-PSMA-PET/CT for the evaluation of pulmonary metastases and opacities in patients with prostate cancer. Cancer Imaging 2018;18(1):20.

27. Damjanovic J, Janssen JC, Prasad V, et al. 68Ga-PSMA-PET/CT for the evaluation of liver metastases in patients with prostate cancer. Cancer Imaging 2019;19(1):37.

28. Donato P, Roberts MJ, Morton A, et al. Improved specificity with 68Ga PSMA PET/CT to detect clinically significant lesions "invisible" on multiparametric MRI of the prostate: a single institution comparative analysis with radical prostatectomy histology. Eur J Nucl Med Mol Imaging 2019; 46(1):20–30.

29. Fendler WP, Calais J, Eiber M, et al. Assessment of 68Ga-PSMA-11 PET accuracy in localizing recurrent prostate cancer: a prospective single-arm clinical trial. JAMA Oncol 2019;5(6):856–63.

30. Ferraro DA, Muehlematter UJ, Garcia Schüler HI, et al. 68Ga-PSMA-11 PET has the potential to improve patient selection for extended pelvic lymph node dissection in intermediate to high-risk prostate cancer. Eur J Nucl Med Mol Imaging 2020;47(1):147–59.

31. Grubmüller B, Baltzer P, Hartenbach S, et al. PSMA ligand PET/MRI for primary prostate cancer: staging performance and clinical impact. Clin Cancer Res 2018;24(24):6300–7.

32. Hamed MAG, Basha MAA, Ahmed H, et al. 68Ga-PSMA PET/CT in patients with rising prostatic-specific antigen after definitive treatment of prostate cancer: detection efficacy and diagnostic accuracy. Acad Radiol 2019;26(4):450–60.

33. Hoffmann MA, Miederer M, Wieler HJ, et al. Diagnostic performance of 68Gallium-PSMA-11 PET/CT to detect significant prostate cancer and comparison with 18FEC PET/CT. Oncotarget 2017; 8(67):111073–83.

34. Hofman MS, Lawrentschuk N, Francis RJ, et al. Prostate-specific membrane antigen PET-CT in

patients with high-risk prostate cancer before curative-intent surgery or radiotherapy (proPSMA): a prospective, randomised, multicentre study. Lancet 2020;395(10231):1208–16.

35. Janssen JC, Meißner S, Woythal N, et al. Comparison of hybrid 68Ga-PSMA-PET/CT and 99mTc-DPD-SPECT/CT for the detection of bone metastases in prostate cancer patients: additional value of morphologic information from low dose CT. Eur Radiol 2018;28(2):610–9.

36. Klingenberg S, Jochumsen MR, Ulhøi BP, et al. 68Ga-PSMA PET/CT for primary NM staging of high-risk prostate cancer [published online ahead of print, 2020 May 22]. J Nucl Med 2020;120: 245605.

37. Kulkarni SC, Sundaram PS, Padma S. In primary lymph nodal staging of patients with high-risk and intermediate-risk prostate cancer, how critical is the role of Gallium-68 prostate-specific membrane antigen positron emission tomography-computed tomography? Nucl Med Commun 2020;41(2): 139–46.

38. Lindenberg L, Mena E, Turkbey B, et al. Evaluating biochemically recurrent prostate cancer: histologic validation of 18F-DCFPyL PET/CT with comparison to multiparametric MRI. Radiology 2020;296(3): 564–72.

39. Lopci E, Lughezzani G, Castello A, et al. Prospective evaluation of 68Ga-labeled prostate-specific membrane antigen ligand positron emission tomography/computed tomography in primary prostate cancer diagnosis. Eur Urol Focus 2020. S2405-4569(20)30092-30094.

40. Pallavi UN, Gogoi S, Thakral P, et al. Incremental value of Ga-68 prostate-specific membrane antigen-11 positron-emission tomography/ computed tomography scan for preoperative risk stratification of prostate cancer. Indian J Nucl Med 2020;35(2):93–9.

41. Radzina M, Tirane M, Roznere L, et al. Accuracy of 68Ga-PSMA-11 PET/CT and multiparametric MRI for the detection of local tumor and lymph node metastases in early biochemical recurrence of prostate cancer. Am J Nucl Med Mol Imaging 2020;10(2):106–18.

42. van Leeuwen PJ, Donswijk M, Nandurkar R, et al. Gallium-68-prostate-specific membrane antigen (68 Ga-PSMA) positron emission tomography (PET)/computed tomography (CT) predicts complete biochemical response from radical prostatectomy and lymph node dissection in intermediate- and high-risk prostate cancer. BJU Int 2019; 124(1):62–8.

43. Yaxley JW, Raveenthiran S, Nouhaud FX, et al. Outcomes of primary lymph node staging of intermediate and high risk prostate cancer with 68Ga-PSMA positron emission tomography/computerized tomography compared to histological correlation of pelvic lymph node pathology. J Urol 2019; 201(4):815–20.

44. Donato P, Morton A, Yaxley J, et al. 68Ga-PSMA PET/CT better characterises localised prostate cancer after MRI and transperineal prostate biopsy: is 68Ga-PSMA PET/CT guided biopsy the future? Eur J Nucl Med Mol Imaging 2020;47(8): 1843–51.

45. Öbek C, Doğanca T, Demirci E, et al. The accuracy of 68Ga-PSMA PET/CT in primary lymph node staging in high-risk prostate cancer. Eur J Nucl Med Mol Imaging 2017;44(11):1806–12.

46. Rahman LA, Rutagengwa D, Lin P, et al. High negative predictive value of 68Ga PSMA PET-CT for local lymph node metastases in high risk primary prostate cancer with histopathological correlation. Cancer Imaging 2019;19(1):86.

47. Zhang J, Shao S, Wu P, et al. Diagnostic performance of 68Ga-PSMA PET/CT in the detection of prostate cancer prior to initial biopsy: comparison with cancer-predicting nomograms. Eur J Nucl Med Mol Imaging 2019;46(4):908–20.

48. Hijazi S, Meller B, Leitsmann C, et al. Pelvic lymph node dissection for nodal oligometastatic prostate cancer detected by 68Ga-PSMA-positron emission tomography/computerized tomography. Prostate 2015;75(16):1934–40.

49. Kaufmann S, Kruck S, Gatidis S, et al. Simultaneous whole-body PET/MRI with integrated multiparametric MRI for primary staging of high-risk prostate cancer. World J Urol 2020;38(10): 2513–21.

50. Kuten J, Fahoum I, Savin Z, et al. Head-to-Head comparison of 68Ga-PSMA-11 with 18F-PSMA-1007 PET/CT in staging prostate cancer using histopathology and Immunohistochemical analysis as a reference standard. J Nucl Med 2020;61(4): 527–32.

51. Lawhn-Heath C, Flavell RR, Behr SC, et al. Single-Center Prospective Evaluation of 68Ga-PSMA-11 PET in biochemical recurrence of prostate cancer. AJR Am J Roentgenol 2019;213(2):266–74.

52. Lengana T, Lawal IO, Boshomane TG, et al. 68Ga-PSMA PET/CT replacing bone scan in the initial staging of skeletal metastasis in prostate cancer: a fait accompli? Clin Genitourin Cancer 2018; 16(5):392–401.

53. Lopci E, Saita A, Lazzeri M, et al. 68Ga-PSMA positron emission tomography/computerized tomography for primary diagnosis of prostate cancer in men with contraindications to or negative multiparametric magnetic resonance imaging: a prospective observational study. J Urol 2018;200(1): 95–103.

54. Sahlmann CO, Meller B, Bouter C, et al. Biphasic 68Ga-PSMA-HBED-CC-PET/CT in patients with

recurrent and high-risk prostate carcinoma. Eur J Nucl Med Mol Imaging 2016;43(5):898–905.

55. de Jong AC, Smits M, van Riet J, et al. 68Ga-PSMA guided bone biopsies for molecular diagnostics in metastatic prostate cancer patients. J Nucl Med 2020;61(11):1607–14.

56. Farolfi A, Ilhan H, Gafita A, et al. Mapping prostate cancer lesions before and after unsuccessful salvage lymph node dissection using repeat PSMA PET. J Nucl Med 2020;61(7):1037–42.

57. Fossati N, Scarcella S, Gandaglia G, et al. Underestimation of positron emission tomography/computerized tomography in assessing tumor burden in prostate cancer nodal recurrence: head-to-head comparison of 68Ga-PSMA and 11C-choline in a large, multi-institutional series of extended salvage lymph node dissections. J Urol 2020;204(2):296–302.

58. Gao J, Zhang C, Zhang Q, et al. Diagnostic performance of 68Ga-PSMA PET/CT for identification of aggressive cribriform morphology in prostate cancer with whole-mount sections. Eur J Nucl Med Mol Imaging 2019;46(7):1531–41.

59. Hinsenveld FJ, Wit EMK, van Leeuwen PJ, et al. Prostate-specific membrane antigen PET/CT combined with sentinel node biopsy for primary lymph node staging in prostate cancer. J Nucl Med 2020;61(4):540–5.

60. Jilg CA, Drendel V, Rischke HC, et al. Detection Rate of 18F-Choline PET/CT and 68Ga-PSMA-HBED-CC PET/CT for prostate cancer lymph node metastases with direct link from PET to histopathology: dependence on the size of tumor deposits in lymph nodes. J Nucl Med 2019;60(7):971–7.

61. Kalapara AA, Nzenza T, Pan HYC, et al. Detection and localisation of primary prostate cancer using 68 gallium prostate-specific membrane antigen positron emission tomography/computed tomography compared with multiparametric magnetic resonance imaging and radical prostatectomy specimen pathology. BJU Int 2020;126(1):83–90.

62. Maurer T, Robu S, Schottelius M, et al. 99mTechnetium-based prostate-specific membrane antigen-radioguided surgery in recurrent prostate cancer. Eur Urol 2019;75(4):659–66.

63. Nandurkar R, van Leeuwen P, Stricker P, et al. 68Ga-HBEDD PSMA-11 PET/CT staging prior to radical prostatectomy in prostate cancer patients: diagnostic and predictive value for the biochemical response to surgery. Br J Radiol 2019;92(1095):20180667.

64. Rauscher I, Düwel C, Wirtz M, et al. Value of 111 In-prostate-specific membrane antigen (PSMA)-radioguided surgery for salvage lymphadenectomy in recurrent prostate cancer: correlation with histopathology and clinical follow-up. BJU Int 2017;120(1):40–7.

65. Siriwardana A, Thompson J, van Leeuwen PJ, et al. Initial multicentre experience of 68 gallium-PSMA PET/CT guided robot-assisted salvage lymphadenectomy: acceptable safety profile but oncological benefit appears limited. BJU Int 2017;120(5):673–81.

66. Thalgott M, Düwel C, Rauscher I, et al. One-Stop-Shop whole-body 68Ga-PSMA-11 PET/MRI compared with clinical nomograms for preoperative T and N staging of high-risk prostate cancer. J Nucl Med 2018;59(12):1850–6.

67. Woythal N, Arsenic R, Kempkensteffen C, et al. Immunohistochemical validation of PSMA expression measured by 68Ga-PSMA PET/CT in primary prostate cancer. J Nucl Med 2018;59(2):238–43.

68. Abufaraj M, Grubmüller B, Zeitlinger M, et al. Prospective evaluation of the performance of [68Ga]Ga-PSMA-11 PET/CT(MRI) for lymph node staging in patients undergoing superextended salvage lymph node dissection after radical prostatectomy. Eur J Nucl Med Mol Imaging 2019;46:2169–77.

69. Berger I, Annabattula C, Lewis J, et al. 68Ga-PSMA PET/CT vs. mpMRI for locoregional prostate cancer staging: correlation with final histopathology. Prostate Cancer Prostatic Dis 2018;21:204–11.

70. Bettermann AS, Zamboglou C, Kiefer S, et al. [68Ga-]PSMA-11 PET/CT and multiparametric MRI for gross tumor volume delineation in a slice by slice analysis with whole mount histopathology as a reference standard - Implications for focal radiotherapy planning in primary prostate cancer. Radiother Oncol 2019;141:214–9.

71. Budäus L, Leyh-Bannurah SR, Salomon G, et al. Initial experience of (68)Ga-PSMA PET/CT imaging in high-risk prostate cancer patients prior to radical prostatectomy. Eur Urol 2016;69:393–6.

72. Cytawa W, Seitz AK, Kircher S, et al. 68Ga-PSMA I&T PET/CT for primary staging of prostate cancer. Eur J Nucl Med Mol Imaging 2020;47:168–77.

73. Dekalo S, Kuten J, Mabjeesh NJ, et al. 68Ga-PSMA PET/CT: does it predict adverse pathology findings at radical prostatectomy? Urol Oncol 2019;37:574.e19-24.

74. Dundee P, Gross T, Moran D, et al. Ga-labeled prostate-specific membrane antigen ligand-positron-emission tomography: still just the tip of the iceberg. Urology 2018;120:187–91.

75. Eiber M, Weirich G, Holzapfel K, et al. Simultaneous 68Ga-PSMA HBED-CC PET/MRI improves the localization of primary prostate cancer. Eur Urol 2016;70:829–36.

76. El Hajj A, Yacoub B, Mansour M, et al. Diagnostic performance of Gallium-68 prostate-specific membrane antigen positron emission tomography-computed tomography in intermediate and high

risk prostate cancer. Medicine (Baltimore) 2019;98: e17491.

77. Fendler WP, Schmidt DF, Wenter V, et al. 68Ga-PSMA PET/CT detects the location and extent of primary prostate cancer. J Nucl Med 2016;57: 1720–5.

78. Gorin MA, Rowe SP, Patel HD, et al. Prostate specific membrane antigen targeted 18F-DCFPyL positron emission tomography/computerized tomography for the preoperative staging of high risk prostate cancer: results of a prospective, phase II, single center study. J Urol 2018;199: 126–32.

79. Gupta M, Choudhury PS, Rawal S, et al. Initial risk stratification and staging in prostate cancer with prostatic-specific membrane antigen positron emission tomography/computed tomography: a first-stop-shop. World J Nucl Med 2018;17:261–9.

80. Hanske J, Ostholt J, Roghmann F, et al. Salvage lymph node dissection in hormone-naïve men: how effective is surgery? Urol Oncol 2019;37:812.e17-24.

81. Herlemann A, Wenter V, Kretschmer A, et al. 68Ga-PSMA positron emission tomography/computed tomography provides accurate staging of lymph node regions prior to lymph node dissection in patients with prostate cancer. Eur Urol 2016;70: 553–7.

82. Hicks RM, Simko JP, Westphalen AC, et al. Diagnostic accuracy of 68Ga-PSMA-11 PET/MRI compared with multiparametric MRI in the detection of prostate cancer. Radiology 2018;289:730–7.

83. Jilg CA, Drendel V, Rischke HC, et al. Diagnostic accuracy of Ga-68-HBED-CC-PSMA-Ligand-PET/CT before salvage lymph node dissection for recurrent prostate cancer. Theranostics 2017;7: 1770–80.

84. Jilg CA, Reichel K, Stoykow C, et al. Results from extended lymphadenectomies with [111In]PSMA-617 for intraoperative detection of PSMA-PET/CT-positive nodal metastatic prostate cancer. EJNMMI Res 2020;10:17.

85. Kopp J, Kopp D, Bernhardt E, et al. 68Ga-PSMA PET/CT based primary staging and histological correlation after extended pelvic lymph node dissection at radical prostatectomy. World J Urol 2020;38(12):3085–90.

86. Kroenke M, Wurzer A, Schwamborn K, et al. Histologically Confirmed diagnostic efficacy of 18F-rhPSMA-7 PET for N-staging of patients with primary high-risk prostate cancer. J Nucl Med 2020; 61:710–5.

87. Liu C, Liu T, Zhang Z, et al. 68Ga-PSMA PET/CT Combined with PET/Ultrasound-Guided Prostate Biopsy Can Diagnose Clinically Significant Prostate Cancer in Men with Previous Negative Biopsy Results. J Nucl Med 2020;61(9):1314–9.

88. Mandel P, Tilki D, Chun FK, et al. Accuracy of 68Ga-prostate-specific membrane antigen positron emission tomography for the detection of lymph node metastases before salvage lymphadenectomy. Eur Urol Focus 2020;6:71–3.

89. Maurer T, Gschwend JE, Rauscher I, et al. Diagnostic Efficacy of (68)Gallium-PSMA positron emission tomography compared to conventional imaging for lymph node staging of 130 consecutive patients with intermediate to high risk prostate cancer. J Urol 2016;195:1436–43.

90. Muehlematter UJ, Burger IA, Becker AS, et al. Diagnostic Accuracy of Multiparametric MRI versus 68Ga-PSMA-11 PET/MRI for extracapsular extension and seminal vesicle invasion in patients with prostate cancer. Radiology 2019;293:350–8.

91. Park SY, Zacharias C, Harrison C, et al. Gallium 68 PSMA-11 PET/MR imaging in patients with intermediate- or high-risk prostate cancer. Radiology 2018; 288:495–505.

92. Petersen LJ, Nielsen JB, Langkilde NC, et al. 68Ga-PSMA PET/CT compared with MRI/CT and diffusion-weighted MRI for primary lymph node staging prior to definitive radiotherapy in prostate cancer: a prospective diagnostic test accuracy study. World J Urol 2020;38:939–48.

93. Pfister D, Porres D, Heidenreich A, et al. Detection of recurrent prostate cancer lesions before salvage lymphadenectomy is more accurate with (68)Ga-PSMA-HBED-CC than with (18)F-Fluoroethylcholine PET/CT. Eur J Nucl Med Mol Imaging 2016;43:1410–7.

94. Rauscher I, Maurer T, Beer AJ, et al. Value of 68Ga-PSMA HBED-CC PET for the assessment of lymph node metastases in prostate cancer patients with biochemical recurrence: comparison with histopathology after salvage lymphadenectomy. J Nucl Med 2016;57:1713–9.

95. Rhee H, Thomas P, Shepherd B, et al. Prostate specific membrane antigen positron emission tomography may improve the diagnostic accuracy of multiparametric magnetic resonance imaging in localized prostate cancer. J Urol 2016;196:1261–7.

96. Scheltema MJ, Chang JI, Stricker PD, et al. Diagnostic accuracy of 68 Ga-prostate-specific membrane antigen (PSMA) positron-emission tomography (PET) and multiparametric (mp)MRI to detect intermediate-grade intra-prostatic prostate cancer using whole-mount pathology: impact of the addition of 68 Ga-PSMA PET to mpMRI. BJU Int 2019;124(Suppl 1):42–9.

97. van Kalmthout LWM, van Melick HHE, Lavalaye J, et al. Prospective validation of gallium-68 prostate specific membrane antigen-positron emission tomography/computerized tomography for primary staging of prostate cancer. J Urol 2020;203: 537–45.

98. van Leeuwen PJ, Emmett L, Ho B, et al. Prospective evaluation of 68Gallium-prostate-specific membrane antigen positron emission tomography/computed tomography for preoperative lymph node staging in prostate cancer. BJU Int 2017;119: 209–15.

99. von Klot CJ, Merseburger AS, Böker A, et al. 68Ga-PSMA PET/CT imaging predicting intraprostatic tumor extent, extracapsular extension and seminal vesicle invasion prior to radical prostatectomy in patients with prostate cancer. Nucl Med Mol Imaging 2017;51:314–22.

100. Yilmaz B, Turkay R, Colakoglu Y, et al. Comparison of preoperative locoregional Ga-68 PSMA-11 PET-CT and mp-MRI results with postoperative histopathology of prostate cancer. Prostate 2019;79: 1007–17.

101. Zhang Q, Zang S, Zhang C, et al. Comparison of 68Ga-PSMA-11 PET-CT with mpMRI for preoperative lymph node staging in patients with intermediate to high-risk prostate cancer. J Transl Med 2017; 15:230.

102. Calais J, Ceci F, Eiber M, et al. 18F-fluciclovine PET-CT and 68Ga-PSMA-11 PET-CT in patients with early biochemical recurrence after prostatectomy: a prospective, single-centre, single-arm, comparative imaging trial. Lancet Oncol 2019;20: 1286–94.

103. Perera M, Papa N, Roberts M, et al. Gallium-68 prostate-specific membrane antigen positron emission tomography in advanced prostate cancer-updated diagnostic utility, sensitivity, specificity, and distribution of prostate-specific membrane antigen-avid lesions: a systematic review and meta-analysis. Eur Urol 2020;77:403–17.

104. Thoeny HC, Froehlich JM, Triantafyllou M, et al. Metastases in normal-sized pelvic lymph nodes: detection with diffusion-weighted MR imaging. Radiology 2014;273:125–35.

105. Sundahl N, Gillessen S, Sweeney C, et al. When what you see is not always what you get: raising the bar of evidence for new diagnostic imaging modalities. Eur Urol 2020. https://doi.org/10.1016/j.eururo.2020.07.029.

106. Fanti S, Minozzi S, Antoch G, et al. Consensus on molecular imaging and theranostics in prostate cancer. Lancet Oncol 2018;19:e696–708.

107. Nanni C, Zanoni L, Pultrone C, et al. 18)F-FACBC (anti1-amino-3-(18)F-fluorocyclobutane-1-carboxylic acid) versus (11)C-choline PET/CT in prostate cancer relapse: results of a prospective trial. Eur J Nucl Med Mol Imaging 2016;43:1601–10.

108. Seierstad T, Hole KH, Tulipan AJ, et al. 18F-fluciclovine PET for assessment of prostate cancer with histopathology as reference standard: a systematic review. PET Clin 2021.

^{18}F-Fluciclovine PET for Assessment of Prostate Cancer with Histopathology as Reference Standard
A Systematic Review

Therese Seierstad, MSc, PhD, MHA[a],*, Knut Håkon Hole, MD, PhD[a,b], Andreas Julius Tulipan, MD[a,b], Hilde Strømme, MSc[c], Wolfgang Lilleby, MD, PhD[d], Mona-Elisabeth Revheim, MD, PhD, MHA[a,b], Eivor Hernes, MD, PhD[a]

KEYWORDS

• Prostate cancer • PSMA • PET/CT • PET/MR imaging • Personalized medicine • Fluciclovine PET
• Histopathology

KEY POINTS

- ^{18}F-fluciclovine PET has high sensitivity, but low specificity for localization of known primary prostate cancer.
- ^{18}F-fluciclovine PET has high specificity, but low sensitivity for detection of primary lymph node metastases.
- Few ^{18}F-fluciclovine studies have systematic sector-based histopathology that allows calculation of sensitivity and specificity.

BACKGROUND

Prostate cancer is the most common cancer in men, and has the second-highest mortality among male malignant carcinomas.[1] At initial diagnosis, the extent and spread of the cancer are key factors in deciding the appropriate treatment. For localized disease, the main treatment modalities are radical prostatectomy, external beam radiotherapy, or brachytherapy. About one-third of patients develop recurrence after primary definitive treatment.[2] Localization of recurrent disease is critical to the subsequent therapeutic strategy and prognosis because focal salvage treatment options are emerging.[3,4]

In the past, the role of PET for prostate cancer imaging has been limited. However, in recent years, several new PET tracers have emerged that offer improved diagnostic performance for detecting localized disease and metastases at initial diagnosis and localize disease recurrence.[5] One of these PET tracers is trans-1-amino-3-^{18}F-fluorocyclobutanecarboxylic acid (anti-^{18}F-FACBC, ^{18}F-fluciclovine). ^{18}F-fluciclovine is a radiolabeled amino acid analogue that exploits the increased demand of amino acids in tumor tissue for prostate cancer imaging[6] (**Fig. 1**). Long half-life and limited urinary excretion are also desirable features of ^{18}F-fluciclovine.[7] At present,

[a] Division of Radiology and Nuclear Medicine, Oslo University Hospital, P.O. Box 4956 Nydalen, 0424 Oslo, Norway; [b] Institute of Clinical Medicine, University of Oslo, P.O. Box 1171 Blindern, 0318 Oslo, Norway; [c] Library of Medicine and Science, University of Oslo, Sognsvannsveien 20, 0372 Oslo, Norway; [d] Department of Oncology, Oslo University Hospital, P.O. Box 4953 Nydalen, 0424 Oslo, Norway
* Corresponding author. Department of Research and Development, Division of Radiology and Nuclear Medicine, Oslo University Hospital, P.O. Box 4956 Nydalen, 0424 Oslo, Norway.
E-mail address: therese@radium.uio.no

PET Clin 16 (2021) 167–176
https://doi.org/10.1016/j.cpet.2020.12.012
1556-8598/21/© 2021 The Authors. Published by Elsevier Inc. This is an open access article under the CC BY license (http://creativecommons.org/licenses/by/4.0/).

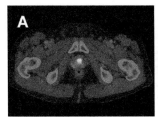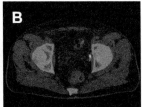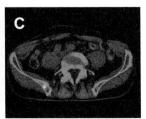

Fig. 1. ^{18}F-fluciclovine PET/CT images showing local recurrence (*A*), a lymph node metastasis (*B*), and a sclerotic bone metastasis (*C*).

^{18}F-fluciclovine is approved in the United States for specific indications: suspected prostate cancer recurrence based on increased prostate-specific antigen (PSA) level.[8]

This article summarizes studies of diagnostic accuracy of ^{18}F-fluciclovine PET for assessment of patients with prostate cancer with systematic sector-based histopathology as reference standard.

EVIDENCE ACQUISITION
Search Strategy

The systematic review followed the Preferred Reporting Items for Systematic Reviews and Meta-Analysis (PRISMA) guidelines.[9] An information specialist (H.S.) planned and performed the systematic literature searches in MEDLINE (Ovid), Embase (Ovid), Cochrane Database of Systematic Reviews (Wiley), Cochrane Central Register of Controlled Trials, including references from ClinicalTrials.gov and The World Health Organization (WHO) International Clinical Trials Registry Platform (Wiley) and Scopus (Elsevier). Search terms were discussed in detail with 2 of the reviewers (A.J.T., T.S.) and the authors searched for a combination of subject headings, where applicable, and text words, including synonyms, for "fluciclovine f 18 AND prostate cancer." The following strategy was used in MEDLINE (Ovid) and adapted to the other databases: "(((((fluciclovine or fluorocyclobutane* or FACBC) adj3 (F-18 or 18F)) or ge-148 or ge148 or F-FACBC or axumin or NMK-36 or NMK36 or NMK-36c or "1-amino-3-fluorocyclobutane-1-carboxylic acid").mp.) OR ((exp Prostatic Neoplasms/or (prostat* adj3 (neoplasm* or cancer* or tumo?r* or carcinom*)).mp.) and FACBC.mp.))." Filters to exclude animal studies were applied in MEDLINE and Embase. All searches were performed on July 14 2020. The complete search strategy for all databases can be obtained from the corresponding author. The results from all searches were imported into EndNote and duplicates were removed. The remaining references were imported in the Rayyan screening software.[10]

Eligibility Criteria

The PICO (patient, intervention, comparator, outcome) framework was used to define the eligibility criteria: the study must consist of patients with prostate cancer (P), the patients must have had ^{18}F-fluciclovine PET (I), the comparator must be systematic sector-based histopathology (C), and the outcome must be diagnostic performance given as sensitivity and specificity (O). Furthermore, the study must report sector-based data either as individual data or as summary diagnostic accuracy and contain at least 10 patients fulfilling all these criteria. In case of studies with mixed settings (primary/recurrence, prostate bed/lymph nodes), each subgroup must fulfill all criteria. Only original articles in English were eligible. Editorials, letters, review articles, comments, conference proceedings, and case reports were excluded, because study quality could not be assessed.

Screening and Study Selection

The screening and article selection was performed by 3 independent evaluators (A.J.T., E.H., T.S.) and conflicts were resolved by consensus. After an initial screening of titles and abstracts, the remaining articles were read in full text and excluded with reasons when appropriate.

Quality Assessment

Two evaluators (E.H., T.S.) in consensus used the Quality Assessment of Diagnostic Accuracy Studies-2 (QUADAS-2) tool[11] to assess the risk of bias in 4 domains: patient selection, index test, reference standard, and reference test timing. For the 3 first domains, applicability concerns were also assessed.

Data Extraction

For each selected study, the following information was collected:

- Basic study characteristics: investigators, year of publication, country, study design (prospective/retrospective), clinical setting

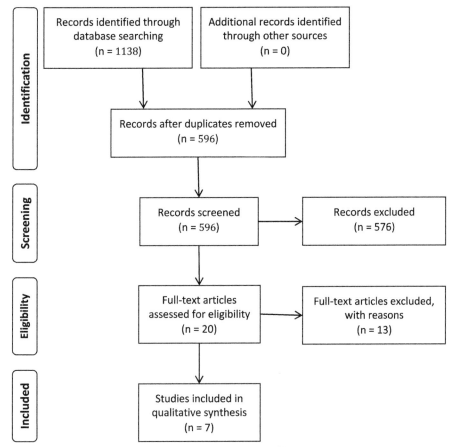

Fig. 2. PRISMA flow chart of studies for the systematic review of ^{18}F-fluciclovine PET for assessment of prostate cancer with systematic sector-based histopathology as reference standard.

(primary/recurrence), anatomy (prostate/lymph nodes), and imaging modality.

- Clinical and pathologic data: number of patients, age, prostate specific antigen (PSA), Gleason score, and tumor stage.
- Diagnostic accuracy data: number of true-positives, true-negatives, false-positives, and false-negatives (2 × 2 contingency tables). Investigators of studies that only reported summary diagnostic data were asked to provide additional data.

Data Synthesis and Analysis

Sensitivity and specificity with 95% confidence interval (CI) were calculated from the 2 × 2 contingency tables for each of the included studies using the MedCalc Diagnostic test evaluator calculator[12] or extracted from studies where 2 × 2 data were not available. Forest plots were drawn to show the variation and explore heterogeneity for sensitivity and specificity.

EVIDENCE SYNTHESIS
Search Results

The results for the identification and selection of studies are shown in **Fig. 2**. Initially, a total of 1138 records were retrieved by the systematic search. The number was reduced to 596 after removal of duplicates. Screening of titles and abstracts excluded 576 records. The remaining 20 records were read in full text and 13 were excluded. The reasons for exclusion were no systematic sector-based histopathology[13–22] or inappropriate study design and/or not within the scope of the review.[23–25]

Table 1
Study characteristics

Author	Journal	Country	Design	Setting	Anatomy	Modality
Alemozaffar, et al,[30] 2020	J Urol	United States	Prospective	Primary	Lymph nodes	PET/CT
Jambor, et al,[32] 2018	EJNMMI	Finland	Prospective	Primary	Prostate	PET/CT + PET/MR imaging
Schuster, et al,[26] 2013	AJNMMI	United States	Prospective	Primary	Prostate	PET/CT
Selnaes, et al,[31] 2018	Eur Radiol	Norway	Prospective	Primary	Lymph nodes	PET/MR imaging
Suzuki, et al,[27] 2016	Jpn J Clin Oncol	Japan	Prospective	Primary	Prostate + lymph nodes	PET/CT
Suzuki, et al,[28] 2019	Jpn J Clin Oncol	Japan	Prospective	Primary	Lymph nodes	PET/CT
Turkbey, et al,[29] 2014	Radiology	United States	Prospective	Primary	Prostate	PET/CT

Description of Included Studies

Study and patient characteristics for the 7 included studies are presented in **Tables 1** and **2**. The 7 eligible studies included a total of 212 patients. All studies were prospective. Five studies used PET/computed tomography (CT),[26–30] 1 study used PET/magnetic resonance (MR) imaging,[31] and 1 study used both PET/CT and PET/MR imaging.[32] The mean age of the study cohorts ranged from 60.8 to 68 years and the mean PSA level ranged from 8.2 to 21.4 ng/mL. The 2 × 2 contingency data for localizing intraprostatic tumors and lymph node metastases are presented in **Tables 3** and **4**.

Table 2
Patient and tumor characteristics

Author	N	Age (y) Mean	Age (y) Range	PSA (ng/mL) Mean	PSA (ng/mL) Range	Gleason Score (%)	Tumor Stage
Alemozaffar, et al,[30] 2020	57	62	7[c]	15.0[a]	7.4–27.6[b]	7a (16), 7b (20), 8 (2), ≤9 (63)	NR
Jambor, et al,[32] 2018	26	65[a]	49–76	12.1[a]	4.1–35.0	7a (38), 7b (35), 8 (4), 9 (23)	pT2 (23), pT3a (38), pT3b (38)
Schuster, et al,[26] 2013	10	61	40–70	8.2	2.3–16.6	6 (27), 7a (22), 7b (11), 8 (25), 10 (15)	NR
Selnaes, et al,[31] 2018	28	66[a]	55–72	14.6[a]	3.7–56.9	7 (42), 8 (31), 9 (27)	pT2 (27), pT3a (27), pT3b (42), pT4 (4)
Suzuki, et al,[27] 2016	42	66	51–74	21.4	3.8–93.9	6 (7), 7 (41), 8 (23), 9 (25), 10 (5)	T1c (14), cT2 (50), cT3a (24), cT3b (14)
Suzuki, et al,[28] 2019	28	68	57–77	17.9	1.2–82.4	≤6 (3), 7 (41), 8 (28), 9 (28)	T1c (14), cT2 (50), cT3a (32), cT3b (5)
Turkbey, et al,[29] 2014	21	62	44–73	13.5	3.6–37.3	6 (14), 7 (57), 8 (24), 9 (5)	NR

Abbreviation: NR, not reported.
[a] Median.
[b] (Q1-Q3).
[c] Standard deviation.

Table 3
Two-by-two contingency data of 18F-fluciclovine for localization of intraprostatic tumor lesions

Author	N	Modality	Sectors	TP	FP	FN	TN	Total
Jambor, et al,[32] 2018	26	PET/CT	12	143	64	22	83	312
		PET/MR imaging	12	138	5	26	143	312
Suzuki, et al,[27] 2016	43	PET/CT	6	173	7	14	64	258
Turkbey, et al,[29] 2014	21	PET/CT	20	NR	NR	NR	NR	420
Schuster, et al,[26] 2013	10	PET/CT, 4 min	12	71	32	8	7	118
		PET/CT, 16 min	12	68	25	13	14	120
		PET/CT, 28 min	12	65	20	15	20	120
		PET/CT, 40 min	12	63	25	17	15	120

Abbreviations: FN, false-negative; FP, false positive; TN, true negative; TP, true positive.

Quality Assessment/Risk of Bias

The quality assessment of the 7 studies regarding risk of bias as indicated by QUADAS-2 analysis is summarized in **Table 5**. The risk of bias regarding patient selection, index test, reference standard, and flow and timing was low except for 1 study that had unclear risk of bias for patient selection and flow and timing.[26] For this study, the risk of bias for patient selection as well as for flow and timing was scored as unclear because of unavailability of data on patient enrollment or time between imaging and surgery. Concerns regarding applicability for index test and reference standard were low in all studies. For 2 studies there was unclear concern of applicability of patient selection because image findings at CT were used for study inclusion.[27,28]

DIAGNOSTIC ACCURACY
Intraprostatic Tumor Localization: Primary Cancer

The accuracy of 18F-fluciclovine PET to localize intraprostatic lesions was investigated by Schuster and colleagues,[26] Suzuki and colleagues,[27] Turkbey and colleagues,[29] and Jambor and colleagues.[32] Those study cohorts consisted of patients with histologically confirmed prostate cancer, and Schuster and colleagues,[26] Turkbey and colleagues,[29] and Jambor and colleagues[32] included lesions with longest diameter greater than 0.5 cm at histopathology. Jambor and colleagues[32] included PET/MR imaging in addition to PET/CT. Three of the studies included dynamic data acquisition,[26,29,32] but the set of images used for lesion detection was different: 1 to 15 minutes summed images in Turkbey and colleagues,[29] 5 frames times 4 minutes in Jambor and colleagues,[32] and acquired at 4, 16, 20, and 28 minutes after injection in Schuster and colleagues.[26] Suzuki and colleagues[27] used whole-body acquisition starting from the thigh immediately after acquisition of CT. Hematoxylin-eosin–stained tissue sections of the resected gland were used as reference standard, with Turkbey and colleagues[29] and Jambor and colleagues[32] using whole-mount histopathology. The prostate gland was divided into 6,[27] 12,[26,32] or 20 sectors.[29] MR-CT coregistration[26,29] or visual assessment[32] was used to allocate the lesions detected on PET to 1 or more of these sectors. Sector-based diagnostic sensitivity and specificity for these 4 studies are summarized in **Fig. 3**.

Table 4
Two-by-two contingency data of 18F-fluciclovine PET for detection of primary lymph node metastases

Author	N	Modality	Sectors	TP	FP	FN	TN	Total
Alemozaffar, et al,[30] 2020	57	PET/CT	4	NR	NR	NR	NR	228
Selnaes, et al,[31] 2018	28	PET/MR imaging	8	6	0	14	185	205
Suzuki, et al,[28] 2019	28	PET/CT	6	4	5	3	28	40[a]
Suzuki, et al,[27] 2016	42	PET/CT	6	0	1	9	234	244

[a] Different from 28 × 6 because only sectors with lymph nodes between 5 and 9 mm at CT were included.

Table 5
Quality of the included studies using the Quality Assessment of Diagnostic Accuracy Studies-2 tool

Study	Risk of Bias				Applicability Concern		
	Patient Selection	Index Test	Reference Standard	Flow and Timing	Patient Selection	Index Test	Reference Standard
Alemozaffar, et al,[30] 2020	Low	Low	Low	Low	Low	Low	Low
Jambor, et al,[32] 2018	Low	Low	Low	Low	Low	Low	Low
Schuster, et al,[26] 2013	Unclear	Low	Low	Unclear	Low	Low	Low
Selnaes, et al,[31] 2018	Low	Low	Low	Low	Low	Low	Low
Suzuki, et al,[27] 2016	Low	Low	Low	Low	Unclear	Low	Low
Suzuki, et al,[28] 2019	Low	Low	Low	Low	Unclear	Low	Low
Turkbey, et al,[29] 2014	Low	Low	Low	Low	Low	Low	Low

Risk of bias and applicability concern are for patient selection, index test, reference standard, and flow and timing.

Schuster and colleagues[26] found the highest combined sensitivity and specificity for 28 minutes. Although there was a significant correlation between ^{18}F-fluciclovine uptake of the malignant sectors and Gleason score, the correlation coefficients for all 4 time points were weak ($r < 0.5$).[29] Both Turkbey and colleagues[29] and Schuster and colleagues[26] reported large overlap between ^{18}F-fluciclovine uptake for malignant and nonmalignant sectors.[26,29] In the FLUCIPRO study, Jambor and colleagues[32] found that PET/CT and PET/MR had similar sensitivity, but that PET/MR had significantly higher specificity (mean, 0.95; 95% CI, 0.91–0.98).[32]

Detection of Primary Lymph Node Metastases

The accuracy of ^{18}F-fluciclovine PET to detect and localize lymph node metastases was investigated by Alemozaffar and colleagues,[30] Selnaes and colleagues,[31] Suzuki and colleagues,[27] and Suzuki and colleagues.[28] All 4 studies recruited among patients referred to prostatectomy and extended lymph node dissection. There were many differences between the studies, including eligibility criteria, data acquisition, data analyses, and percentage of patients with nodal disease. Selnaes and colleagues[31] included high-risk patients, Alemozaffar and colleagues[30] included patients with unfavorable intermediate-risk to very-high-risk cancer without definitive findings of systemic

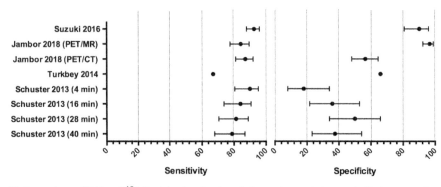

Fig. 3. Sensitivity and specificity of ^{18}F-fluciclovine for localizing primary intraprostatic tumor extent. The dots mark mean values and the whiskers are 95% CIs.

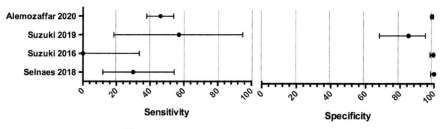

Fig. 4. Sensitivity and specificity of ^{18}F-fluciclovine for detection of primary lymph nodes. The dots mark mean values and the whiskers are 95% CIs.

metastases on conventional imaging, whereas the requirement of Suzuki and colleagues[27] was no findings indicating metastases at conventional imaging. Lymph nodes with longest diameters between 5 and 9 mm at CT were required in Suzuki and colleagues.[28] Acquisition time per bed ranged from 2 to 5 minutes. For the detection of lymph nodes Alemozaffar and colleagues[30] used acquisition at 5 minutes in addition to early (immediately after injection) and delayed pelvic imaging (22.5 minutes), Selnaes and colleagues[31] used 5 to 10 minutes summed images, Suzuki and colleagues[28] used images acquired at 10 minutes, and Suzuki and colleagues[27] used whole-body imaging completed by 30 minutes after injection. The number of lymph node sectors was 4[30] 6,[27,28] or 8[31]. Alemozaffar and colleagues,[30] Selnaes and colleagues,[31] and Suzuki and colleagues[28] included all sectors in their analyses and defined a sector as true-positive if 1 or more lymph nodes were positive in that sector on imaging and 1 or more nodes were positive on histopathology, whereas Suzuki and colleagues[27] only included sectors with lymph nodes within the predefined size range at CT in the analyses and defined the sector as positive if the node identified at CT was positive at histopathology. This approach yielded a total of 40 sectors in the study cohort of 28 patients. The percentage of patients with nodal disease was 16.7% (7 out of 42) in Suzuki and colleagues,[27] 54% (31 out of 57) in Alemozzafar and colleagues,[30] 38% (10 out of 26) in Selnaes and colleagues,[31] and 21% (6 out of 28) in Suzuki and colleagues.[28] The sector-based sensitivity and specificity for the 4 included studies are shown in **Fig. 4**.

DISCUSSION

The literature search identified 7 studies of patients with prostate cancer in which systematic sector-based histopathology had been used to confirm findings at ^{18}F-fluciclovine PET. For all studies, ^{18}F-fluciclovine PET was performed as part of the preoperative assessment of primary prostate cancer: 3 for intraprostatic lesion detection, 3 for lymph nodes detection, and 1 investigating both intraprostatic lesion and lymph node detection. There was a large variation in sensitivity and specificity among the included studies.

In this systematic review, only studies that had systematic sector-based histopathology as reference standard are included. This limitation is necessary in order to complete a 2 × 2 contingency table with true-positives, true-negatives, false-positives, and false-negatives that enable calculation of sensitivity and specificity. The use of other end points than systematic sector-based histopathology is problematic. The authors found 3 categories of such end points that are frequently used: first, comparison between 2 tracers or modalities without reference standard. Second, the term detection rate, where any positive findings are considered as true-positives. Third, altered treatment based on image findings, which by nature is self-affirming.

All 7 studies that fulfilled the inclusion criteria for this systematic review were performed in patients with known primary prostate cancer. The main finding from the 4 studies investigating intraprostatic tumor localization was high sensitivity and large variation in specificity. However, there are some factors that contribute to the high sensitivity that may limit the transferability to other cohorts. First, the readers knew that all patients had prostate cancer. Second, benign hyperplasia, commonly present in this age group, has similar ^{18}F-fluciclovine uptake to tumor (**Fig. 5**). Defining the cutoff for pathologic uptake is a trade-off between false-positives and false-negatives and thus is decisive for sensitivity and specificity. In a different setting such as screening for prostate cancer, the reader would probably use a higher cutoff for pathologic uptake in order to reduce false-positives and thereby reduce the sensitivity. Two of the studies[27,32] reported specificity greater than 80%. The study cohort of Suzuki and colleagues[27] consisted of overall large primary tumors and divided the prostate into only 6 sectors. This approach led to nearly 70% true-

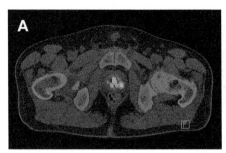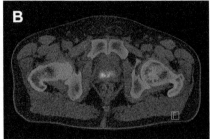

Fig. 5. Images in a 66-year-old-man with a serum PSA level of 12.0 ng/mL. High ^{18}F-fluciclovine uptake in a focus in the left peripheral zone (A) histopathologically confirmed to be Gleason 4 + 3. Similarly high ^{18}F-fluciclovine in the right side of the transitional zone (B) histologically confirmed to be benign hyperplasia.

positive sectors, which, in combination with few false-positive sectors, contributed to the high specificity. Jambor and colleagues[32] reported high specificity for PET/MR imaging only, not for PET/CT, indicating that the additional information from MR imaging probably was the reason for the high accuracy.

The main finding from the 4 studies investigating primary lymph node metastases was high specificity but very low sensitivity. This indicates that a certain amount of tumor is needed in order for the lymph node metastases to be detected at 18F-fluciclovine PET/CT. This is supported by Alemozaffar and colleagues,[30] who found that the detection rate was closely linked to the diameter of the metastatic foci: 83.3% for foci greater than 9 mm compared with 23.7% for foci of 3 mm or less. Selnaes and colleagues[31] also reported a relationship between size and detectability. In a large study of 4686 lymph nodes, Thoeny and colleagues[33] showed that most metastases were 3 mm or less. This finding may explain why Suzuki and colleagues[27] did not detect any of the 7 lymph node metastases in their cohort of 42 patients.

At present, the US Food and Drug Administration (FDA)–approved indication for ^{18}F-fluciclovine PET is men with biochemical recurrence after local treatment.[8] During the past decade, several studies have evaluated use of ^{18}F-fluciclovine PET in this setting and found it to offer a reliable cancer detection rate both for locally persistent disease (prostate/bed) and extraprostatic disease.[14,16–18,20,22] The diagnostic performance has been reported to be superior to that of CT,[19] multiparametric MR imaging,[14] choline PET,[18] and ^{111}In–capromab pendetide single-photon emission CT/CT.[20] The lack of systematic sector-based histopathology as reference standard made these studies ineligible for the current systematic review.

In the clinical setting of biochemical recurrence, it is difficult to obtain systematic histopathology:

For local recurrence in the prostate/prostate bed, biopsies are seldom performed. Early PSA recurrence after prostatectomy is considered as recurrence within the prostatic bed and treated with salvage radiation therapy, often without image investigation or biopsies. Intraprostatic recurrence after primary radiation therapy often leads to systemic oncologic treatment without systematic prostate biopsies. Salvage prostatectomy, which would provide histopathologic reference, is seldom performed because of risk of serious side effects. However, for pelvic lymph nodes, it is feasible to obtain the required 2 × 2 contingency table using extended pelvic lymph node dissection as reference standard. The authors found no such studies in the recurrence setting, but 4 in the primary setting (see **Table 1**). Two major studies of ^{18}F-fluciclovine in the recurrence setting[18,20] reported divergent findings that exemplify this challenge, and how dependent the findings are on study cohort and reference standard. Whereas Schuster and colleagues[20] reported high sensitivity and specificity, Nanni and colleagues[18] reported negative imaging in more than half of the patients.

For distant metastases (M+) it is impossible to assess the rate of false-negatives. In this context, imaging is mainly used to evaluate treatment response of systemic disease and to identify oligometastatic patients suited for image-guided focal treatment. The clinical usefulness of imaging cannot be assessed by sensitivity and specify in these settings. Clinical follow-up and survival are needed.

A recent review in *Lancet Oncology* concluded that the PET radioligand Ga-68- prostate-specific membrane antigen (PSMA) increasingly has replaced both fluciclovine and choline for prostate cancer assessment because of its higher sensitivity and specificity over a range of PSA levels.[34] The authors performed an equivalent systematic literature search for PSMA[35] to their search for fluciclovine. The search yielded 14 studies for primary prostate, 13 for primary lymph nodes, and 8 for lymph node recurrence. To our knowledge, there are only 2 studies that compare fluciclovine and PSMA in the same patients, both in recurrence settings.[36,37] Pernthaler and colleagues[36] found in a study of 58 patients that ^{18}F-fluciclovine had a superior detection rate for local recurrence, whereas the results for nodal disease and bone metastases were similar to 68Ga-PSMA-11. In another study of 50 patients, Calais and colleagues[37] found a similar detection rate for local recurrence, but more than twice as high for lymph nodes and for extrapelvic metastasis for ^{68}Ga-PSMA-11. None of these studies met the inclusion criteria of our reviews because of the lack of systematic sector-based histopathology. The authors therefore conclude that there is little evidence for superiority of any of the 2 tracers; however, the body of evidence for PSMA is substantially larger than for ^{18}F-fluciclovine.

In conclusion, our literature search, investigating the PET tracer ^{18}F-fluciclovine in patients with prostate cancer, identified only a few studies that had systematic sector-based histopathology allowing calculation of sensitivity and specificity. In primary prostate, the sensitivity was high, but the specificity was limited. In primary lymph nodes, the sensitivity was low.

DISCLOSURE

The authors declare that they have no conflicts of interest that relates to the subject matter of the present review.

REFERENCES

1. Bray F, Ferlay J, Soerjomataram I, et al. Global cancer statistics 2018: GLOBOCAN estimates of incidence and mortality worldwide for 36 cancers in 185 countries. CA Cancer J Clin 2018;68:394–424.
2. Kishan AU, Chu FI, King CR, et al. Local failure and survival after definitive radiotherapy for aggressive prostate cancer: an individual patient-level meta-analysis of six randomized trials. Eur Urol 2020;77:201–8.
3. Duijzentkunst DA, Peters M, van der Voort van Zyp JR, et al. Focal salvage therapy for local prostate cancer recurrences after primary radiotherapy: a comprehensive review. World J Urol 2016;34:1521–31.
4. Zdrojowy R, Dembowski J, Malkievwicz B, et al. Salvage local therapy for radiation-recurrent prostate cancer - where are we? Cent Eur J Urol 2016; 69:264–70.
5. Walker SM, Lim I, Lindenberg L, et al. Positron emission tomography (PET) radiotracers for prostate cancer imaging. Abdom Radiol 2020;45:2165–75.
6. Schuster DM, Votaw JR, Nieh PT, et al. Initial experience with the radiotracer anti-1-amino-3-18F-fluorocyclobutane-1-carboxylic acid with PET/CT in prostate carcinoma. J Nucl Med 2007;48(1):56–63.
7. Asano Y, Inoue Y, Ikeda Y, et al. Phase I clinical study of NMK36: a new PET tracer with the synthetic amino acid analogue anti-[18F]FACBC. Ann Nucl Med 2011;25:414–8.
8. US Food and Drug Administration FDA Approves new diagnostic imaging agent to detect recurrent prostate cancer. Available at: https://fda.gov/news-events/press-announcements/fda-approves-new-di agnostic-imaging-agent-detect-recurrent-prostate-cancer. Accessed August 21, 2020.
9. Moher D, Liberati A, Tetzlaff J, et al. Preferred reporting items for systematic reviews and meta-analyses: the PRISMA statement. PLoS Med 2009;6: e1000097.
10. Ouzzani M, Hammady H, Fedorowicz Z, et al. Rayyan – a web and mobile app for systematic reviews. Syst Rev 2016;5:210.
11. Whiting PF, Rutjes AWS, Westwood ME, et al. QUADAS-2: a revised tool for the quality assessment of diagnostic accuracy studies. Ann Intern Med 2011; 155:529–36.
12. MedCalc Diagnostic test evaluation calculator. Available at: https://www.medcalc.org/calc/diagnostic_test.php.
13. Abiodun-Ojo OA, Akintayo A, Akin-Akintayo OO, et al. 18F -fluciclovine parameters on targeted prostate biopsy associated with true positivity in recurrent prostate cancer. J Nucl Med 2019;60:1531–6.
14. Akin-Akintayo O, Tade F, Mittal P, et al. Prospective evaluation of fluciclovine 18F PET-CT and MRI in detection of recurrent prostate cancer in non-prostatectomy patients. Eur J Radiol 2018;102: 1–8.
15. Bach-Gansmo T, Nanni C, Nieh PT, et al. Multisite experience of the safety, detection rate and diagnostic performance of fluciclovine 18F positron emission tomography/computerized tomography Imaging in the staging of biochemically recurrent prostate cancer. J Urol 2017;197:676–8.
16. Kairemo K, Rasulova N, Partanen K, et al. Preliminary clinical experience of trans-1-Amino-3-(18)F-fluorocyclobutanecarboxylic Acid (anti-(18)F-FACBC) PET/CT imaging in Prostate Cancer Patients. Biomed Res Int 2014;2014:305182.
17. Miller MP, Kostakoglu L, Pryma D, et al. Reader training for the restaging of biochemically recurrent prostate cancer using 18F-fluciclovine PET/CT. J Nucl Med 2017;58:1596–602.
18. Nanni C, Zanoni L, Pultrone C, et al. 18)F-FACBC (anti1-amino-3-(18)F-fluorocyclobutane-1-carboxylic acid) versus (11)C-choline PET/CT in prostate cancer relapse: results of a prospective trial. Eur J Nucl Med Mol Imaging 2016;43:1601–10.

19. Odewole OA, Tade FI, Nieh PT, et al. Recurrent prostate cancer detection with anti-3-(18)F FACBC PET/CT: comparison with CT. Eur J Nucl Med Mol Imaging 2016;43:1773–83.

20. Schuster DM, Nieh PT, Jani AB, et al. Anti-3-(18F) FACBC positron emission tomography-computerized tomography and 111In-Capromab pendetide single photon emission computerized tomography-computerized tomography for recurrent prostate carcinoma: results of a prospective clinical trial. J Urol 2014;191:1446–53.

21. Schuster DM, Savir-Baruch B, Nieh PT, et al. Detection of recurrent prostate carcinoma with anti-1-amino-3-18F-fluorocyclobutane-1-carboxylic acid PET/CT and 111In-capromab pendetide SPECT/CT. Radiology 2011;259(3):852–61.

22. Tulipan AJ, Hole KH, Vlatkovic L, et al. Localization of radio-recurrence within the prostate: anti-3-18F-FACBC PET/CT compared with multiparametric MRI using histopathology as reference standard. Acta Oncol 2019;60:1028–38.

23. Esmaeili M, Tayari N, Scheenen T, et al. Simultaneous 18F-fluciclovine positron emission tomography and magnetic resonance spectroscopic imaging of prostate cancer. Front Oncol 2018;8:516.

24. Fei B, Abiodun-Ojo OA, Akintayo AA, et al. Feasibility and initial results: fluciclovine positron emission tomography/ultrasound fusion targeted biopsy of recurrent prostate cancer. J Urol 2019;202:413–21.

25. Elschot M, Selnaes KM, Sandsmark E, et al. A PET/MRI study towards finding the optimal 18F fluciclovine PET protocol for detection and characterization of primary prostate cancer. Eur J Nucl Med Mol Imaging 2017;44:695–703.

26. Schuster DM, Taleghani PA, Nieh PT, et al. M. Characterization of primary prostate carcinoma by anti-1-amino-2-(18)F-fluorocyclobutane-1-carboxylic acid (anti-3- (18)F FACBC) uptake. Am J Nucl Med Mol Imaging 2013;3:85–96.

27. Suzuki H, Inoue Y, Fujimoto, et al. Diagnostic performance and safety of NMK36 (trans-1-amino-3- 18F fluorocyclobutanecarboxylic acid)-PET/CT in primary prostate cancer: multicenter Phase IIb clinical trial. Jpn J Clin Oncol 2016;46:152–62.

28. Suzuki H, Jinnouchi S, Kaji Y, et al. Diagnostic performance of 18F-fluciclovine PET/CT for regional lymph node metastases in patients with primary prostate cancer: a multicenter phase II clinical trial. Jpn J Clin Oncol 2019;49:803–11.

29. Turkbey B, Mena E, Shih J, et al. Localized prostate cancer detection with 18F FACBC PET/CT: comparison with MR imaging and histopathologic analysis. Radiology 2014;270:849–56.

30. Alemozaffar M, Akintayo AA, Abiodun-Ojo OA, et al. 18F fluciclovine PET/CT for preoperative staging in patients with intermediate to high risk primary prostate cancer. J Urol 2020;204:1–7.

31. Selnaes KM, Kruger-Stokke B, Elschot M, et al. 18F-Fluciclovine PET/MRI for preoperative lymph node staging in high-risk prostate cancer patients. Eur Radiol 2018;28(8):3151–9.

32. Jambor I, Kuisma A, Kahkonen E, et al. Prospective evaluation of 18F-FACBC PET/CT and PET/MRI versus multiparametric MRI in intermediate- to high-risk prostate cancer patients (FLUCIPRO trial). Eur J Nucl Med Mol Imaging 2018;45:355–64.

33. Thoeny HC, Froehlich JM, Triantafyllou M, et al. Metastases in normal-sized pelvic lymph nodes: detection with diffusion-weighted MR imaging. Radiology 2014;273:125–35.

34. Fanti S, Minozzi S, Antoch G, et al. Consensus on molecular imaging and theranostics in prostate cancer. Lancet Oncol 2018;19:e696–708.

35. Hernes E, Revheim ME, Hole KH, et al. Prostate-Specific Membrane Antigen (PSMA) PET for assessment of primary and recurrent prostate cancer with histopathology as reference standard – a systematic review and meta-analysis. PET Clin 2021.

36. Pernthaler B, Kulnik R, Gstettner C, et al. A prospective head-to-head comparison of 18F-fluciclovine with 68Ga-PSMA-11 in biochemical recurrence of prostate cancer in PET/CT. Clin Nucl Med 2019;44:e566–73.

37. Calais J, Ceci F, Eiber M, et al. 18F-fluciclovine PET-CT and 68Ga-PSMA-11 PET-CT in patients with early biochemical recurrence after prostatectomy: a prospective, single-centre, single-arm, comparative imaging trial. Lancet Oncol 2019;20:1286–94.

Critical Role of 2-[18F]-fluoro-2-deoxy-glucose in Hormonally Active Malignancies

Divya Yadav, MD[a], Rakesh Kumar, MD, PhD[b],*

KEYWORDS

• FDG • Hormonally active malignances • NET • Prostate cancer

KEY POINTS

- Many newer tracers targeting hormonal receptors introduced for imaging in breast cancer, prostate cancer, neuroendocrine tumors, and thyroid cancers might be more specific than 2-[18F]-fluoro-2-deoxyglucose (FDG) .
- FDG continues to remain a more widely available radiotracer and highly sensitive for diagnosis, response assessment, and prognostication in these malignancies.
- Personalized use of specific radiotracers in conjunction with FDG can optimize characterization of tumor and aid in holistic patient management.

INTRODUCTION

PET has revolutionized the study of various biologic processes and opened new possibilities in both fundamental research and the day-to-day practice of medicine. Currently, 2-[18F]-fluoro-2-deoxyglucose (FDG) is one of the most commonly used tracers for PET imaging worldwide. FDG is a radiolabeled analog of glucose and can detect altered glucose metabolism in both physiologic and pathologic states, for example, cancer cells. The hypermetabolism in malignant tissue is based on the Warburg effect, overexpression of cellular membrane glucose transporters (GLUT-1), and enhanced hexokinase enzymatic activity in tumors.[1] The role of FDG-PET in the initial staging, monitoring response to the therapy, and management of many types of cancer has been well documented.[2] In recent years, however, with the introduction of other PET radiotracers targeting hormonal receptors, such as 18F-16α-17β-fluoroestradiol (18F-FES) in breast cancer, Gallium-68 [68Ga]-PSMA [Prostate-specific membrane antigen] in prostate cancer, and so forth, the role of FDG has been undermined. These radiotracers, however, often can be false negative, especially in the undifferentiated tumors. FDG-PET in these undifferentiated subtypes of tumors is highly positive.[3] This review article focuses on the importance of FDG-PET imaging in hormonally active malignancies, including breast, thyroid, prostate, and neuroendocrine tumors.

BREAST CANCER

Several PET tracers have been used for targeted imaging of breast cancer, including FDG, [18F]-fluoro-3'-deoxy-3'-L-fluorothymidine (18F-FLT), 18F-FES, 11C-choline, and so forth, but FDG has been the most extensively studied.[4] The intensity of FDG uptake is variable in different tumor types and sites[5] and is influenced by the phenotype, grade, and Ki-67 index.[6,7] Changes in metabolic activity generally occur earlier than changes in

[a] Department of Nuclear Medicine, All India Institute of Medical Sciences, New Delhi, India; [b] Diagnostic Nuclear Medicine Division, Department of Nuclear Medicine, AIIMS, Ansari nagar, New Delhi 110029, India
* Corresponding author. Apt 32302, 1885 El Passeo St, Houston, TX 77054, USA
E-mail address: rkphulia@yahoo.com

PET Clin 16 (2021) 177–189
https://doi.org/10.1016/j.cpet.2020.12.007

tumor size. The metabolic information provided by FDG-PET has been shown valuable for the early assessment of the response to chemotherapy in both neoadjuvant and metastatic settings.[8] One of the most advocated advantage to the use of PET/CT is its ability to evaluate different sites of metastases in a single examination.

Staging and Prognostication

Proper staging is critical in selecting appropriate treatment modalities for breast cancer treatment. FDG-PET/CT is indicated in breast cancer staging for its role in detection of internal mammary nodal and distant metastases. Skeletal system is one of the most common sites of metastases and FDG-PET is shown to be superior than radiographic imaging, including MR and bone scan, in detecting osseous metastases.[9–11] Also, FDG has proved a good predictive as well as prognostic imaging biomarker.[12] Several quantitative parameters, such as maximum standardized uptake value (SUVmax), mean standardized uptake value, metabolic tumor volume, and total lesion glycolysis have been used for prognostication of breast cancer.[8] The degree of FDG uptake inversely correlates with prognosis.[13,14] FDG-PET/CT also can predict molecular subtype of breast cancer. Kitajima and coworkers[15] found that an SUVmax cutoff value of 3.60 yielded 70.1% sensitivity and 66.1% specificity for predicting luminal A, and cutoff value 6.75 yielded 65.4% sensitivity and 75.2% specificity for predicting a Her2-positive subtype.

Response Assessment

Early response of treatment also is important in the metastatic setting to use the most efficient drugs and to timely stop ineffective chemotherapy. Changes in metabolic activity generally occur earlier than changes in tumor size. FDG-PET/CT has shown excellent performances to assess the response in metastatic patients with high accuracy. PET/CT is helpful to detect a heterogeneous response, which is the coexistence of responding and nonresponding lesions within the same patient.[16] Approximately 20% of breast tumors are Her2 positive—which activates phosphatidylinositol 3-kinase/AKT pathway, up-regulating glucose uptake. Effective Her2 blockade decreases glucose uptake and hence FDG-PET/CT can be useful in predicting response to anti-Her therapy, as demonstrated by Lin and colleagues.[17] In metastatic breast cancer patients treated with lapatinib and trastuzumab, it was observed that patients who did not have a metabolic response on FDG-PET/CT at the end of week 1 failed to achieve an objective response (by

Response Evaluation Criteria in Solid Tumors [RECIST]), with a negative predictive value of 91%.[17] FDG-PET/CT also can predict response to neoadjuvant therapy. In the NeoALTTO trial, mean SUVmax reductions in patients with a pathologic complete response (pCR) were 54.3% versus 32.8% in non-pCR group at week 2 and 61.5% versus 34.1% at week 6, respectively.[18]

18F-16α-17β-Fluoroestradiol

Many other agents apart from FDG have emerged recently. More than 70% of the breast tumors are estrogen receptor (ER) positive, and adjuvant endocrine therapy in such patients has led to increased survival and better outcomes. Among these, 18F-FES, with target to background tissue activities exceeding 80:1, has shown promising results.[19] Intensity of FES uptake in primary and metastatic tumor showed good correlation with immunohistochemistry of biopsy material, that is, tumor ER concentration.[20] The same can be used to predict response to tamoxifen therapy as well as aid in selection of refractory patients to antiestrogen therapy.[21]

Limitations of 18F-16α-17β-Fluoroestradiol–PET/Computed Tomography

FES-PET/CT, however, is an excellent tool of radiomic histology in revealing ER expression heterogeneity with high specificity. But it has lower sensitivity and can miss lesions with no ER expression (**Fig. 1**). Gupta and colleagues[22] compared the diagnostic strength of FES-PET/CT and FDG-PET/CT prospectively in 12 patients and found that FDG has overall better sensitivity than FES-PET/CT. Out of a total of 154 lesions considered as disease sites, FDG picked up 142 lesions (sensitivity 92.21%), whereas FES picked up 116 lesions (sensitivity 75.32%). Another limitation of FES is very high physiologic tracer uptake in liver (liver background SUVmax range: 12.5–18.7) and, hence, most liver lesions appear relatively cold.

Limitations of 2-[18F]-Fluoro-2-Deoxyglucose–PET/Computed Tomography

The ambitious use of PET/CT is hampered by the cost of imaging, the potential for delaying care, the risk of invasive procedures stimulated by false-positive results, the exposure to ionizing radiation, and the lack of proof that changing treatment early improves patients' survival. Other important limitations for the use of PET/CT are the absence of consensus of the criteria to use to assess the response, of the number of metastatic sites to analyze, and of the optimal time to

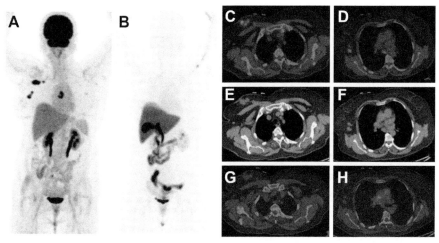

Fig. 1. In a 36-year-old woman with right breast carcinoma, maximum intensity projection images of (*A*) 18F-FDG–PET/CT and (*B*) 18F-FES–PET/CT showing (*C*) primary right breast lesion, (*D*) right axillary and subcarinal lymph nodes in axial fused PET/CT, and (*E*) and (*F*) CT images with increased FDG uptake (*C*) and (*D*) and no 18F-FES uptake (*G*) and (*H*).

perform PET during treatment. A major limitation of using SUVmax is its reproducibility, which depends on a long list of factors.[23]

False positivity in inflammatory conditions is a major limitation of FDG-PET/CT scan; hence, characterization of lung lesions and mediastinal lymph nodes on FDG alone is not easy. FES scan helps in the characterization of these lesions to a great extent. FES-PET/CT should be used along with FDG-PET/CT in strongly ER-expressing patients for better specificity, evaluation of the disease extent, and impact on treatment.

THYROID CANCER

Differentiated thyroid cancer (DTC), including papillary cancer (classic and follicular variant) and follicular cancer, usually possesses the ability to concentrate radioiodine with the exception of aggressive variants, such as sclerosing, columnar, or tall cell variants, and Hürthle cell variant. So the standard care in patients with DTC include I-131 radioiodine whole-body scan (WBS) for metastatic evaluation.

Staging

The FDG-PET/CT is recommended in DTC, when patients present with elevated thyroglobulin (Tg) levels (>10 ng/mL) and negative radioactive iodine WBS (TENIS).[24,25] In patients who present with Thyroglobulin elevated negative iodine scintigraphy (TENIS), elevated Tg, and negative iodine WBS (**Fig. 2**), the reported overall sensitivity of 18F-FDG–PET/CT ranges from 50% to 75%, with

specificity ranging from 41.7% to 100%.[25] Bertagna and colleagues[26] demonstrated that there was a significant positive correlation between FDG-PET/CT positive results and Tg levels with highest accuracy when Tg was greater than 21 ng/mL, but they did not note any statistically significant correlation between PET/CT results and TSH levels. Iagaru and colleagues[27] suggested that FDG-PET/CT may not be as accurate in patients with Tg levels below 2 ng/dL. FDG-PET/CT also can detect new radioiodine-negative metastases in advanced DTC patients with unchanged positive WBS and increasing Tg levels.[28] It also may be considered as a part of initial staging in poorly DTCs and invasive Hürthle cell carcinomas (**Fig. 3**).[25] FDG uptake represents less DTC cells or dedifferentiated cells and PET-positive lesions are more likely to be resistant to I-131 treatment.

Prognostication and Response Assessment

FDG-PET scanning also can be considered as a prognostic tool in patients with metastatic disease to identify lesions and patients at highest risk for rapid disease progression and disease-specific mortality.[25,29] A high FDG uptake suggests dedifferentiated, more aggressive, and metabolically active tumor cells and thereby indicates poorer prognosis and reduced survival. In a study with 50 DTC patients, Esteva and colleagues[30] found that tumor size ($P<.05$) and thyroid capsular invasion ($P<.05$) were significantly associated with positive FDG-PET studies. The volume of FDG-avid lesions, SUVmax, and number and location of metastases can correlate with outcome and

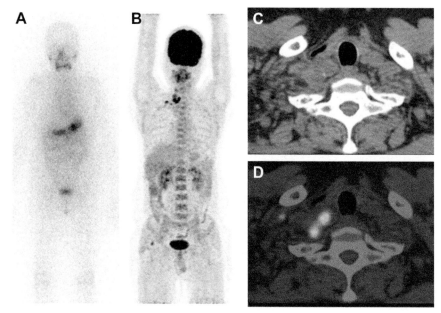

Fig. 2. After a month of total thyroidectomy, a 28-year-old man with papillary thyroid cancer presented with elevated thyroglobulin level and (*A*) negative I-131 WBS. (*B*) Maximum intensity projection image of FDG–PET/CT showed hypermetabolic right cervical level III/IV and supraclavicular lymph nodes, also seen in (*C*) axial CT and (*D*) fused PET/CT image with increased FDG uptake.

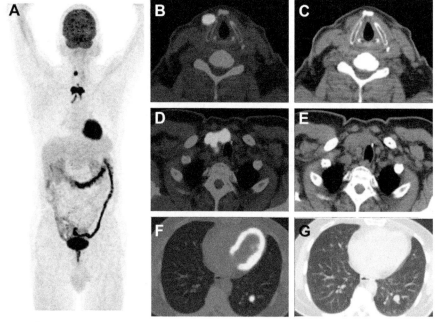

Fig. 3. A 40-year-old man diagnosed with thyroid cancer of aggressive histology, post–total thyroidectomy underwent FDG–PET/CT scan (*A*), which revealed hypermetabolic cervical lymph node (*B, C*), thyroid bed remnant (*D, E*), and lung metastases (*F, G*).

survival in univariate and multivariate analyses.[31,32] Similarly, Wang and colleagues[33] found that the total volume of FDG-avid disease correlated with prognosis and was the strongest single factor for predicting survival in 125 patients with elevated Tg and negative WBS who were monitored for up to 41 months. Patients with extensive metastatic involvement, radioactive iodine–refractory disease, and positive FDG-PET/CT scans are more likely to have progressive disease and to have a median survival of less than 5 years.[31] In addition, FDG-PET/CT may enable early evaluation of posttreatment response following systemic or local therapy for metastatic or locally invasive disease.[25] Recently, multitargeted tyrosine kinase inhibitors (TKIs) have been used in DTC but their use is limited because of their toxicities. FDG-PET/CT can provide a basis for more uniform patient selection for TKI initiation and continuation.[34]

Evaluation of Thyroid Nodule with Indeterminate Cytology

FDG-PET imaging is not recommended routinely for the evaluation of thyroid nodules with indeterminate cytology.[25] A recent meta-analysis showed sensitivity and specificity of FDG-PET were 89% and 55%, respectively, resulting in a 41% positive predictive value and 93% negative predictive value.[35] Vriens and colleagues[36] showed that FDG-PET was more cost effective than surgery, or mutational testing. A recent prospective analysis showed that FDG-PET/CT represents a great preoperative, noninvasive tool when combined with sonographic features to further evaluate indeterminate nodules at low risk for malignancy.[37] A review by Castellana and colleagues[38] showed that FDG-PET/CT has a moderate ability to correctly discriminate malignant from benign lesions in patients with thyroid nodules with indeterminate FNA and could represent a reliable option to reduce unnecessary diagnostic surgeries.

Thyroid Incidentalomas

With the increasing clinical use of FDG-PET/CT for the staging and restaging of various malignancies, increasing number of thyroid incidentalomas are being reported. Most thyroid incidentalomas are benign; diffuse FDG uptake usually indicates chronic or acute thyroiditis, whereas a focal area of FDG uptake has 30% to 40% chance of being cancer, either primary or metastasis from the known nonthyroidal cancer, for example, melanoma, hypernephroma, or lung, bowel, or breast cancer.[39] A proportion meta-analysis performed by Bertagna and colleagues,[40] with a total of 147,505 subjects from 27 studies, revealed a pooled incidence and a malignancy ratio of 2.46% (95% CI, 1.68-3.39) and 34.6% (95% CI, 29.3-40.2), respectively. An FDG-PET/CT report should suggest further evaluation when focal thyroid incidentalomas are described because these findings are associated with a significant risk of cancer.[41] Moreover, it is not clear whether there are differences in the management of patients diagnosed by PET/CT and patients diagnosed when the nodular thyroid disease is clinically evident.[42]

Medullary and Anaplastic Thyroid Cancer

FDG-PET/CT also can be used in the management of patients with medullary thyroid cancer (MTC) and anaplastic thyroid cancer.[25] PET/CT is the more sensitive compared with conventional imaging in detecting metastases of recurrent MTC in patients with increased serum calcitonin levels.[43,44] 68Ga-DOTANOC (DOTA-1-Nal3-octreotide) is mainly used for this purpose because of better tumor-to-background ratio, but FDG-PET/CT also can be used as effectively (Fig. 4). A meta-analysis by Cheng and colleagues[45] obtained sensitivity of FDG-PET/CT ranging from 0.47 to 0.96, and pooled sensitivity of 0.69 (95% CI, 0.64–0.74). Poisson and colleagues[46] evaluated 20 patients with ATC and found that FDG-PET/CT caused a change in treatment in 25% of the participants. The high FDG uptake in the lesions and the FDG uptake volume both were highly prognostic for a bad outcome.[47] FDG-PET/CT also may permit an early assessment of the response to therapy and a reliable method to follow patients after therapy.

NEUROENDOCRINE TUMORS

Neuroendocrine tumors (NETs) arise from neuroendocrine cells exhibiting uniform histologic features but different biological behavioral characteristics. The gastrointestinal tract and pancreas are common sites and these tumors are grouped as gastroenteropancreatic (GEP) neuroendocrine neoplasias (NENs).[48,49] The World Health Organization classification defines 3 categories of NETs based on mitotic count and Ki-67 proliferative index (G1, mitotic count <2 cells/10 high-power fields or Ki-67 index <3%; G2, mitotic count 2–20 cells/10 high-power fields or Ki-67 index 3%–20%; and G3, mitotic count >20 cells/10 high-power fields or Ki-67 index >20%).[50]

G1/G2 tumors consists of well-differentiated neuroendocrine cells whereas G3 tumors exhibit significant malignant characteristics and have poorer prognoses compared with G1/G2 tumors.

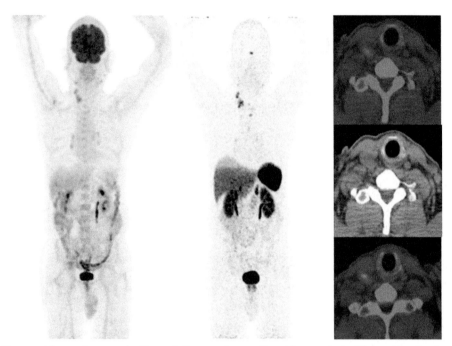

Fig. 4. A 44-year-old man diagnosed with medullary carcinoma thyroid presented with persistently elevated calcitonin levels post–total thyroidectomy. (*A*) FDG–PET/CT and (*B*) 68Ga-DOTANOC–PET/CT images showed (*C*) increased FDG uptake in (*D*) right cervical level IV lymph nodes with (*E*) increased 68Ga-DOTANOC uptake.

Hence, the preoperative differentiation between G1/G2 and G3 tumors can aid in the prognostication. Also, pancreatic neuroendocrine tumors exhibit intratumoral heterogeneity, preoperative grading based on diagnostic imaging modalities offer attractive benefit.[51] A majority of these tumors express somatostatin receptors (SSTR) on tumor cell surface. SSTR imaging previously has been performed with a gamma camera using Indium (In) 111 or Technetium (TC) 99mc-labeled compounds, whereas 68Ga-DOTA-somatostatin receptor targeting peptide (SST) analogs PET/CT imaging has recently become the gold standard for the diagnosis of these tumors as well as during follow-up.[52] FDG-PET/CT has been suggested as an alternative tool for tissue sampling for the assessment of the aggressiveness of tumors, and it has shown prognostic value in NENs.[53]

Well-Differentiated Neuroendocrine Tumors

Overall, approximately 90% of G1/G2 GEP-NENs present a positive finding due to the high SSTR expression on cell surface of these tumors. A meta-analysis by Treglia and colleagues[54] showed high sensitivity and specificity of 68Ga-DOTA-SST PET/CT, which are reported to vary between 91% to 95% and 82% to 97%, respectively. Newer chelator-like 68Ga-DATA-d-Phe1-Tyr3-octreotide also showed similar diagnostic efficacy in GEP-

NENs.[55] Recently, a negative correlation between tumor proliferative activity, expressed by Ki67, and 68Ga-DOTA-0-Tyr3-Octreotate, expressed as SUVmax, has been observed in a retrospective analysis, including 126 GEP-NENs.[56] FDG-PET/CT plays a very small role and has low sensitivity in small growing well differentiated neuroendocrine tumors (G1 and G2), but its role is emerging in the evaluation and management of high-grade NENs (G3). FDG-PET/CT sensitivity in G1/G2 GEP-NENs is reported to range between 40% and 60%, whereas it increases to approximately 95% in G3 tumors.[57,58] Kayani and colleagues[57] evaluated the distribution of 68Ga-DOTA-TATE PET/CT in NENs and compared its performance with FDG-PET/CT in 38 patients affected by primary or recurrent NEN. A significant correlation between FDG tumoral uptake and proliferation and tumor grade was observed; and tumor size was not found to affect tracer uptake significantly.

Poorly Differentiated Neuroendocrine Tumor

It is postulated that well-differentiated NETs may show dedifferentiation with time, losing their ability to express SSTRs and increasing their metabolism and FDG avidity. Many studies have demonstrated a positive correlation between Ki67 expression and FDG SUVmax.[59,60] FDG-PET/CT has emerged as an important tool to define tumor aggressiveness and give relevant prognostic information, particularly when coupled with 68Ga-labeled SST analogs PET/CT. Several investigators have suggested combining both FDG and 68Ga-DOTA-0-Tyr3-Octreotate PET/CT for the management of neuroendocrine tumors, in particularly G2 and G3.[61–64] The flip-flop phenomenon between 68Ga-DOTANOC and FDG uptake is common in lesions, particularly in G2 NETs (**Fig. 5**). This combined analysis can provide useful information on tumor heterogeneity, the characterization of SSTRs expression, and tumor grade, thus guiding clinicians to the proper treatment options.[65]

PROSTATE CANCER

Prostate cancers usually are treated with radical prostatectomy or a combination of radiation therapy, chemotherapy, and/or hormonal therapy. Optimal treatment depends on the accurate staging of the disease at the time of presentation. Conventional imaging techniques, including CT, transrectal ultrasonography, and MR imaging, show excellent anatomic details and sensitivity in detecting cancer in the prostate but cannot distinguish benign from malignant tissues and identify metastatic disease in small lymph nodes. In addition, CT cannot differentiate postsurgical or radiation-induced changes from recurrence. PET as a functional imaging modality improves sensitivity and specificity of other diagnostic procedures for better management of

the disease. Apart from FDG-PET/CT, several other radiolabeled tracers have demonstrated efficacy in various clinical settings, including 18F-fluoride, choline, fluciclovine, and PSMA PET/CT.[66]

Staging

There appears to be a general misconception that FDG-PET/CT is not useful in prostate cancer.[67] Further experience suggests, however, that FDG-PET/CT is useful in diagnosis and initial staging of aggressive/high-risk primary prostate tumors, in particular those with Gleason score greater than 7 (**Fig. 6**).[68] FDG-PET/CT also may be useful in the detection of local and metastatic disease in biochemical recurrence with scan sensitivity that increases with increasing serum prostate-specific antigen (PSA) level.[69]

Incidentaloma

Sometimes, incidental high FDG uptake is seen in prostate of patients who undergo FDG-PET/CT for a condition unrelated to prostate pathology (**Fig. 7**). A meta-analysis of 47,935 patients reported a pooled prevalence of 1.8% for incidental high FDG uptake in the prostate gland and the pooled risk of malignancy with biopsy verification was 62%.[70] It has been suggested that incidental prostate uptake on FDG-PET/CT scans should be evaluated further with at least serum PSA measurement correlation.[71,72]

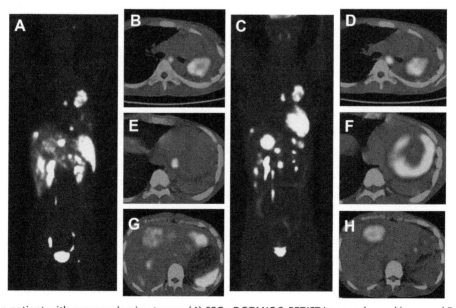

Fig. 5. In a patient with neuroendocrine tumor, (*A*) 68Ga-DOTANOC–PET/CT images showed increased DOTANOC uptake in (*B*) left bronchial mass, which also is seen equally in (*C, D*) FDG–PET/CT. (*E, G*) Some lesions, however, show mild 68Ga-DOTANOC uptake, better seen in (*F, H*) FDG–PET/CT images with increased FDG uptake.

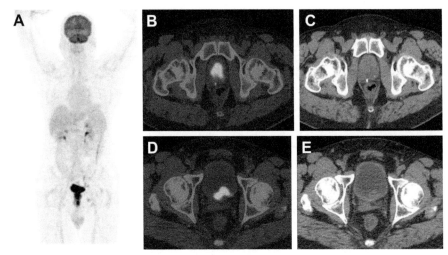

Fig. 6. (*A*) An FDG–PET/CT scan done for staging of high-risk prostate cancer with Gleason score of 9 and serum PSA of 21 ng/mL. (*B*) Increased FDG uptake is seen in (*C*) primary prostate lesion and (*D*) delayed post–diuretic view revealed (*E*) increased FDG uptake in lesion invading posterior bladder wall.

Response Assessment

Further evidence suggests that FDG-PET/CT has its application in the assessment of extent of metabolically active metastatic castrate-resistant prostate cancer (mCRPC), in prognostication and in monitoring response to androgen deprivation therapy (ADT) and other treatments.[73–76] Although it is not indicated in naïve prostate cancer, because they have low FDG-avidity, mCRPC patients, in particular patients with chemotherapy-refractory mCRPC, are characterized by higher FDG uptake. Because there are a growing number of novel drug regimens for mCRPC therapy (eg, enzalutamide, abiratirone, cabazitaxel, and 223Ra dichloride), FDG-PET/CT may have scope in therapy response assessment in this clinical space. Evidence suggests that FDG-PET/CT might represent an effective tool for measuring disease burden and aggressiveness at baseline and for assessing the treatment response to nuclide therapy like 223Ra

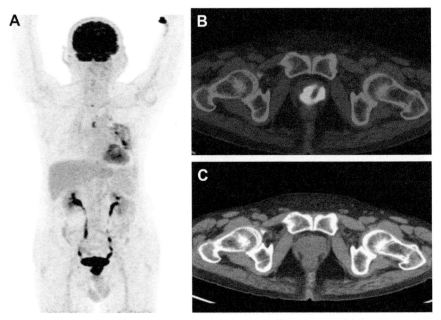

Fig. 7. (*A*) An FDG–PET/CT was done for post–treatment evaluation of lung cancer; (*B*) focal intense FDG uptake in (*C*) prostate gland suggested further evaluation and prostate cancer was diagnosed incidentally.

in mCRPC.[77] But additional studies are needed to decipher the optimal combination of investigations that can reflect the effect of various current and novel therapies most accurately.

A major issue in assessing therapy response in metastatic prostate cancer is that the most common site for metastases is bone, considered nontarget lesions for the structurally based response criteria, such as RECIST, and therefore metabolically based criteria, such as PERCIST, may best serve such task. 18F-NaF (sodium fluoride)–PET/CT binds to osteoblastic sites and has shown efficacy in detecting bone metastases with high sensitivity but relatively low specificity. Although it is superior to bone scintigraphy because it can detect both osteolytic and osteoblastic osseous lesions, it cannot differentiate between active and healing lesions.[78] For this reason, FDG-PET/CT has been proposed as a tool that has high potential for the evaluation of response in mCRPC patients with bone involvement.[74,79]

Other Tracers

Choline PET/CT has been the most extensively studied tracer for detection of prostate cancer. Choline analogs radiolabeled with C11 and F18 both have shown clear superiority over FDG.[80] Although having superior specificity, choline PET/CT suffers from low sensitivity, especially at low PSA levels.[81,82] Newer methods using 18F-fluciclovine and PSMA-targeted radiotracers have preliminarily demonstrated great promise in primary and recurrent staging of prostate cancer. 18F-fluciclovine takes a favorable biodistribution, and it has proved valuable for detection of recurrent cancer after treatment failure, with sensitivity and specificity of 90.2% and 40%, respectively, for recurrence within the prostatic fossa, and 55% and 96.7%, respectively, for nodal and distant recurrences.[83]

Both 68Ga-labeled and 18F-labeled PSMA are highly specific for prostate cancer cells and have rapid nontarget clearance.[84] PSMA expression has been linked to increasing cancer aggressiveness as well as progression to androgen independence.[85] 68Ga-PSMA is better in detecting recurrence/metastases than choline PET/CT, especially in patients with PSA under 2 ng/mL (detection rates for PSA 0.5–2 ng/mL: 69% vs 31% and for PSA<0.5 ng/mL: 50% vs 12.5%, respectively).[86,87] It also can detect rare visceral metastases.[88] But up to 10% of prostate cancers do not overexpress PSMA[89] and PSMA expression in the primary tumor and lymph node metastases are higher than in bone metastases.[90]

PSMA expression can be used as a surrogate marker to monitor androgen receptor signaling; hence, has a potential to act as a noninvasive marker for response to ADT.[91] In mCRPC, PET/CT imaging with FDG and 16β-[18F]-Fluoro-5α Dihydrotestosterone also can be used before treatment with second-generation ADT or chemotherapy. Disease burden, as represented by lesion number, and 18F-FDG SUVmax greater than 7.6 as an indicator of Warburg effect are powerful prognostic biomarkers.[92]

SUMMARY

Even with the advent of several specific tracers, the role of FDG-PET/CT has been unbiased in management of aggressive hormonally sensitive malignancies. It still is a promising modality for staging, prognostication, and response assessment in poorly differentiated malignancies. Newer tracers have increased detection accuracies for small, incipient tumor foci. But the clinical implications of FDG-PET/CT require organized application in high-risk patients with aggressive histology and is always relied on for disease evaluation and prognostication. Efforts should be aimed at defining their natural behavior as well as responsiveness and impact of personalized therapy to achieve maximum benefits from this mainstream functional imaging.

DISCLOSURE

The authors have nothing to disclose. The authors have no conflict of interest. No financial aid was provided for this project.

REFERENCE

1. Vander Heiden MG, Cantley LC, Thompson CB. Understanding the warburg effect: the metabolic requirements of cell proliferation. Science 2009;324: 1029–33.
2. Kumar R, Bhargava P, Bozkurt MF, et al. Positron emission tomography imaging in evaluation of cancer patients. Indian J Cancer 2003;40:87–100.
3. Kostakoglu L, Agress H, Goldsmith SJ. Clinical role of FDG PET in evaluation of cancer patients. RadioGraphics 2003;23:315–40.
4. Lebron L, Greenspan D, Pandit-Taskar N. PET imaging of breast cancer: role in patient management. PET Clin 2015;10:159–95.
5. García Vicente AM, Soriano Castrejón Á, León Martín A, et al. Molecular subtypes of breast cancer: metabolic correlation with 18F-FDG PET/CT. Eur J Nucl Med Mol Imaging 2013;40:1304–11.
6. Buck A, Schirrmeister H, Kühn T, et al. FDG uptake in breast cancer: correlation with biological and

clinical prognostic parameters. Eur J Nucl Med Mol Imaging 2002;29:1317–23.

7. Tchou J, Sonnad SS, Bergey MR, et al. Degree of tumor FDG uptake correlates with proliferation index in triple negative breast cancer. Mol Imaging Biol 2010;12:657–62.

8. Groheux D. Role of fludeoxyglucose in breast cancer: treatment response. PET Clin 2018;13:395–414.

9. Koolen BB, VranckenPeeters M-JTFD, Aukema TS, et al. 18F-FDG PET/CT as a staging procedure in primary stage II and III breast cancer: comparison with conventional imaging techniques. Breast Cancer Res Treat 2012;131:117–26.

10. Hahn S, Heusner T, Kümmel S, et al. Comparison of FDG-PET/CT and bone scintigraphy for detection of bone metastases in breast cancer. Acta Radiol 2011;52:1009–14.

11. Niikura N, Costelloe CM, Madewell JE, et al. FDG-PET/CT compared with conventional imaging in the detection of distant metastases of primary breast cancer. Oncologist 2011;16:1111–9.

12. Groheux D, Giacchetti S, Moretti J-L, et al. Correlation of high 18F-FDG uptake to clinical, pathological and biological prognostic factors in breast cancer. Eur J Nucl Med Mol Imaging 2011;38:426–35.

13. Koo HR, Park JS, Kang KW, et al. 18F-FDG uptake in breast cancer correlates with immunohistochemically defined subtypes. Eur Radiol 2014;24:610–8.

14. Koolen BB, VranckenPeeters MJTFD, Wesseling J, et al. Association of primary tumour FDG uptake with clinical, histopathological and molecular characteristics in breast cancer patients scheduled for neoadjuvant chemotherapy. Eur J Nucl Med Mol Imaging 2012;39:1830–8.

15. Kitajima K, Murphy RC, Nathan MA, et al. Detection of recurrent prostate cancer after radical prostatectomy: comparison of 11C-choline PET/CT with pelvic multiparametric MR imaging with endorectal coil. J Nucl Med 2014;55:223–32.

16. Huyge V, Garcia C, Alexiou J, et al. Heterogeneity of metabolic response to systemic therapy in metastatic breast cancer patients. Clin Oncol 2010;22: 818–27.

17. Lin NU, Guo H, Yap JT, et al. Phase II study of lapatinib in combination with trastuzumab in patients with human epidermal growth factor receptor 2-positive metastatic breast cancer: clinical outcomes and predictive value of early [18F]fluorodeoxyglucose positron emission tomography imaging (TBCRC 003). J Clin Oncol 2015;33:2623–31.

18. Baselga J, Bradbury I, Eidtmann H, et al. Lapatinib with trastuzumab for HER2-positive early breast cancer (NeoALTTO): a randomised, open-label, multicentre, phase 3 trial. Lancet 2012;379:633–40.

19. Kiesewetter DO, Kilbourn MR, Landvatter SW, et al. Preparation of four fluorine- 18-labeled estrogens and their selective uptakes in target tissues of immature rats. J Nucl Med 1984;25:1212–21.

20. Mintun MA, Welch MJ, Siegel BA, et al. Breast cancer: PET imaging of estrogen receptors. Radiology 1988;169:45–8.

21. Mortimer JE, Dehdashti F, Siegel BA, et al. Metabolic flare: indicator of hormone responsiveness in advanced breast cancer. J Clin Oncol 2001;19: 2797–803.

22. Gupta M, Datta A, Choudhury PS, et al. Can 18F-Fluoroestradiol positron emission tomography become a new imaging standard in the estrogen receptor-positive breast cancer patient: a prospective comparative study with 18F-Fluorodeoxyglucose positron emission tomography? World J Nucl Med 2017;16:133–9.

23. Suresh Malapure S, Das KJ, Kumar R. PET/computed tomography in breast cancer: can it aid in developing a personalized treatment design? PET Clin 2016;11:297–303.

24. Fletcher JW, Djulbegovic B, Soares HP, et al. Recommendations on the use of 18F-FDG PET in oncology. J Nucl Med 2008;49:480–508.

25. Haugen BR, Alexander EK, Bible KC, et al. 2015 American thyroid association management guidelines for adult patients with thyroid nodules and differentiated thyroid cancer: the American thyroid association guidelines task force on thyroid nodules and differentiated thyroid cancer. Thyroid 2015;26: 1–133.

26. Bertagna F, Bosio G, Biasiotto G, et al. F-18 FDG-PET/CT evaluation of patients with differentiated thyroid cancer with negative I-131 total body scan and high thyroglobulin level. Clin Nucl Med 2009;34: 756–61.

27. Iagaru A, Masamed R, Singer PA, et al. 2-Deoxy-2-[18F]fluoro-D-glucose-positron emission tomography and positron emission tomography/computed tomography diagnosis of patients with recurrent papillary thyroid cancer. Mol Imaging Biol 2006;8: 309–14.

28. Piccardo A, Foppiani L, Morbelli S, et al. Could ^{18}F-fluorodeoxyglucose PET/CT change the therapeutic management of stage IV thyroid cancer with positive (131)I whole body scan? Q J Nucl Med Mol Imaging 2011;55:57–65.

29. Vural GU, Akkas BE, Ercakmak N, et al. Prognostic significance of FDG PET/CT on the follow-up of patients of differentiated thyroid carcinoma with negative 131I whole-body scan and elevated thyroglobulin levels: correlation with clinical and histopathologic characteristics and long-term follow-up data. Clin Nucl Med 2012;37:953–9.

30. Esteva D, Muros MA, Llamas-Elvira JM, et al. Clinical and pathological factors related to 18F-FDG-PET positivity in the diagnosis of recurrence and/or

metastasis in patients with differentiated thyroid cancer. Ann Surg Oncol 2009;16:2006–13.

31. Robbins RJ, Wan Q, Grewal RK, et al. Real-time prognosis for metastatic thyroid carcinoma based on 2-[18F]fluoro-2-deoxy-D-glucose-positron emission tomography scanning. J Clin Endocrinol Metab 2006;91:498–505.

32. Deandreis D, Al Ghuzlan A, Leboulleux S, et al. Do histological, immunohistochemical, and metabolic (radioiodine and fluorodeoxyglucose uptakes) patterns of metastatic thyroid cancer correlate with patient outcome? Endocr Relat Cancer 2011;18: 159–69.

33. Wang W, Larson SM, Fazzari M, et al. Prognostic value of [18F]fluorodeoxyglucose positron emission tomographic scanning in patients with thyroid cancer. J Clin Endocrinol Metab 2000;85:1107–13.

34. Haugen BR, Sherman SI. Evolving approaches to patients with advanced differentiated thyroid cancer. Endocr Rev 2013;34:439–55.

35. Wang N, Zhai H, Lu Y. Is fluorine-18 fluorodeoxyglucose positron emission tomography useful for the thyroid nodules with indeterminate fine needle aspiration biopsy? a meta-analysis of the literature. J Otolaryngol Head Neck Surg 2013;42:38.

36. Vriens D, Adang EMM, Netea-Maier RT, et al. Cost-effectiveness of FDG-PET/CT for cytologically indeterminate thyroid nodules: a decision analytic approach. J Clin Endocrinol Metab 2014;99: 3263–74.

37. Merten MM, Castro MR, Zhang J, et al. Examining the role of preoperative positron emission tomography/computerized tomography in combination with ultrasonography in discriminating benign from malignant cytologically indeterminate thyroid nodules. Thyroid 2017;27:95–102.

38. Castellana M, Trimboli P, Piccardo A, et al. Performance of 18F-FDG PET/CT in selecting thyroid nodules with indeterminate fine-needle aspiration cytology for surgery. a systematic review and a meta-analysis. J Clin Med 2019;8:1333.

39. Chen W, Li G, Parsons M, et al. Clinical significance of incidental focal versus diffuse thyroid uptake on FDG-PET imaging. PET Clin 2007;2:321–9.

40. Bertagna F, Treglia G, Piccardo A, et al. Diagnostic and clinical significance of F-18-FDG-PET/CT thyroid incidentalomas. J Clin Endocrinol Metab 2012; 97:3866–75.

41. Treglia G, Muoio B, Giovanella L, et al. The role of positron emission tomography and positron emission tomography/computed tomography in thyroid tumours: an overview. Eur Arch Otorhinolaryngol 2012;270:1783–7.

42. Soelberg KK, Bonnema SJ, Brix TH, et al. Risk of malignancy in thyroid incidentalomas detected by 18F-fluorodeoxyglucose positron emission tomography: a systematic review. Thyroid 2012;22:918–25.

43. de Groot JWB, Links TP, Jager PL, et al. Impact of 18F-fluoro-2-deoxy-D-glucose positron emission tomography (FDG-PET) in patients with biochemical evidence of recurrent or residual medullary thyroid cancer. Ann Surg Oncol 2004;11:786–94.

44. Rubello D, Rampin L, Nanni C, et al. The role of 18F-FDG PET/CT in detecting metastatic deposits of recurrent medullary thyroid carcinoma: a prospective study. Eur J Surg Oncol 2008;34:581–6.

45. Cheng X, Bao L, Xu Z, et al. ^{18}F-FDG-PET and ^{18}F-FDG-PET/CT in the detection of recurrent or metastatic medullary thyroid carcinoma: a systematic review and meta-analysis. J Med Imaging Radiat Oncol 2012;56:136–42.

46. Poisson T, Deandreis D, Leboulleux S, et al. 18F-fluorodeoxyglucose positron emission tomography and computed tomography in anaplastic thyroid cancer. Eur J Nucl Med Mol Imaging 2010;37: 2277–85.

47. Bogsrud TV, Karantanis D, Nathan MA, et al. 18F-FDG PET in the management of patients with anaplastic thyroid carcinoma. Thyroid 2008;18: 713–9.

48. Modlin IM, Oberg K, Chung DC, et al. Gastroenteropancreatic neuroendocrine tumours. Lancet Oncol 2008;9:61–72.

49. Dasari A, Shen C, Halperin D, et al. Trends in the incidence, prevalence, and survival outcomes in patients with neuroendocrine tumors in the United States. JAMA Oncol 2017;3:1335–42.

50. Bosman FT, Carneiro F, Hruban RH, et al. 4th edition. WHO classification of tumours of the digestive system. WHO classification of tumours, vol. 3. IARC Publication; 2010. Available at: https://publications.iarc.fr/Book-And-Report-Series/Who-Classification-Of-Tumours/Digestive-System-Tumours-2019. Accessed July 10, 2020.

51. Panzuto F, Campana D, Fazio N, et al. Risk factors for disease progression in advanced jejunoileal neuroendocrine tumors. Neuroendocrinology 2012; 96:32–40.

52. Sundin A, Arnold R, Baudin E, et al. ENETS consensus guidelines for the standards of care in neuroendocrine tumors: radiological, nuclear medicine & hybrid imaging. Neuroendocrinology 2017; 105:212–44.

53. Binderup T, Knigge U, Loft A, et al. 18F-fluorodeoxyglucose positron emission tomography predicts survival of patients with neuroendocrine tumors. Clin Cancer Res 2010;16:978–85.

54. Treglia G, Castaldi P, Rindi G, et al. Diagnostic performance of Gallium-68 somatostatin receptor PET and PET/CT in patients with thoracic and gastroenteropancreatic neuroendocrine tumours: a meta-analysis. Endocrine 2012;42:80–7.

55. Yadav D, Ballal S, Yadav MP, et al. Evaluation of [68Ga]Ga-DATA-TOC for imaging of neuroendocrine

tumours: comparison with [68Ga]Ga-DOTA-NOC PET/CT. Eur J Nucl Med Mol Imaging 2020;47: 860–9.

56. Ambrosini V, Campana D, Polverari G, et al. Prognostic value of 68Ga-DOTANOC PET/CT SUVmax in patients with neuroendocrine tumors of the pancreas. J Nucl Med 2015;56:1843–8.

57. Kayani I, Bomanji JB, Groves A, et al. Functional imaging of neuroendocrine tumors with combined PET/CT using 68Ga-DOTATATE (DOTA-DPhe1,Tyr3-octreotate) and 18F-FDG. Cancer 2008;112:2447–55.

58. Rinzivillo M, Partelli S, Prosperi D, et al. Clinical usefulness of 18F-fluorodeoxyglucose positron emission tomography in the diagnostic algorithm of advanced entero-pancreatic neuroendocrine neoplasms. Oncologist 2018;23:186–92.

59. Panagiotidis E, Alshammari A, Michopoulou S, et al. Comparison of the impact of 68Ga-DOTATATE and 18F-FDG PET/CT on clinical management in patients with neuroendocrine tumors. J Nucl Med 2017;58:91–6.

60. Sharma P, Naswa N, Kc SS, et al. Comparison of the prognostic values of 68Ga-DOTANOC PET/CT and 18F-FDG PET/CT in patients with well-differentiated neuroendocrine tumor. Eur J Nucl Med Mol Imaging 2014;41:2194–202.

61. Chan DL, Pavlakis N, Schembri GP, et al. Dual somatostatin receptor/FDG PET/CT imaging in metastatic neuroendocrine tumours: proposal for a novel grading scheme with prognostic significance. Theranostics 2017;7:1149–58.

62. Naswa N, Sharma P, Gupta SK, et al. Dual tracer functional imaging of gastroenteropancreatic neuroendocrine tumors using 68Ga-DOTA-NOC PET-CT and 18F-FDG PET-CT: competitive or complimentary? Clin Nucl Med 2014;39:27–34.

63. Cingarlini S, Ortolani S, Salgarello M, et al. Role of combined 68Ga-DOTATOC and 18F-FDG positron emission tomography/computed tomography in the diagnostic workup of pancreas neuroendocrine tumors: implications for managing surgical decisions. Pancreas 2017;46:42–7.

64. Hindié E. The NETPET score: combining FDG and somatostatin receptor imaging for optimal management of patients with metastatic well-differentiated neuroendocrine tumors. Theranostics 2017;7: 1159–63.

65. Carideo L, Prosperi D, Panzuto F, et al. Role of combined [68Ga]Ga-DOTA-SST Analogues and [18F] FDG PET/CT in the Management of GEP-NENs: a systematic review. J Clin Med 2019;8:1032.

66. Jadvar H. Molecular imaging of prostate cancer: PET radiotracers. AJR Am J Roentgenol 2012;199: 278–91.

67. Salminen E, Hogg A, Binns D, et al. Investigations with FDG-PET scanning in prostate cancer show limited value for clinical practice. Acta Oncol 2002; 41:425–9.

68. Oyama N, Akino H, Suzuki Y, et al. The increased accumulation of [18F]fluorodeoxyglucose in untreated prostate cancer. Jpn J Clin Oncol 1999;29: 623–9.

69. Jadvar H, Desai B, Ji L, et al. Prospective evaluation of 18F-NaF and 18F-FDG PET/CT in detection of occult metastatic disease in biochemical recurrence of prostate cancer. Clin Nucl Med 2012;37: 637–43.

70. Bertagna F, Sadeghi R, Giovanella L, et al. Incidental uptake of 18F-fluorodeoxyglucose in the prostate gland. Systematic review and meta-analysis on prevalence and risk of malignancy. Nuklearmedizin 2014;53:249–58.

71. Kang PM, Seo WI, Lee SS, et al. Incidental abnormal FDG uptake in the prostate on 18-fluoro-2-deoxyglucose positron emission tomography-computed tomography scans. Asian Pac J Cancer Prev 2014; 15:8699–703.

72. Seino H, Ono S, Miura H, et al. Incidental prostate 18F-FDG uptake without calcification indicates the possibility of prostate cancer. Oncol Rep 2014;31: 1517–22.

73. Jadvar H, Desai B, Ji L, et al. Baseline 18F-FDG PET/CT parameters as imaging biomarkers of overall survival in castrate-resistant metastatic prostate cancer. J Nucl Med 2013;54:1195–201.

74. Vargas HA, Wassberg C, Fox JJ, et al. Bone metastases in castration-resistant prostate cancer: associations between morphologic CT patterns, glycolytic activity, and androgen receptor expression on PET and overall survival. Radiology 2014;271:220–9.

75. Morris MJ, Akhurst T, Larson SM, et al. Fluorodeoxyglucose positron emission tomography as an outcome measure for castrate metastatic prostate cancer treated with antimicrotubule chemotherapy. Clin Cancer Res 2005;11:3210–6.

76. Jadvar H. Is there use for FDG-PET in prostate cancer? Semin Nucl Med 2016;46:502–6.

77. Bauckneht M, Capitanio S, Donegani MI, et al. Role of baseline and post-therapy 18F-FDG PET in the prognostic stratification of metastatic castration-resistant prostate cancer (mCRPC) patients treated with Radium-223. Cancers 2019;12:31.

78. Langsteger W, Rezaee A, Pirich C, et al. 18F-NaF-PET/CT and 99mTc-MDP bone scintigraphy in the detection of bone metastases in prostate cancer. Semin Nucl Med 2016;46:491–501.

79. Zukotynski KA, Kim CK, Gerbaudo VH, et al. 18F-FDG-PET/CT and 18F-NaF-PET/CT in men with castrate-resistant prostate cancer. Am J Nucl Med Mol Imaging 2014;5:72–82.

80. Picchio M, Messa C, Landoni C, et al. Value of [11C] choline-positron emission tomography for re-staging prostate cancer: a comparison with [18F] fluorodeoxyglucose-positron emission tomography. J Urol 2003;169:1337–40.

81. Martorana G, Schiavina R, Corti B, et al. 11C-choline positron emission tomography/computerized tomography for tumor localization of primary prostate cancer in comparison with 12-core biopsy. J Urol 2006;176:954–60.

82. Evangelista L, Guttilla A, Zattoni F, et al. Utility of choline positron emission tomography/computed tomography for lymph node involvement identification in intermediate- to high-risk prostate cancer: a systematic literature review and meta-analysis. Eur Urol 2013;63:1040–8.

83. Schuster DM, Nieh PT, Jani AB, et al. Anti-3-[(18)F]FACBC positron emission tomography-computerized tomography and (111)In-capromab pendetide single photon emission computerized tomography-computerized tomography for recurrent prostate carcinoma: results of a prospective clinical trial. J Urol 2014;191:1446–53.

84. Maurer T, Eiber M, Schwaiger M, et al. Current use of PSMA-PET in prostate cancer management. Nat Rev Urol 2016;13:226–35.

85. Perner S, Hofer MD, Kim R, et al. Prostate-specific membrane antigen expression as a predictor of prostate cancer progression. Hum Pathol 2007;38:696–701.

86. Afshar-Oromieh A, Haberkorn U, Schlemmer HP, et al. Comparison of PET/CT and PET/MRI hybrid systems using a 68Ga-labelled PSMA ligand for the diagnosis of recurrent prostate cancer: initial experience. Eur J Nucl Med Mol Imaging 2014;41:887–97.

87. Morigi JJ, Stricker PD, van Leeuwen PJ, et al. Prospective comparison of 18F-fluoromethylcholine versus 68Ga-PSMA PET/CT in prostate cancer patients who have rising PSA after curative treatment and are being considered for targeted therapy. J Nucl Med 2015;56:1185–90.

88. Chakraborty PS, Kumar R, Tripathi M, et al. Detection of brain metastasis with 68Ga-labeled PSMA ligand PET/CT: a novel radiotracer for imaging of prostate carcinoma. Clin Nucl Med 2015;40:328–9.

89. Maurer T, Gschwend JE, Rauscher I, et al. Diagnostic efficacy of (68)Gallium-PSMA positron emission tomography compared to conventional imaging for lymph node staging of 130 consecutive patients with intermediate to high risk prostate cancer. J Urol 2016;195:1436–43.

90. Sweat SD, Pacelli A, Murphy GP, et al. Prostate-specific membrane antigen expression is greatest in prostate adenocarcinoma and lymph node metastases. Urology 1998;52:637–40.

91. Evans MJ, Smith-Jones PM, Wongvipat J, et al. Noninvasive measurement of androgen receptor signaling with a positron-emitting radiopharmaceutical that targets prostate-specific membrane antigen. Proc Natl Acad Sci U S A 2011;108:9578–82.

92. Fox JJ, Gavane SC, Blanc-Autran E, et al. Positron emission tomography/computed tomography–based assessments of androgen receptor expression and glycolytic activity as a prognostic biomarker for metastatic castration-resistant prostate cancer. JAMA Oncol 2018;4:217–24.

Somatostatin Receptor Imaging PET in Neuroendocrine Neoplasm

Camilla Bardram Johnbeck, MD, PhD[a,b], Jann Mortensen, MD, DMSc[a,b,c],*

KEYWORDS

- Meta-analysis • Head-to-head studies • Gallium-68 • Cobber-64 • DOTATATE • DOTATOC
- DOTANOC • Somatostatin Receptor Antagonist

KEY POINTS

- Several somatostatin receptor imaging PET tracers are highly sensitive and clinically used. The pursuit towards the perfect theranostic pair is ongoing.
- All approved somatostatin receptor imaging tracers so far are agonists. Recent promising studies show high tumor accumulation in liver-lesions and a low background using antagonists.
- Gallium-68 tracers can be generator-produced local. Cobber-64 tracers demand a cyclotron, but due to long shelf-life they can be centrally distributed.
- ^{64}Cu-DOTATATE enables a flexible scan-time (1-3 hours p.i) in comparison to ^{68}Ga-based tracers, but at the cost of a higher radiation dose to the patient.

INTRODUCTION

In the era of personalized medicine, neuroendocrine neoplasms (NENs) have paved the way in nuclear medicine. The connection between diagnostics and consequent therapy—theranostics—has been widely used in NENs, and the pursuit for the most perfect theranostic pair—a highly specific and sensitive NEN imaging tracer and its subsequent therapeutic drug for peptide receptor radionuclide therapy (PRRT)—is ongoing.

NEUROENDOCRINE NEOPLASMS

NENs can arise in tissue consisting of neuroendocrine cells, nerve structures, endocrine organs, or structures hosting the diffuse neuroendocrine cell system. Most NENs, however, arise from gastroenteropancreatic (GEP) sites and the lungs. Disease manifestations, progression rates, and life expectancy are highly heterogeneous. The treatment algorithms for NENs are numerous, emphasizing exact diagnosis, determination of extent of disease, and prognostic subgrouping of patients into categories from, on one side the group of patients needing urgent treatment to on the other side the group of patients with NENs of an almost benign nature. The common feature of NEN is the neuroendocrine phenotype expressing general markers of neuroendocrine cell differentiation, mainly chromogranin A and synaptophysin. Furthermore, most NENs express somatostatin receptors (SSTRs), paving the way for molecular imaging for diagnostic purposes as well as treatment with somatostatin analogs and PRRT.

Although NENs comprise a very heterogenous group, a general classification system is attempted independent of site of origin. NEN as a cancer category is divided based on morphology into well-differentiated neuroendocrine tumors (NETs) and poorly differentiated neuroendocrine carcinomas (NECs). NETs are divided further by

[a] Department of Clinical Physiology, Nuclear Medicine and PET, Rigshospitalet, Copenhagen, Denmark;
[b] European Neuroendocrine Tumor Society Center of Excellence, Rigshospitalet, Copenhagen, Denmark;
[c] Medical Faculty, University of Copenhagen, Denmark
* Corresponding author. Department of Clinical Physiology, Nuclear Medicine and PET, Rigshospitalet, Blegdamsvej 9, Copenhagen DK-2100, Denmark.
E-mail address: jann.mortensen@regionh.dk

PET Clin 16 (2021) 191–203
https://doi.org/10.1016/j.cpet.2020.12.011

a proliferation-based grading system based on immunohistochemical assessment, Ki67, into low grade (G1, Ki67 ≤2%), intermediate grade (G2, Ki67 3%–20%), and high grade (G3, Ki67 >20%) whereas NECs always are high grade.[1,2]

SOMATOSTATIN RECEPTORS

SSTRs have been identified in a variety of most neuroendocrine human tumors, especially in tumors with amine precursor uptake and decarboxylation characteristics like pituitary tumors, medullary thyroid carcinomas, paragangliomas, small cell lung cancers, endocrine pancreatic tumors and carcinoids, but also in meningiomas, astrocytomas, neuroblastoma and some breast cancers.[3]

Five different subtypes of SSTRs have been described: sst1–sst5. Two subtypes of sst2 exist: sst2a and sst2b. Sst2a is the most abundantly expressed followed by sst3 and sst1, both in GEP NENs and lung NENs.[4–6] It is well established that the expression of SSTRs correlates inversely to the tumor grade, having the most abundant expression in low-grade tumors and the lowest expression in high-grade tumors or poorly differentiated NECs.[7–9] A recent study evaluated SSTR-2a expression in high grade (ki67 >20 %) GEP NENs and found 26 % of the 163 included patients to be strongly positive for SSTR-2a.[10] Low SSTR-2a expression was seen on the poorly differentiated most proliferative NECs.

SOMATOSTATIN RECEPTOR IMAGING

SSTR imaging (SRI) with radiolabeled somatostatin analogs has been used for more than 30 years and gone from a γ-camera–based to a PET-based technique (**Fig. 1**).

The first scintigraphy of SSTR was by ^{123}I-Tyr2-octreotide.[11] Afterwards, more than 1000 patients were scanned in Rotterdam using this or ^{111}In-diethylenetriaminepentaacetic acid (DTPA)-octreotide, and sensitivity of 80% to 95% for determining pancreatic NET and carcinoids was found.[3] Also, a technetium-based tracer, allowing same-day scintigraphy, is available.[12] Yet, the most used tracer for SSRT scintigraphy has been ^{111}In-DTPA-octreotide (^{111}In-pentreotide), with a 2-day protocol.

Labeling peptides with radioisotopes of other members of the metal group, such as ^{68}Ga, ^{64}Cu, ^{90}Y, and ^{177}Lu, moved a big step further with the introduction of a universal chelator, 1,4,7,10-tetraazacyclodecane-1,4,7,10-tetraacetic acid (DOTA).[13] In the past 2 decades, new tracers have been developed using the DOTA-chelator to combine mainly PET isotopes with somatostatin analogs.

Changing small parts of the somatostatin peptide readily changes the affinity for the different SSTR subtypes (sst1–sst5).

The most used octreotide modifications are Tyr[3]-octreotide, Tyr[3]-octreotate, and I-Nal[3]-octreotide and, when combined with gallium and the DOTA chelator, they are named ^{68}Ga-DOTATATE, ^{68}Ga-DOTATOC, ^{68}Ga-DOTANOC, respectively. The highest affinity for the most abundant sst2 is by ^{68}Ga-DOTATATE that binds exclusively to sst2 with a 10-fold higher affinity than both ^{68}Ga-DOTATOC and ^{68}Ga-DOTANOC at least in vitro. ^{68}Ga-DOTATOC, however, also has some affinity for sst5, and ^{68}Ga-DOTANOC has affinity for both sst5 and sst3.[14,15] A fourth less often used combination showing affinity

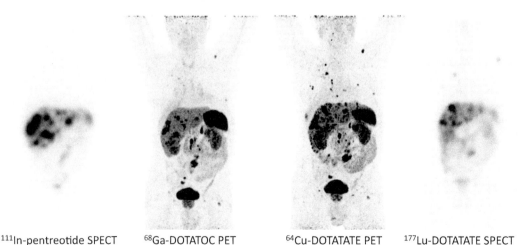

| ^{111}In-pentreotide SPECT | ^{68}Ga-DOTATOC PET | ^{64}Cu-DOTATATE PET | ^{177}Lu-DOTATATE SPECT |

Fig. 1. The same NEN patient scanned over 6 years with SPECT and PET SRI tracers. The first scan (*left*) was an ^{111}In-pentrotide SPECT scan in 2013. Later PET tracers became available and the patient was scanned with ^{68}Ga-DOTATOC and subsequent ^{64}Cu-DOTATATE PET. Recently the patient was treated with peptide radionuclide therapy and a post treatment SPECT was done using the 177Lu-DOTATATE (*right*).

towards sst2 and sst5 is the somatostatin analog lanreotide in combination with ^{68}Ga-DOTA called ^{68}Ga-DOTALAN. In addition, the affinity of each peptide to the different SSTRs also varies with the radioisotope chosen for labeling; hence, labeling DOTATOC and DOTATATE with gallium shows binding affinity to sst2 that is a factor 4-8 times higher compared with the corresponding yttrium or indium derivatives.[14]

Several studies have proved superiority of PET NET imaging in comparison to γ-emitting tracers, with significantly higher sensitivity and greater clinical impact.[16–19]

The additional value of SSTR PET/computed tomography (CT) after ^{111}In-DTPA-octreotide was evaluated in a review of 3 ^{68}Ga-DOTATATE studies and 1 ^{68}Ga-DOTANOC study. A total of 278 patients were included and, in 39% of the cases, additional findings with impact on patient management were found.[20]

In Europe, the shift from ^{111}In-DTPA-octreotide to mainly ^{68}Ga-based SRI PET is well established. Yet, it is with the rather recent approvals from the US Food and Drug Administration of ^{68}Ga-DOTATATE NETSPOT (June 2016) and ^{68}Ga-DOTATOC (August 2019) that the United States also is changing the NET imaging approach toward PET-based tracers.

Mostly, ^{68}Ga has been used, because it is widely available being produced from a generator. The amount of generator produced gallium-68 at one time is limited and therefore cyclotrone production of the radioisotope has been exploited and was FDA approved in october 2020. However the half-time of 68 minutes sets certain demands for the clinical set-up. A third SRI PET tracer, 64CU-DOTATATE, which has been used oustside the United States for some years was also recently FDA approved.[21,22] Also, labeling DOTATOC with ^{64}Cu recently has been published in a study of 33 patients.[23] Using ^{64}Cu instead of ^{68}Ga, despite the higher amount of β-radiation, has the benefit of a half-time of 12.7 hours and at least in theory a better spatial resolution due to the lower positron energy and hence shorter positron range.

ANTAGONISTS

All clinically available tracers for SRI depend on somatostatin agonists. An exciting development within the field is the recent introduction of SSTR antagonists.[24–27] Receptor internalization, after binding to the somatostatin analog, formerly was considered crucial for both imaging and therapy. Lately, it has been shown that somatostatin antagonists, even though their internalization rates are very low compared with the agonists, show operational tumor

uptake and favorable pharmacokinetics.[28,29] The theory behind this phenomenon is the binding of antagonists to a larger number of binding sites and a slower dissociation rate and has encouraged further development and the design of potent SSTR antagonist radiotracers for PET imaging and therapy.

Several combinations of the sst2 antagonists LM3 (p-Cl-Phe-cyclo [D-Cys-Tyr-D-Aph(Cbm)-Lys-Thr-Cys]D-Tyr-NH2), JR10 (p-NO2-Phe-c[D-Cys-Tyr- D-Aph(Cbm)-Lys-Thr-Cys]-D-Tyr-NH2), and JR11 (Cpa-c[D-Cys-Aph(Hor)-D-Aph(Cbm)-Lys-Thr-Cys]-D-Tyr-NH2) with the chelators (DOTA, NODAGA, and CB-TE2A) and different isotopes (^{68}Ga, ^{64}Cu, ^{177}Lu, ^{111}In, and ^{90}Y) have been studied.[30,31] The antagonists are highly sensitive to modifications of both the chelator and the radiometal, and significantly higher tumor uptakes have been found with low-affinity antagonists compared with high-affinity agonists, at least preclinically.[30]

In the preclinical settings, the analog JR11 seemed the most promising and further clinical studies are ongoing with PET tracer ^{68}Ga-NODAGA-JR11 or [68]Ga -DOTA-JR11 for imaging and ^{177}Lu-DOTA-JR11 for therapy as a new promising theranostic pair in NEN.

Nicolas and colleagues[32,33] compared the sensitivity of ^{68}Ga-NODAGA-JR11 with ^{68}Ga-DOTATOC PET/CT in patients with NET and found the antagonist superior in sensitivity, image contrast, and lesion detection.

Krebs and colleagues[34] demonstrated good safety, rapid tumor uptake, and high tumor/background ratios in patients with metastatic NET, using [68]Ga -DOTA-JR11.

PERFORMANE OF THE SOMATOSTATIN RECEPTOR PET IMAGING TRACERS

Four meta-analysis comprising overlapping studies has been done. Treglia and colleagues[35] analyzed 16 studies comprising 567 patients with thoracic and/or GEP-NET and found pooled sensitivity of 93% (95% CI, 91%–95%) and specificity of 91% (95% CI, 82%–97%), respectively, on a per-patient–based analysis.

Geijer and Breimer[36] analyzed 22 articles, published through December 2012, on 2105 patients with different NET grades, stages, and locations studied with ^{68}Ga-DOTATOC (11 studies), ^{68}Ga-DOTATATE PET/CT (8 studies), or ^{68}Ga-DOTANOC (3 studies). Pooled sensitivity on a per-patient basis was 93%, specificity was 96%, and area under summary receiver operating characteristic curve was 98%.

Yang and colleagues[37] analyzed 10 articles published through April 2013 on 416 patients with different NET grades, stages, and locations studied with either ^{68}Ga-DOTATOC (6 studies, 1 being prospective) or ^{68}Ga-DOTATATE PET/CT (4 studies). Pooled sensitivities on per-patient basis were 93% and 96% and specificities were 85% and 100%, respectively. Too few DOTANOC studies were accepted to be included.

In 2014, the authors looked at the performance of the tracers individually. For ^{68}Ga-DOTATATE (6 studies), the ^{68}Ga sensitivity ranged from 72% to 96% and specificity was 100% (only reported in 1 study). For DOTATOC (6 studies), sensitivity was 92% to 100% and specificity 83% to 100% (reported in 3 studies). For ^{68}Ga-DOTANOC (9 studies), sensitivity was 68% to 100% and specificity 93% to 100% (reported in 5 studies).[38]

These seem excellent results in general for SRI PET/CT, but because NENs comprise a very heterogenous group of patients, the optimal evaluation is prospective head-to-head comparisons of different tracers in the same patients.

In **Table 1**, 9 head-to-head studies of the SRI PET tracers are summarized.

Poeppel and colleagues[39] compared ^{68}Ga-DOTATOC with ^{68}Ga-DOTATATE and found significantly higher tumor uptake and more lesions with ^{68}Ga-DOTATOC versus ^{68}Ga-DOTATATE. Tumor uptake of the tracers varied considerably, however, within and between patients. Overall, the diagnostic accuracies of ^{68}Ga-DOTATOC and ^{68}Ga-DOTATATE were comparable. Hence, the approximately 10-fold higher affinity for the sst2 of DOTATATE does not prove clinically relevant, and presence of sst5 might explain the small differences in some tumors.

Two studies have compared ^{68}Ga-DOTANOC with ^{68}Ga-DOTATATE.[40,41] Kabasakal and colleagues[40] found significantly higher uptake in tumor lesions by ^{68}Ga-DOTATATE versus ^{68}Ga-DOTANOC but comparable diagnostic accuracy. In the other study, by Wild and colleagues,[41] ^{68}Ga-DOTANOC had a higher liver and pancreas lesion detection rate, whereas ^{68}Ga-DOTATATE found more bone lesions.

^{68}Ga-DOTALAN was compared with ^{68}Ga-DOTATOC in 1 study.[42] A significantly higher lesion detection rate and higher tumor uptake was shown for ^{68}Ga-DOTATOC. Likewise, in another study of ^{68}Ga-DOTALAN, a lower sensitivity of only 44% was found compared with 94% for ^{68}Ga-DOTATATE.[43]

[64]Cu-DOTATATE studied head-to-head with ^{68}Ga-DOTATOC in 59 NET patients had comparable patient-based diagnostic accuracy. ^{64}Cu-DOTATATE detected more additional true positive lesions (>2 years of follow-up) and had higher maximum SUV (SUVmax) in tumor lesions as well as in background organs. Tumor-to-background ratio (TBR) was comparable for liver and lymph nodes but higher for bones using ^{68}Ga-DOTATOC, even though more bone lesions were found by ^{64}Cu-DOTATATE.[44] Hicks and colleagues[45] used the tracer ^{64}Cu-MeCOSar-Tyr[3]-octreotate (^{64}Cu-SARTATE) in comparison with ^{68}Ga-DOTATATE. Higher uptake and retention of ^{64}Cu-SARTATE in tumors provided high-contrast diagnostic images until at least 24 hours after injection. Comparison of ^{64}Cu-SARTATE PET/CT obtained at 4 hours to ^{68}Ga-DOTATATE PET/CT obtained at 1 hour indicated comparable or superior lesion detection with ^{64}Cu-SARTATE in all patients, especially in the liver.

Recently the first head-to-head prospective comparison of the antagonistic ^{68}Ga-DOTA-JR11 and ^{68}Ga-DOTATATE PET/CT in 29 patients with metastatic NET was published.[46] The background organ uptakes were much lower on ^{68}Ga-DOTA-JR11 than on ^{68}Ga-DOTATATE PET/CT and the antagonist tracer detected significantly more liver lesions (539 vs 356; $P = .002$) than the agonist. The TBR of liver lesions also was significantly higher with ^{68}Ga-DOTA-JR11. The antagonist PET scan, however, detected fewer bone lesions than the agonist ^{68}Ga-DOTATATE PET (156 vs 374; $P = .031$) and the 2 scans performed equally for primary tumors and lymph node metastases.

Interpretation of the studies: ^{68}Ga-DOTALAN was inferior compared with ^{68}Ga-DOTATATE and ^{68}Ga-DOTATOC in 2 head-to head studies; hence, ^{68}Ga-DOTALAN should not be used as first choice if alternatives are available.

Comparisons of the other agonist tracers—[68]Ga-DOTATATE versus ^{68}Ga-DOTANOC and ^{68}Ga-DOTATATE versus ^{68}Ga-DOTATOC and ^{64}Cu-DOTATATE and ^{68}Ga-DOTATOC—showed equal diagnostic accuracy on a per-patient basis, indicating that their clinical value is comparable most likely because all have affinity to the most abundant sst2. There were some differences, however, favoring 1 of the tracers in some studies and the other tracer in other studies when analyzed on a per-lesion basis. Thus, in some patients and tumors, 1 specific tracer may be more favorable, which likely is the case in the few tumors where sst2 is not the most abundant SSTR.

[64]Cu-labeling has some pros and cons compared with ^{68}Ga labeling. The pros include better spatial resolution due to the lower positron range and better logistics on the PET scanner through the day due to the long half-life of 12.7 hours and the flexible scan time, which can be from 1 hour to 3 hours postinjection without significant loss of lesion detection.[47]

Table 1
Summary of 9 head-to-head studies of the somatostatin receptor imaging PET tracers

Tracer	Patients	Days Between Scans	Tumor-to-Background Ratio	Lesion Detection/ Sensitivity	Conclusion	Author
^{68}Ga-DOTATOC vs ^{68}Ga-DOTATATE	40 verified GEP/or lung NET, 1 paraganglioma	<14	Normalized SUVmax for liver metastases (SD): 2.5 (1.4) vs 2.4 (2.7)	262 lesions detected 254 lesions detected (P = .012)	Significantly higher SUV max in lesions by ^{68}Ga-DOTATOC vs ^{68}Ga-DOTATATE but comparable diagnostic value	Poeppel et al,[39] 2011
^{68}Ga-DOTANOC vs ^{68}Ga-DOTATATE	20 verified GEP and lung NET, 2 paragangliomas	0–7	TBR not reported Significant higher uptake in normal liver and in lesions for ^{68}Ga-DOTATATE	^{68}Ga-DOTANOC detected only 116 (89%) of the 130 lesions detected by ^{68}Ga-DOTATATE	Significantly higher uptake in tumor lesions by ^{68}Ga-DOTATATE vs ^{68}Ga-DOTANOC. Comparable diagnostic accuracy but more lesions by ^{68}Ga-DOTATATE	Kabasakal et al,[40] 2012
^{68}Ga-DOTANOC vs ^{68}Ga-DOTATATE	18 verified GEPNET	0–2	Liver TBR: ^{68}Ga-DOTANOC > ^{68}Ga-DOTATATE Bone TBR: ^{68}Ga-DOTANOC < ^{68}Ga-DOTATATE	232 of 248/93.5% 212 of 248/85.5% (P = .005)	^{68}Ga-DOTANOC had a higher liver and pancreas lesion detection rate. ^{68}Ga-DOTATATE found more bone lesions	Wild et al,[41] 2013
^{68}Ga-DOTALAN vs ^{68}Ga-DOTATOC	38 NET with low or no uptake on ^{68}Ga-DOTATOC	7–90	Tumor-to-liver ratio: higher for ^{68}Ga-DOTATOC (P<.02)	53 vs 106 overall lesions Compared with CT sensitivity, specificity, and accuracy was: ^{68}Ga-DOTALAN; 63%, 50%, and 62% ^{68}Ga-DOTATOC: 78%, 50%, and 76%	Overall higher SUVmax for ^{68}Ga-DOTATOC and higher lesion detection ^{68}Ga-DOTALAN should only serve as a second-choice tracer in patients without uptake of ^{68}Ga-DOTATOC	Putzer et al,[42] 2013

(continued on next page)

Table 1
(continued)

Tracer	Patients	Days Between Scans	Tumor-to-Background Ratio	Lesion Detection/ Sensitivity	Conclusion	Author
68Ga-DOTALAN vs 68Ga-DOTATATE	12 verified NET	0–2	Not reported Significantly higher uptake in both tumor lesions and organs by 68Ga-DOTATATE	23/67 (44%) 63/67 (94%)	68Ga-DOTATATE is a better radioligand than 68Ga-DOTALAN in the diagnosis of NETs. High uptake in bone marrow of 68Ga-DOTALAN.	Demirci et al,[43] 2013
68Ga-DOTATOC vs 64Cu-DOTATATE	59 GEP or lung NET	1–5	Liver TBR (SEM): 4.60 (0.52) vs 5.49 (0.45) ($P = .13$).	701 lesions detected by both scans. 64Cu-DOTATATE detected 33 additional true-positive lesions. 68Ga-DOTATOC detected 7 additional true-positive lesions.	Patient based sensitivity the same Significantly more true discordant lesions were detected by 64Cu-DOTATATE	Johnbeck et al,[44] 2017
64Cu-SARTATE vs 68Ga-DOTATATE	10 NET positive on 68Ga-DOTATATE	6–27	Progressive increase in lesion to liver ratio over time (up to 24 h) with 64Cu-SARTATE	Comparison of 64Cu-SARTATE PET/CT obtained at 4 h to 68Ga-DOTATATE PET/CT obtained at 1 h indicated comparable or superior lesion detection with 64Cu-SARTATE in all patients, especially in the liver.	High uptake and retention of 64Cu-SARTATE in tumors provides high-contrast diagnostic images until at least 24 h after injection, increasing flexibility in the usage.	Hicks et al,[45] 2019
68Ga-NODAGA-JR11 high and low peptide vs 68Ga-DOTATOC	12 GEP NET G1+G2	27.5–135	Liver TBR (CI): 5.3 (2.9–5.7) and 4.3 (3.4–6.3) vs 1.9 (1.4–2.9)	68Ga-NODAGA-JR11 high and low peptide had higher sensitivity than 68Ga-DOTATOC (94% and 88% vs 59%) ($P<.001$)	Mainly liver lesions, no report of bone metastases. No significant difference in tumor uptake (high inter-reader differences)	Nicolas et al,[33] 2018

68Ga-DOTA-JR11 vs 68Ga-DOTATATE	31 metastatic well-differentiated NET	1	Liver TBR: 7.7 ± 5.4 vs 3.4 ± 2.0 (P<.001) Low or no uptake of 68Ga-DOTA-JR11 in spleen, pituitary and adrenal glands	552 liver lesions 158 bone lesions vs 365 liver lesions (P = .001) 388 bone lesions (P = .016)	68Ga-DOTA-JR11 detects most liver lesions and has better TBR in liver but an overall lower tumor uptake. 68Ga-DOTATATE detected most bone metastases	Zhu et al,[46] 2020

Abbreviations: EM, standard error of mean; CI, confidence Interval 95 %.

The cons are higher dosimetry and less availability because it is not generator based. Yet, the long shelf-life, greater than 24 hours, enables central distribution.

More head-to-head comparative studies in NEN patients are needed to evaluate if the antagonist tracers should replace the traditional agonists in the clinical diagnostic setting.

VALUE OF SOMATOSTATIN RECEPTOR IMAGING PET VERSUS OTHER ANATOMIC IMAGING

In a study of 38 NET patients with cancer of unknown primary, ^{68}Ga-DOTATATE PET/CT compared with contrast-enhanced CT (ceCT) alone provided an improvement in sensitivity of 50% and an improvement in accuracy of 30% in primary tumor detection.[48]

Similar results were seen comparing ^{68}Ga-DOTATATE PET/ceCT to standalone ceCT in 54 NET patients and significantly more bone and lymph node metastases were found adding PET.[49]

The added value from PET often changes patient management. In a study of 22 patients, ^{68}Ga-DOTATATE PET/CT imaging could detect NET in 41% (9 of 22) symptomatic patients with negative anatomic imaging on 3-phase CT and endoscopy and changed the treatment in a majority of these patients.[50]

In a comparative imaging study of 131 patients with unknown primary and metastatic GEPNET ^{68}Ga-DOTATATE PET/CT changed the management for 33% of the patients compared with multiphasic CT and/or MR.[51]

Conventional MR imaging, especially with the use of diffusion-weighted images, is highly sensitive in detecting liver metastases and pancreas lesions whereas CT is more sensitive for lung lesions.[52] The high amount of liver and pancreatic lesions in NEN makes PET/MR scanners for SRI interesting.

Two studies found similar lesion detection rates using PET/CT and PET/MR and the same PET tracers ^{68}Ga-DOTATOC (n = 8) and ^{68}Ga-DOTA-NOC (n = 28), respectively.[53,54]

Lesion-based analysis of 30 NET patients showed a higher proportion of correctly rated NET lesions on PET/MR imaging than on PET/CT using ^{68}Ga-DOTATOC (90.8% vs 86.7%, respectively; P = .031), whereas on PET/CT there was a higher proportion of correctly rated non-NET lesions (94.5% vs 83.6%, respectively; P = .031).[55]

Pros for using PET/MR imaging is the lower radiation dose to the patient but cons are the long acquisition time. Seith and colleagues,[56] however, reported comparable performance in lesion detection in a shortened version of PET/MR compared with PET/CT. The intravenous contrast was eliminated and a nonenhanced ^{68}Ga-DOTA-SSTR PET/MR imaging comprised only 3 MR imaging sequences (T2-weigted half-Fourier single-shot turbo spin-echo, T2-weighted fast spin-echo sequence, and diffusion-weighted imaging) was performed. This set-up shortens the scan time to 35 minutes, which still is longer than the average SRI PET/CT scan time, in particular with the spread of digital PET/CT scanners enabling whole-body SRI PET/CT in less than 10 minutes.[57]

PROGNOSTIC VALUE OF SOMATOSTATIN RECEPTOR IMAGING

In addition to diagnosis and staging, prognostic information might be obtained by SRI PET.

Total tumor volume of ^{68}Ga-DOTATATE avidity was found a prognostic factor for progression-free survival (PFS) in a prospective study of 184 patients with various locations, stages, and grades of NET after median 18 months' follow-up. An inverse correlation was found between quartiles of tumor volume and PFS and overall survival (OS).[58]

Uptake values of PET SRI as a measure of SSTR density might contain information on prognosis due to the quantitative nature of PET.

In a group of 47 NET patients scanned with ^{68}Ga-DOTANOC, the SUVmax greater than 19.3 was a significant positive prognostic factor,[59] whereas in another group of 43 pancreatic NET patients, ^{68}Ga-DOTANOC SUVmax below 37.8 was the cutoff for significant risk (hazard ratio 3.09; $P<.003$) and median PFSs were, respectively, 16 months versus 27 months (P = .002) for patients with SUVmax lower and greater than 38.[60]

In well-differentiated NET patients treated with somatostatin analog (octreotide acetate), patients with ^{68}Ga-DOTATATE SUVmax greater than 29.4 had significantly higher PFS than those with lower SUVmax; and for 128 NEN patients, SUVmax greater than 43.3 for ^{64}Cu-DOTATATE was associated with half the likelihood of progression compared with patients with lower SUVmax.[61,62]

In conclusion, different prognostic cutoff values for SRI PET SUVmax have been found in NEN patients groupwise; however, low sensitivity and specificity are found on an individual basis. Also, SRI PET SUVs for predicting outcome of PRRT have not been convincing so far.[63]

OTHER IMAGING TRACERS FOR NEUROENDOCRINE NEOPLASMS
[18]F-fluorodeoxyglucose PET

The latest guidelines from ENETS recommend ^{18}F-fluorodeoxyglucose PET/CT for NEN patients with no uptake on SRI-PET, because ^{18}F-FDG PET/CT has a higher sensitivity than SRI for G3 NEN.[64] In 252 bronchopulmonary NENs (typical and atypical carcinoids and large cell NECs), 95% were ^{18}F-FDG positive, confirming that ^{18}F-FDG PET/CT should be part of the diagnostic work-up for these patients.[65]

A prognostic grading scheme (NETPET) was proposed for PET/CT with dual SSTR/^{18}F-FDG, from analyzing retrospective data from 62 metastatic NET patients, from the most benign group with positive SRI and negative ^{18}F-FDG PET, to groups with varying positivity of both SRI and ^{18}F-FDG PET, and to the most aggressive group with negative SRI and very positive ^{18}F-FDG PET. The NETPET grading was correlated significantly with survival ($P = .0018$), whereas the World Health Organization grading system at the time of diagnosis did not correlate with survival.[66]

^{18}F-FDG PET/CT alone provides prognostic information of PFS and OS for NEN patients.[67]

[18]F-dihydroxyphenylalanine PET

Several studies have found SRI PET/CT with ^{68}Ga-DOTATATE and ^{68}Ga-DOTANOC more accurate in detecting NET than ^{18}F-dihydroxyphenylalanine (^{18}F-DOPA) PET/CT.

PET/CT using both ^{68}Ga-DOTANOC and ^{18}F-DOPA was performed in 13 patients with biopsy-proved GEP and pulmonary NET (10 NEN and 3 NEC).[68] ^{68}Ga-DOTANOC was positive in 13/13 and ^{18}F-DOPA was positive in 9/13 patients—on a lesion basis: 71 versus 45, respectively. Likewise, ^{68}Ga-DOTATATE PET proved clearly superior to ^{18}F-DOPA PET for detection and staging of NET in 25 patients with histologically proven metastatic NET.[69] A majority of the patients with elevated serotonin were ^{18}F-DOPA PET positive, so the examination may be used especially in serotonin-positive patients with a negative SRI PET/CT.

[123]I-metaiodobenzylguanidin Single-photon Emission Computed Tomography

If no uptake on SRI-PET is seen, ^{123}I-metaiodo-benzylguanidin (^{123}I-MIBG) compels another theranostic team with ^{131}I-MIBG and may be useful in neuroblastomas, paragangliomas, and pheochromocytomas.[70]

In conclusion, additional tracers to SRI are ^{18}F-FDG for staging, follow-up, and prognosis of NECs and high-grade NETs and furthermore also containing prognostic information for low-grade NET. ^{18}F-DOPA and ^{123}I-MIBG must be part of the toolbox for NENs if SRI-PET is negative.

DISCUSSION

The perfect tracer for SRI is specific for and accumulates quickly and solely in NEN, preferably in a quantitative manner, correlating to grade or differentiation of the disease. Further preferences are no (or low) uptake in normal tissue, rapid clearing from the blood, no side effects, reliable few-step synthesis, wide availability, low bone marrow and renal accumulation, low overall radiation burden, low costs, and preferably part of a theranostic pair with a corresponding drug for PRRT (**Box 1**).

The change from single-photon emission computed tomography (SPECT) to PET tracers has added to the specificity by obtaining higher affinity to SSTRs with the ^{68}Ga-DOTA or ^{64}Cu-DOTA combination compared with SPECT imaging isotopes. In addition, the tracer uptake can be measured quantitatively and is shown to correlate to tumor grade and differentiation. Head to head studies have shown tracers with high affinity towards sst2 to be the most sensitive in NEN lesion detection overall. In special cases radionuclide with different affinities may be useful. For instance, in pulmonary carcinoids Vesterinen and colleagues[6] found that

---

Box 1
Ideal characteristics of a radionuclide for neuroendocrine neoplasms

- Specific for NENs
- Accumulation in NENs
- Quantitative uptake (PET isotope)
- No/low uptake in normal tissue and organs
- Fast clearing from blood
- No side effects
- Availability
- Easy, reliable synthesis
- Flexible scan time
- Low cost
- Low dose
- Low marrow and renal accumulation
- Part of a theranostic pair

approximetaly 25 % did not express sst2, whereas 85% of these expressed another sub-type of SSTRs, mainly sst3 and sst4. Low back-ground accumulation is achieved the best by the antagonists of the SRI PET tracers available and results in higher TBR primarily for liver lesions. Unfortunately, tumor accumulation tends not to be reliable for all types of NEN lesions, for example, bone lesions are not detected as well by the antagonists. At present, generator-pro-duced ^{68}Ga SRI PET is the most available tracer but, due to the long shelf life of ^{64}Cu-DOTA-TATE, widespread distribution is possible. Radi-ation burden is most favorable using ^{68}Ga, but it comes with the cost of less clinical flexibility. The optimal scan window is small compared to ^{64}Cu tracers. The digital PET scanners enable a high throughput of PET patients due to the low scan-time or maybe lower dosage to the pa-tients may be traded instead. A recent head to head study reported a low inter-reader repro-ducibility for the description of SRI PET.[33] A seldom reported parameter, which challenges the sensitivity of the procedure and emphasizes the value of a well-known tracer.

SUMMARY

The main workhorse in NEN imaging is a stable, available and reliable tracer with high affinity to sst2 and maybe additional sst5 or sst3 affinity as DOTATATE, DOTATOC or DOTANOC labeled to either ^{68}Ga or ^{64}Cu. There are several PET-based SSTR tracers with comparable perfor-mances and all three FDA approved SRI PET tracers ^{68}Ga-DOTATATE, ^{68}Ga-DOTATOC and ^{64}Cu-DOTATATE are well suited as the main clin-ical NEN-imaging tool. In addition to these tracers, centers scanning a high number of NEN patients, especially centers of excellence, could benefit of having additional work-zebras for those special cases that are negative on the usual SRI. Tracers based on STTR antagonists seem to have a favorable liver-to-tumor ratio and some may show a very low physiologic up-take in the uncinate process, pituitary and adre-nal glands, and the spleen, which usually have a high SRI uptake. In patients known to have liver metastases only or suspicious of splenic lesions, an antagonist tracer could be of value. With ongoing SSTR affinity refinement, higher tumor to background ratios and better technology evolving, soon the biggest drawback is in the hands of the interpreter. Maybe the next impor-tant step will come from artificial intelligence helping to delineate tumor lesions in a reprodu-ible matter.

CLINICS CARE POINTS

- Somatostatin receptor imaging PET in NEN in addition to contrast enhanced CT or MR alone alters patient management.
- The FDA approved tracers 68Ga-DOTATATE, 68Ga-DOTATOC and 64Cu-DOTATATE have comparable high diagnostic performances.
- High SUV max in SRI DOTA PET is a positive prognostic factor in NEN, however FDG PET is more prognostic.
- SRI PET/MR imaging and SRI PET/CT have com-parable performance in lesion detection.
- Pros for PET/MR is markedly reduced radia-tion dose to the patient. Cons are a three-fold increase in scan-time and less availability.

DISCLOSURE OF COMMERCIAL OR FINANCIAL CONFLICTS OF INTEREST AND ANY FUNDING SOURCES

The authors have nothing to disclose.

REFERENCES

1. Rindi G, Inzani F. Neuroendocrine neoplasm update: toward universal nomenclature. Endocr Relat Can-cer 2020;27(6):R211–8.
2. Rindi G, Klimstra DS, Abedi-Ardekani B, et al. A common classification framework for neuroendo-crine neoplasms: an International Agency for Research on Cancer (IARC) and World Health Orga-nization (WHO) expert consensus proposal. Mod Pathol 2018;31(12):1770–86.
3. Krenning EP, Kwekkeboom DJ, Oei HY, et al. So-matostatin-receptor scintigraphy in gastroentero-pancreatic tumors. An overview of European results. Ann N Y Acad Sci 1994;733:416–24.
4. Kanakis G, Grimelius L, Spathis A, et al. Expression of somatostatin receptors 1-5 and dopamine recep-tor 2 in lung carcinoids: implications for a therapeu-tic role. Neuroendocrinology 2015;101(3):211–22.
5. Remes SM, Leijon HL, Vesterinen TJ, et al. Immuno-histochemical expression of somatostatin receptor subtypes in a panel of neuroendocrine neoplasias. J Histochem Cytochem 2019;67(10):735–43.
6. Vesterinen T, Leijon H, Mustonen H, et al. Somato-statin receptor expression is associated with metas-tasis and patient outcome in pulmonary carcinoid tumors. J Clin Endocrinol Metab 2019;104(6):2083–93.

7. Righi L, Volante M, Tavaglione V, et al. Somatostatin receptor tissue distribution in lung neuroendocrine tumours: a clinicopathologic and immunohistochemical study of 218 'clinically aggressive' cases. Ann Oncol 2010;21(3):548–55.

8. Srirajaskanthan R, Watkins J, Marelli L, et al. Expression of somatostatin and dopamine 2 receptors in neuroendocrine tumours and the potential role for new biotherapies. Neuroendocrinology 2009;89(3):308–14.

9. Wang Y, Wang W, Jin K, et al. Somatostatin receptor expression indicates improved prognosis in gastroenteropancreatic neuroendocrine neoplasm, and octreotide long-acting release is effective and safe in Chinese patients with advanced gastroenteropancreatic neuroendocrine tumors. Oncol Lett 2017;13(3):1165–74.

10. Nielsen K, Binderup T, Langer SW, et al. P53, Somatostatin receptor 2a and Chromogranin A immunostaining as prognostic markers in high grade gastroenteropancreatic neuroendocrine neoplasms. BMC Cancer 2020;20(1):27.

11. Krenning EP, Bakker WH, Breeman WA, et al. Localisation of endocrine-related tumours with radioiodinated analogue of somatostatin. Lancet 1989;1(8632):242–4.

12. Gabriel M, Decristoforo C, Donnemiller E, et al. An intrapatient comparison of 99mTc-EDDA/HYNIC-TOC with 111In-DTPA-octreotide for diagnosis of somatostatin receptor-expressing tumors. J Nucl Med 2003;44(5):708–16. Available at: https://www.ncbi.nlm.nih.gov/pubmed/12732671.

13. Al-Nahhas A, Win Z, Szyszko T, et al. Gallium-68 PET: a new frontier in receptor cancer imaging. Anticancer Res 2007;27(6B):4087–94. Available at: https://www.ncbi.nlm.nih.gov/pubmed/18225576.

14. Antunes P, Ginj M, Zhang H, et al. Are radiogallium-labelled DOTA-conjugated somatostatin analogues superior to those labelled with other radiometals? Eur J Nucl Med Mol Imaging 2007;34(7):982–93.

15. Reubi JC, Schar JC, Waser B, et al. Affinity profiles for human somatostatin receptor subtypes SST1-SST5 of somatostatin radiotracers selected for scintigraphic and radiotherapeutic use. Eur J Nucl Med 2000;27(3):273–82.

16. Buchmann I, Henze M, Engelbrecht S, et al. Comparison of 68Ga-DOTATOC PET and 111In-DTPAOC (Octreoscan) SPECT in patients with neuroendocrine tumours. Eur J Nucl Med Mol Imaging 2007;34(10):1617–26.

17. Gabriel M, Decristoforo C, Kendler D, et al. 68Ga-DOTA-Tyr3-octreotide PET in neuroendocrine tumors: comparison with somatostatin receptor scintigraphy and CT. J Nucl Med 2007;48(4):508–18.

18. Krausz Y, Freedman N, Rubinstein R, et al. 68Ga-DOTA-NOC PET/CT imaging of neuroendocrine tumors: comparison with (1)(1)(1)In-DTPA-octreotide (OctreoScan(R)). Mol Imaging Biol 2011;13(3):583–93.

19. Srirajaskanthan R, Kayani I, Quigley AM, et al. The Role of Ga-68-DOTATATE PET in patients with neuroendocrine tumors and negative or equivocal findings on In-111-DTPA-octreotide scintigraphy. J Nucl Med 2010;51(6):875–82.

20. Barrio M, Czernin J, Fanti S, et al. The impact of somatostatin receptor-directed PET/CT on the management of patients with neuroendocrine tumor: a systematic review and meta-analysis. J Nucl Med 2017;58(5):756–61.

21. Pfeifer A, Knigge U, Mortensen J, et al. Clinical PET of neuroendocrine tumors using 64Cu-DOTATATE: first-in-humans study. J Nucl Med 2012;53(8):1207–15.

22. Sunderland JJ. The Academic NDA: justification, process, and lessons learned. J Nucl Med 2020;61(4):480–7.

23. Mirzaei S, Revheim ME, Raynor W, et al. (64)Cu-DOTATOC PET-CT in patients with neuroendocrine tumors. Oncol Ther 2020;8(1):125–31.

24. Bass RT, Buckwalter BL, Patel BP, et al. Identification and characterization of novel somatostatin antagonists. Mol Pharmacol 1996;50(4):709–15. Available at: https://www.ncbi.nlm.nih.gov/pubmed/8863814.

25. Cescato R, Erchegyi J, Waser B, et al. Design and in vitro characterization of highly sst2-selective somatostatin antagonists suitable for radiotargeting. J Med Chem 2008;51(13):4030–7.

26. Fani M, Nicolas GP, Wild D. Somatostatin receptor antagonists for imaging and therapy. J Nucl Med 2017;58(Suppl 2):61S–6S.

27. Reubi JC, Schaer JC, Wenger S, et al. SST3-selective potent peptidic somatostatin receptor antagonists. Proc Natl Acad Sci U S A 2000;97(25):13973–8.

28. Ginj M, Zhang H, Waser B, et al. Radiolabeled somatostatin receptor antagonists are preferable to agonists for in vivo peptide receptor targeting of tumors. Proc Natl Acad Sci U S A 2006;103(44):16436–41.

29. Wild D, Fani M, Behe M, et al. First clinical evidence that imaging with somatostatin receptor antagonists is feasible. J Nucl Med 2011;52(9):1412–7.

30. Fani M, Braun F, Waser B, et al. Unexpected sensitivity of sst2 antagonists to N-terminal radiometal modifications. J Nucl Med 2012;53(9):1481–9.

31. Fani M, Del Pozzo L, Abiraj K, et al. PET of somatostatin receptor-positive tumors using 64Cu- and 68Ga-somatostatin antagonists: the chelate makes the difference. J Nucl Med 2011;52(7):1110–8.

32. Nicolas GP, Beykan S, Bouterfa H, et al. Safety, biodistribution, and radiation dosimetry of (68)Ga-OPS202 in patients with gastroenteropancreatic neuroendocrine tumors: a prospective phase imaging study. J Nucl Med 2018;59(6):909–14.

33. Nicolas GP, Schreiter N, Kaul F, et al. Sensitivity Comparison of (68)Ga-OPS202 and (68)Ga-DOTA-TOC PET/CT in patients with gastroenteropancreatic neuroendocrine tumors: a prospective phase II imaging study. J Nucl Med 2018;59(6):915–21.

34. Krebs S, Pandit-Taskar N, Reidy D, et al. Biodistribution and radiation dose estimates for (68)Ga-DOTA-JR11 in patients with metastatic neuroendocrine tumors. Eur J Nucl Med Mol Imaging 2019;46(3):677–85.

35. Treglia G, Castaldi P, Rindi G, et al. Diagnostic performance of Gallium-68 somatostatin receptor PET and PET/CT in patients with thoracic and gastroenteropancreatic neuroendocrine tumours: a meta-analysis. Endocrine 2012;42(1):80–7.

36. Geijer H, Breimer LH. Somatostatin receptor PET/CT in neuroendocrine tumours: update on systematic review and meta-analysis. Eur J Nucl Med Mol Imaging 2013;40(11):1770–80.

37. Yang J, Kan Y, Ge BH, et al. Diagnostic role of Gallium-68 DOTATOC and Gallium-68 DOTATATE PET in patients with neuroendocrine tumors: a meta-analysis. Acta Radiologica 2014;55(4):389–98.

38. Johnbeck CB, Knigge U, Kjaer A. PET tracers for somatostatin receptor imaging of neuroendocrine tumors: current status and review of the literature. Future Oncol 2014;10(14):2259–77.

39. Poeppel TD, Binse I, Petersenn S, et al. 68Ga-DOTATOC versus 68Ga-DOTATATE PET/CT in functional imaging of neuroendocrine tumors. J Nucl Med 2011;52(12):1864–70.

40. Kabasakal L, Demirci E, Ocak M, et al. Comparison of (6)(8)Ga-DOTATATE and (6)(8)Ga-DOTANOC PET/CT imaging in the same patient group with neuroendocrine tumours. Eur J Nucl Med Mol Imaging 2012;39(8):1271–7.

41. Wild D, Bomanji JB, Benkert P, et al. Comparison of 68Ga-DOTANOC and 68Ga-DOTATATE PET/CT within patients with gastroenteropancreatic neuroendocrine tumors. J Nucl Med 2013;54(3):364–72.

42. Putzer D, Kroiss A, Waitz D, et al. Somatostatin receptor PET in neuroendocrine tumours: 68Ga-DOTA0,Tyr3-octreotide versus 68Ga-DOTA0-lanreotide. Eur J Nucl Med Mol Imaging 2013;40(3):364–72.

43. Demirci E, Ocak M, Kabasakal L, et al. Comparison of Ga-68 DOTA-TATE and Ga-68 DOTA-LAN PET/CT imaging in the same patient group with neuroendocrine tumours: preliminary results. Nucl Med Commun 2013;34(8):727–32.

44. Johnbeck CB, Knigge U, Loft A, et al. Head-to-Head Comparison of (64)Cu-DOTATATE and (68)Ga-DOTATOC PET/CT: a prospective study of 59 patients with neuroendocrine tumors. J Nucl Med 2017;58(3):451–7.

45. Hicks RJ, Jackson P, Kong G, et al. (64)Cu-SARTATE PET imaging of patients with neuroendocrine tumors demonstrates high tumor uptake and retention, potentially allowing prospective dosimetry for peptide receptor radionuclide therapy. J Nucl Med 2019;60(6):777–85.

46. Zhu W, Cheng Y, Wang X, et al. Head-to-Head comparison of (68)Ga-DOTA-JR11 and (68)Ga-DOTA-TATE PET/CT in patients with metastatic, well-differentiated neuroendocrine tumors: a prospective study. J Nucl Med 2020;61(6):897–903.

47. Loft M, Carlsen EA, Johnbeck CB, et al. (64)Cu-DO-TATATE PET in patients with neuroendocrine neoplasms:prospective, head-to-head comparison of imaging at 1 hour and 3 hours post-injection. J Nucl Med 2020;62(1):73–80.

48. Kazimierszak PM, Rominger A, Wenter V et al. The added value of 68 Ga-DOTA-TATE-PET to contrast-enhanced CT for primary site detection in CUP of neuroendocrine origin. Eur Radiol. 2017;27(4):1676-84.

49. Albanus DR, Apitzsch J, Erdem Z, et al. Clinical value of (6)(8)Ga-DOTATATE-PET/CT compared to stand-alone contrast enhanced CT for the detection of extra-hepatic metastases in patients with neuroendocrine tumours (NET). Eur J Radiol 2015;84(10):1866–72.

50. Shell J, Keutgen XM, Millo C, et al. 68-Gallium DOTATATE scanning in symptomatic patients with negative anatomic imaging but suspected neuroendocrine tumor. Int J Endocr Oncol 2018;5(1):IJE04.

51. Sadowski SM, Neychev V, Millo C, et al. Prospective Study of 68Ga-DOTATATE positron emission tomography/computed tomography for detecting gastro-entero-pancreatic neuroendocrine tumors and unknown primary sites. J Clin Oncol 2016;34(6):588–96.

52. Bodei L, Sundin A, Kidd M, et al. The status of neuroendocrine tumor imaging: from darkness to light? Neuroendocrinology 2015;101(1):1–17.

53. Beiderwellen KJ, Poeppel TD, Hartung-Knemeyer V, et al. Simultaneous 68Ga-DOTATOC PET/MRI in patients with gastroenteropancreatic neuroendocrine tumors: initial results. Invest Radiol 2013;48(5):273–9.

54. Berzaczy D, Giraudo C, Haug AR, et al. Whole-body 68Ga-DOTANOC PET/MRI versus 68Ga-DOTANOC PET/CT in patients with neuroendocrine tumors: a prospective study in 28 patients. Clin Nucl Med 2017;42(9):669–74.

55. Sawicki LM, Deuschl C, Beiderwellen K, et al. Evaluation of (68)Ga-DOTATOC PET/MRI for whole-body staging of neuroendocrine tumours in comparison with (68)Ga-DOTATOC PET/CT. Eur Radiol 2017;27(10):4091–9.

56. Seith F, Schraml C, Reischl G, et al. Fast non-enhanced abdominal examination protocols in PET/MRI for patients with neuroendocrine tumors

(NET): comparison to multiphase contrast-enhanced PET/CT. Radiol Med 2018;123(11):860–70.

57. Loft M, Johnbeck CB, Carlsen E et al. Initial Experiences of 64Cu-DOTATATE Digital PET of Patients with Neuroendocrine Neoplasms: Comparison with Analog PET. Under submission.

58. Tirosh A, Papadakis GZ, Millo C, et al. Prognostic utility of total (68)Ga-DOTATATE-Avid tumor volume in patients with neuroendocrine tumors. Gastroenterology 2018;154(4):998–1008.e1.

59. Campana D, Ambrosini V, Pezzilli R, et al. Standardized uptake values of (68)Ga-DOTANOC PET: a promising prognostic tool in neuroendocrine tumors. J Nucl Med 2010;51(3):353–9.

60. Ambrosini V, Campana D, Polverari G, et al. Prognostic Value of 68Ga-DOTANOC PET/CT SUVmax in patients with neuroendocrine tumors of the pancreas. J Nucl Med 2015;56(12):1843–8.

61. Bhanat E, Koch CA, Parmar R, et al. Somatostatin receptor expression in non-classical locations - clinical relevance? Rev Endocr Metab Disord 2018; 19(2):123–32.

62. Carlsen EA, Johnbeck CB, Binderup T, et al. (64)Cu-DOTATATE PET/CT and prediction of overall and progression-free survival in patients with neuroendocrine neoplasms. J Nucl Med 2020;61(10):1491–7.

63. Gabriel M, Oberauer A, Dobrozemsky G, et al. 68Ga-DOTA-Tyr3-octreotide PET for assessing response to somatostatin-receptor-mediated radionuclide therapy. J Nucl Med 2009;50(9):1427–34.

64. Knigge U, Capdevila J, Bartsch DK, et al. ENETS consensus recommendations for the standards of care in neuroendocrine neoplasms: follow-up and documentation. Antibes consensus conference. Neuroendocrinology 2017;105(3):310–9.

65. Grondahl V, Binderup T, Langer SW, et al. Characteristics of 252 patients with bronchopulmonary neuroendocrine tumours treated at the Copenhagen NET Centre of Excellence. Lung Cancer 2019;132:141–9.

66. Chan DL, Pavlakis N, Schembri GP, et al. Dual somatostatin receptor/FDG PET/CT imaging in metastatic neuroendocrine tumours: proposal for a novel grading scheme with prognostic significance. Theranostics 2017;7(5):1149–58.

67. Binderup T, Knigge U, Johnbeck CB, et al. 18 F-FDG-PET is superior to WHO grading as prognostic tool in neuroendocrine neoplasms and useful in guiding peptide receptor radionuclide therapy: a prospective 10-year follow-up study of 166 patients. J Nucl Med 2020. https://doi.org/10.2967/jnumed. 120.244798.

68. Ambrosini V, Tomassetti P, Castellucci P, et al. Comparison between 68Ga-DOTA-NOC and 18F-DOPA PET for the detection of gastro-entero-pancreatic and lung neuro-endocrine tumours. Eur J Nucl Med Mol Imaging 2008;35(8):1431–8.

69. Haug A, Auernhammer CJ, Wangler B, et al. Intraindividual comparison of 68Ga-DOTA-TATE and 18F-DOPA PET in patients with well-differentiated metastatic neuroendocrine tumours. Eur J Nucl Med Mol Imaging 2009;36(5):765–70.

70. Kroiss AS. Current status of functional imaging in neuroblastoma, pheochromocytoma, and paraganglioma disease. Wien Med Wochenschr 2019; 169(1–2):25–32.

Imaging of Insulinoma by Targeting Glucagonlike Peptide-1 Receptor

Yaping Luo, MD[a,b], Xiaoyuan Chen, PhD[c],*

KEYWORDS

- Insulinoma • Glucagonlike peptide-1 receptor • Exendin-4

KEY POINTS

- Somatostatin receptors are insufficiently expressed in many insulinomas, instead, glucagonlike peptide-1 (GLP-1) receptor is highly overexpressed on benign insulinoma cell surface with very high incidence and extremely high density.
- GLP-1 receptor imaging, using radiolabeled exendin-4, is a sensitive and specific method for preoperative localization of insulinoma.
- It is worth further investigating GLP-1 receptor imaging in localizing nesidioblatosis in adult patients with hyperinsulinemic hypoglycemia, assessment of viability of transplanted functional islets, β cell mass quantification in diabetes mellitus, and intraoperative imaging-guided surgery of insulinoma.

INTRODUCTION OF INSULINOMA

Insulinoma is a rare neuroendocrine tumor arising from pancreatic β cells with an incidence of 0.4 per 100,000 people per year.[1] It is the most common cause of endogenous hyperinsulinemic hypoglycemia in adult patients without diabetes. Insulinoma was first reported in 1927 in a patient with malignant pancreatic islet-cell tumor who had episodes of severe hypoglycemia[2]; meanwhile, the first cure of hypoglycemia caused by insulinoma by surgical removal of the tumor was reported in 1929.[3] Although insulinoma has been recognized for nearly a century, it still presents a diagnostic dilemma for the clinicians. The most common clinical manifestation of an insulinoma is fasting hypoglycemia, with discrete episodes of neuroglycopenia, whereas some patients may predominantly present with postprandial hypoglycemia.

The diagnosis of insulinoma was initially based on demonstrating inappropriately high serum insulin concentration during a spontaneous or induced episode of hypoglycemia, for example, 72-hour fast for a patient with fasting hypoglycemia, or the mixed-meal test in the case of postprandial hypoglycemia. Then imaging techniques are used to localize the tumor, which is critical for diagnosis and surgical planning. Conventional imaging procedures include contrast-enhanced computed tomography (CT), MRI, and endoscopic ultrasonography. In contrast-enhanced CT and MRI, insulinomas are typically small and sharply delineated, and are best visualized as contrast-enhancing tumors in the portal venous inflow phase and in the pancreatic contrast-enhancement phase. The accuracy of contrast-enhanced CT and MRI in localizing insulinoma is 60% to 70%, and the detection of tumor is

Conflict of Interest and Source of Funding: This work is supported by the National University of Singapore start-up fund (R-180-000-017-133, R-180-000-017,731, and R-180-000-017-733).

[a] Department of Nuclear Medicine, Chinese Academy of Medical Sciences and Peking Union Medical College Hospital, #1 Shuaifuyuan Wangfujing, Dongcheng District, Beijing 100730, P. R. China; [b] Beijing Key Laboratory of Molecular Targeted Diagnosis and Therapy in Nuclear Medicine; [c] Yong Loo Lin School of Medicine and Faculty of Engineering, National University of Singapore, Singapore 117597, Singapore

* Corresponding author.

E-mail address: chen.shawn@nus.edu.sg

pet.theclinics.com

hampered in those with mild enhancement or in transiently enhanced tumors.[4,5] The sensitivity of endoscopic ultrasonography in detecting insulinoma was reported to be 80% to 90%; however, it was limited to tumors localized in the head and body of the pancreas. Moreover, this technique is observer-dependent and requires specialized expertise.[5–7] Selective arterial calcium stimulation test with hepatic venous sampling, based on the observation that calcium stimulates the release of insulin from hyperfunctional β cells but not from normal β cells, enables the surgeon to limit the intraoperative search of the insulinoma to the corresponding arterial territory. It had a sensitivity of more than 90% in patients with insulinomas that were not localized using conventional imaging procedures.[8] However, this method does not determine the insulinoma itself but only the arterial territory. Moreover, it is an invasive procedure with the associated risk of complications.

Nuclear medicine imaging based on peptide receptor targeting has been successfully introduced for decades. For instance, somatostatin receptor imaging is considered the most sensitive method for detecting neuroendocrine tumors due to the marked overexpression of somatostatin receptors. However, somatostatin receptors are insufficiently expressed in many insulinomas (less than 60%),[9] thus the sensitivity of somatostatin receptor scintigraphy for detecting insulinoma is only 20% to 60%.[10–13] In recent years, a new receptor-targeted imaging technique, glucagonlike peptide-1 (GLP-1) receptor imaging, for detecting Insulinoma has been established. GLP-1 receptor is highly overexpressed on benign insulinoma cell surface with very high incidence and extremely high density. No other peptide receptor has been found to exhibit such high expression levels in insulinoma.[14,15] This review mainly summarizes the development, clinical research, and perspective of GLP-1 receptor imaging in insulinoma.

GLUCAGONLIKE PEPTIDE-1 RECEPTOR

Physiologically, the GLP-1 receptor is expressed in pancreas, duodenum, neurohypophysis, intestines, breast, thyroid gland, kidney, and lung in humans. Most tissues express GLP-1 receptor at a low level, whereas the most striking receptor expression is found in the neurohypophysis. In the pancreas, both islets and acini express GLP-1 receptors, with much higher receptor level in the islets.[16] Besides the β cells in pancreatic islets, some studies showed that the GLP-1 receptor was also found in α and δ cells.[17,18] However, a more recent study identified that GLP-1 receptor was restricted to the pancreatic β cells, as GLP-1

receptor messenger RNA was detectable only in the β cells.[19]

In tumors, the highest density of GLP-1 receptor expression was found in insulinoma, and virtually all benign insulinomas highly overexpress GLP-1 receptors with an approximately fivefold higher density over normal β cells.[14–16] GLP-1 receptors are also expressed in various endocrine tumors, such as pheochromocytomas and gastrinomas, as well as in brain tumors and embryonic tumors at a low density and/or with low incidence, whereas GLP-1 receptors are virtually absent in carcinomas and lymphomas.[16] Therefore, the GLP-1 receptor has a high potential for targeting insulinoma, and it is reasonable to achieve successful imaging of insulinoma with radiolabeled GLP-1 receptor selective analogues. Moreover, due to the extraordinarily high GLP-1 receptor density in insulinoma, the use of GLP-1 receptor targeting also permits successful radionuclide therapy.[14]

EXENDIN-4: ANALOGUE OF GLUCAGONLIKE PEPTIDE-1

The GLP-1 receptor, mainly expressed in the alimentary tract, mediates the actions of GLP-1 released from the enteroendocrine L cells in the small intestines in response to food intake. GLP-1 is one of the most important glucose-dependent insulin secretagogues. It stimulates glucose-dependent insulin synthesis and secretion, promotes β-cell proliferation, and inhibits apoptosis. It also controls glycemia via inhibition of gastric emptying, food intake, and glucagon secretion from pancreatic α cells.[20,21] Native GLP-1 is rapidly degraded by the endogenous enzyme dipeptidyl peptidase IV with a biological half-life of only 1 to 2 minutes.[22] Therefore, it is necessary to develop stable peptide analogues in clinical applications including imaging.

Exendin-4 is a biologically active peptide isolated from venom of the Gila monster lizards. It is a 39-amino acid peptide that shares 53% sequence homology with GLP-1.[23,24] Exendin-4 is a GLP-1 receptor agonist with similar binding affinity to GLP-1 receptor.[16,25] It has a specific internalization in β-cell tumor cells after binding with GLP-1 receptor, and shows a high metabolic stability in β-cell tumor cells.[26–28] It is also resistant to dipeptidyl peptidase IV cleavage, and more than 70% of the intact peptide remains in human blood serum after 24 hours.[28–30] In addition to exendin-4, other exendin peptides also were discovered, such as exendin-3 and exendin(9–39).[31,32] As exendin-3 and exendin(9–39) showed lower binding affinity for GLP-1 receptor, less in vivo stability, internalization, or cellular retention as compared with exendin-4[26]; moreover, exendin(9–39) can target GLP-1 receptor in mice but not in human pancreatic β cells or insulinomas,[33] exendin-4 is therefore an optimal candidate for the development of radiolabeled GLP-1 receptor ligands.

GLUCAGONLIKE PEPTIDE-1 RECEPTOR IMAGING IN INSULINOMAS

The first tested radiolabeled peptides targeting GLP-1 receptor were ^{125}I-GLP-1(7–36)amide and ^{125}I-exendin-3.[27] However, the low stability of GLP-1 and the low efficiency of radio-iodination of exendin-4 limit the clinical use. Then ^{111}In-labeled exendin-4 peptides were developed.[28,34] (Lys[40][Ahx-DTPA]-NH$_2$)-exendin-4 labeled with [111]In (^{111}In-DTPA-exendin-4) was the first compound based on a GLP-1 analogue checked under clinical conditions. In 2008, Wild and colleagues[35] reported the first clinical application of GLP-1 receptor imaging using ^{111}In-DTPA-exendin-4 in 2 patients to localize occult insulinomas that were not shown with conventional imaging methods (**Fig. 1**). The GLP-1 receptor imaging enabled the surgeon to localize and resect the tumor. This report was a proof-of-concept that GLP-1 receptor imaging may offer a new diagnostic approach that permits the successful localization of small insulinomas. Subsequently, Christ and colleagues[36] reported a prospective open-label investigation of (Lys[40][Ahx-DOTA-^{111}In]NH$_2$)-exendin-4 (^{111}In-DOTA-exendin-4) for localization of insulinomas in 6 patients with proven biochemical endogenous hyperinsulinemic hypoglycemia. In all 6 patients, GLP-1 receptor scintigraphy successfully detected the insulinomas (including 1 patient with ectopic insulinoma); however, CT and MRI detected the tumor in only 1 case, and endoscopic ultrasonography identified the tumor in 4 cases. Furthermore, within a time frame of 2 to 14 days after injection of ^{111}In-DOTA-exendin-4, intraoperative use of a γ-probe for GLP-1 receptor detection permitted successful surgical removal of the tumors in all these patients. In 2013, Christ and colleagues[37] reported the result of a prospective multicenter phase II clinical trial in GLP-1 receptor imaging with ^{111}In-DTPA-exendin-4 for the localization of insulinomas. The trial included 30 patients with biochemically proven endogenous hyperinsulinemic hypoglycemia and no evidence of metastasis on conventional imaging. The sensitivity of ^{111}In-DTPA-exendin-4 single-photon emission CT (SPECT)/CT in localizing benign insulinoma (95% confidence interval [CI] 74–100) was higher than CT/MRI (47% [95% CI 27–68];

$P = .011$), and ^{111}In-DTPA-exendin-4 SPECT/CT yielded a positive predictive value of 83% (95% CI 62–94). In that study, 23% of the patients showed evidence of insulinoma only on ^{111}In-DTPA-exendin-4 SPECT/CT, which changed the clinical management by reinforcing the recommendation for surgery. GLP-1 receptor imaging is also crucial for planning the resection of insulinoma. A report of 3 cases of insulinoma showed preoperative GLP-1 receptor imaging with ^{111}In-DOTA-exendin-4 allowed a more precise resection of the tumor, thereby reducing surgical trauma, loss of healthy pancreatic tissue, and increasing safety and quality of the surgical intervention.[38]

Owing to the advantageous physical properties of ^{99m}Tc in comparison with ^{111}In, GLP-1 receptor scintigraphy with ^{99m}Tc-labeled exendin-4 has also been investigated. Sowa-Staszczak and colleagues[39] reported the result of (Lys[40][Ahx-HYNIC-^{99m}Tc/EDDA]NH2)-exendin-4 (^{99m}Tc-HYNIC-exendin-4) in the diagnosis of insulinoma in 11 patients with negative results for all available conventional imaging. In that study, both sensitivity and specificity of GLP-1 receptor imaging were 100% in patients with benign insulinoma. They further reported the result of ^{99m}Tc-HYNIC-exendin-4 in detecting occult insulinoma in a larger cohort of 40 patients with hyperinsulinemic hypoglycemia and negative/inconclusive result of conventional imaging.[40] Positive results of GLP-1 receptor imaging were observed in 28 patients, and 18 patients had confirmed diagnosis of insulinoma with postsurgical histopathological examination (**Fig. 2**). Similarly, Senica and colleagues[41] reported that ^{99m}Tc-HYNIC-exendin-4 successfully detected the insulinomas in 8 patients with negative or inconclusive conventional imaging by CT, MRI, endoscopic ultrasonography, and somatostatin receptor scintigraphy. Although the results presented in these studies showed scintigraphy with ^{99m}Tc-HYNIC-exendin-4 was able to detect insulinoma with high sensitivity,[39–41] it is noteworthy that the tumor uptake of ^{99m}Tc-HYNIC-exendin-4 is lower due to the significantly less efficient internalization compared with ^{111}In-DOTA-exendin-4.[25]

Due to the small size of insulinoma (usually <2 cm), GLP-1 receptor imaging with PET may offer an advantage over SPECT with higher spatial resolution, sensitivity, and imaging contrast in localizing insulinoma. Exendin-based PET tracers labeled with ^{68}Ga,[30,42–45] [18]F,[46–51] [64]Cu,[43,52–55] and [89]Zr[56] have been successfully prepared. For human use, generator-produced positron-emitting [68]Ga ($t_{1/2}$ = 68 minutes, 89% positron emission [β^+], electron capture 11%) is a preferred candidate due to its availability, low

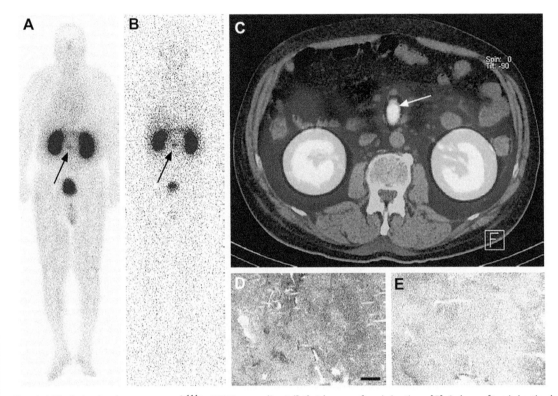

Fig. 1. Whole-body planar scans of ^{111}In-DTPA-exendin-4 ([A] 4 hours after injection; [B] 4 days after injection) and SPECT/CT image (C) detected an ectopic insulinoma located between the duodenum and the superior mesenteric artery (*arrows*) that was not shown in conventional imaging. GLP-1 receptor autoradiograph (D) shows total binding of ^{125}I-labeled GLP-1(7–36) amide in tumor tissue. Autoradiograph with nonspecific binding (E) is shown for comparison. (*From* Wild, D., et al., Glucagon-like peptide 1-receptor scans to localize occult insulinomas. N Engl J Med, 2008. 359(7): p. 766-8.)

price, and short physical half-life. Several studies have reported the clinical application of ^{68}Ga-labeled exendin-4 in localizing insulinoma since 2015.[57–65] We have performed a prospective cohort study including 52 patients with endogenous hyperinsulinemic hypoglycemia on the diagnostic value of ^{68}Ga-NOTA-MAL-cys^{40}-exendin-4

(^{68}Ga-NOTA-exendin-4) PET/CT for detecting localized insulinoma[60] (example in **Fig. 3**). The sensitivity of ^{68}Ga-NOTA-exendin-4 PET/CT in localizing insulinoma was 97.7% (95% CI 87.7–99.9), which was significantly higher than contrast-enhanced CT with pancreatic perfusion scan (74.4% [95% CI 58.8–86.5]), MRI (56.0%

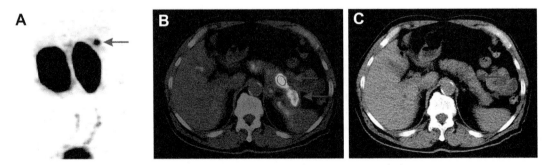

Fig. 2. ^{99m}Tc-HYNIC-exendin-4 SPECT/CT ([A] MIP; [B] SPECT/CT fusion; [C] CT) revealed 2 insulinomas in the pancreatic body and tail (*arrows*) that were not detected by other diagnostic methods. (*From* Sowa-Staszczak, A., et al., 99mTc Labeled Glucagon-Like Peptide-1-Analogue (99mTc-GLP1) Scintigraphy in the Management of Patients with Occult Insulinoma. PLoS One, 2016. 11(8): p. e0160714.)

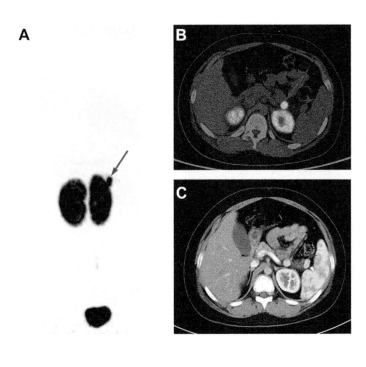

Fig. 3. ^{68}Ga-NOTA-exendin-4 PET/CT ([*A*] MIP; [*B*] PET/CT fusion; [*C*] CT) shows an insulinoma in the body of the pancreas with intense radioactivity (*arrows*). Another photopenic lesion in the pancreatic tail (*arrowhead*) was an intrapancreatic accessory spleen. (*From* Luo, Y., et al., Glucagon-Like Peptide-1 Receptor PET/CT with 68Ga-NOTA-Exendin-4 for Detecting Localized Insulinoma: A Prospective Cohort Study. J Nucl Med, 2016. 57(5): p. 715-20.)

[95% CI 34.9–75.6]), endoscopic ultrasonography (84.0% [95% CI 63.9–95.5]), and somatostatin receptor scintigraphy with ^{99m}Tc-HYNIC-TOC (19.5% [95% CI 8.8–34.9]). In contrast to the positive predictive value reported in the clinical trial of ^{111}In-DTPA-exendin-4 (83% [95% CI 62–94]),[37] there was no false-positive result with ^{68}Ga-NOTA-exendin-4, yielding a positive predictive value of 100% (95% CI 92–100).[60] The discrepancy can be explained by less partial-volume effect and higher spatial resolution in PET. Consistently, a randomized crossover study comparing (Nle[14],Lys[40][Ahx-DOTA-^{68}Ga]NH2) exendin-4 (^{68}Ga-DOTA-exendin-4) PET/CT with ^{111}In-DOTA-exendin-4 SPECT/CT showed superior performance of PET over SPECT imaging.[57,63] The accuracies for ^{68}Ga-DOTA-exendin-4 PET/CT and ^{111}In-DOTA-exendin-4 SPECT/CT were 93.9% (95% CI 87.8–97.5), and 67.5% (95% CI 58.1–76.0), respectively (example in **Fig. 4**). Moreover, with higher tumor-to-background ratios (faster blood clearance of ^{68}Ga-DOTA-exendin-4 than ^{111}In-DOTA-exendin-4), and higher spatial resolution in PET, ^{68}Ga-DOTA-exendin-4 PET/CT enabled a more confident diagnosis of insulinoma with fewer equivocal interpretations compared with ^{111}In-DOTA-exendin-4 SPECT/CT (percentage of reading agreement, 89.5% vs 75.7%).[63] These findings are encouraging and suggest that GLP-1 receptor imaging defines a new noninvasive diagnostic approach to successfully localize small benign insulinomas; furthermore, GLP-1

receptor PET is favored over SPECT imaging and should be considered in patients with insulinoma where localization fails with conventional imaging.

In addition to preoperative localization of insulinoma, GLP-1 receptor imaging also might be used for dynamic evaluation of response to nonsurgical treatment of insulinoma. A case report presented a patient with insulinoma who was not a candidate for surgery underwent endoscopic ultrasound-guided ethanol ablation of the insulinoma. Compared with the baseline ^{68}Ga-exendin-4 PET/CT, postablation PET/CT showed markedly decreased radioactivity of the tumor, which was consistent with his clinical outcome and biochemical response.[66] It might be interesting to further investigate the role of GLP-1 receptor imaging in such indication of insulinoma.

Besides sporadic insulinoma, GLP-1 receptor imaging is also useful for patients with multiple endocrine neoplasia type-1 (MEN-1) and may guide the surgical procedure. In patients with MEN-1, aggressive resection of pancreatic neuroendocrine tumors identified by conventional imaging was previously proposed,[67] but it was associated with significant mortality and long-term morbidity.[68] Recent studies showed that nonfunctioning pancreatic neuroendocrine tumors smaller than 20 mm rarely develop metastases, and studies have not shown any survival benefit for those patients who received surgery compared with patients who underwent watchful waiting.[69,70] Therefore, it is recommended only to resect

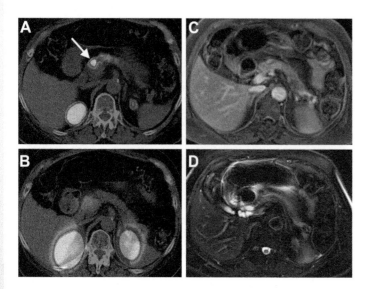

Fig. 4. ^{68}Ga-DOTA-exendin-4 PET/CT. (A) An insulinoma in the pancreatic head (arrow), but ^{111}In-DOTA-exendin-4 SPECT/CT (B) and MRI ([C] contrast-enhanced T1-weighted image; [D] T2-weighted image) did not show the tumor. (From Antwi, K., et al., Comparison of glucagon-like peptide-1 receptor (GLP-1R) PET/CT, SPECT/CT and 3T MRI for the localisation of occult insulinomas: evaluation of diagnostic accuracy in a prospective crossover imaging study. Eur J Nucl Med Mol Imaging, 2018. 45(13): p. 2318-2327.)

symptomatic insulinomas to control hypoglycemia, and to resect nonfunctioning pancreatic neuroendocrine tumors ≥20 mm due to the increased risk for progression.[71] A recent study showed that the sensitivity, specificity, and accuracy of ^{68}Ga-DOTA-exendin-4 PET/CT in detecting clinically relevant lesions (insulinoma or nonfunctioning pancreatic neuroendocrine tumor ≥20 mm) in patients with endogenous hyperinsulinemic hypoglycemia in MEN-1 were 84.6% (95% CI 54.6–98.1), 100% (95% CI 85.8–100), and 94.6% (95% CI 81.8–99.3), respectively, which was superior to the diagnostic value of MRI.[72] The careful interpretation of a morphologic modality in combination with GLP-1 receptor imaging may guide the surgical strategy and avoid unnecessary pancreatic resections.

Malignant insulinomas constitute less than 10% of all insulinomas. As opposed to benign insulinomas, malignant insulinomas often lack GLP-1 receptors. In a study on GLP-1 receptor and somatostatin receptor expression in malignant insulinomas, only a low percentage of malignant insulinomas express GLP-1 receptor; instead, most of the malignant insulinomas express somatostatin receptor subtype 2 (36% vs 73%).[73] However, the successful localization of multiple distant metastases of malignant insulinoma by ^{68}Ga-exendin-4 PET/CT was also reported.[60,74] Recently, ^{177}Lu-labeled exendin-4 peptides have been developed and their biological behaviors have been evaluated in small animal models.[75,76] Thus, patients with GLP-1 receptor–positive tumors, if somatostatin receptor expression is low or absent, may be eligible for exendin-4–based peptide receptor radionuclide therapy (PRRT). A recent study reported the preliminary estimation of the insulinoma absorbed dose and predicted that a dose between 30.3 and 127.8 Gy could be safely delivered to the insulinoma with ^{177}Lu-labeled exendin-4, an absorbed dose range shown to induce tumor shrinkage in pancreatic neuroendocrine tumors treated with ^{177}Lu-DOTATATE.[77] However, as radiation nephropathy after PRRT with somatostatin analogues have been reported previously,[78] and renal damage with thickening and necrosis of tubular basal lamina and glomerulosclerosis was also noted in mice several weeks after injection of 35 to 43 MBq ^{111}In-DTPA-exendin-4,[79] the high renal uptake and the potential associated renal toxicity are an important issues to consider.[77] As a result, research to further reduce accumulation of high-energy isotope radiolabeled exendin-4 in the kidneys, which is the dose-limiting organ, may improve the feasibility of exendin-4-based PRRT.

PITFALLS OF GLUCAGONLIKE PEPTIDE-1RECEPTOR IMAGING

There are some pitfalls of GLP-1 receptor imaging. First, due to the high physiologic expression of GLP-1 receptor in the Brunner glands located in the proximal duodenum,[16,80] the physiologic uptake of radiolabeled exendin-4 in the Brunner gland may cause false interpretation of GLP-1 receptor imaging (false-positive reading or falsely interpreted as physiologic uptake in the Brunner gland instead of an insulinoma)[36,37,58,80,81] (Fig. 5). A recent study showed that the percentage of false-negative readings of GLP-1 receptor PET/CT and SPECT/CT due to false interpretation

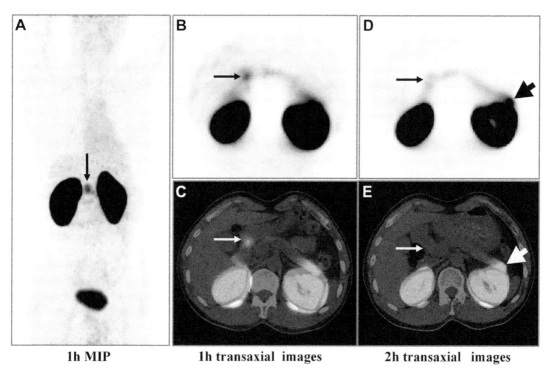

1h MIP **1h transaxial images** **2h transaxial images**

Fig. 5. ^{68}Ga-exendin-4 PET/CT imaged 1 hour (*A–C*) and 2 hours after injection (*D–E*). Arrowheads showed an insulinoma in the distal pancreatic tail that was detected only in the 2-hour scan. Arrows showed the uptake in the proximal duodenum that was possibly caused by the GLP-1 receptor expressed in the Brunner's gland. (*From* Luo, Y., et al., (68)Ga-NOTA-exendin-4 PET/CT in detection of occult insulinoma and evaluation of physiological uptake. Eur J Nucl Med Mol Imaging, 2015. 42(3): p. 531-2.)

of uptake in the pancreaticoduodenal region were 0.6% and 9.0%, respectively.[81]

Second, it is recognized that the highly radioactive kidneys owing to renal excretion of radiolabeled exendin-4 ligand may interfere with the detection of insulinomas in the distal pancreas tail located next to the left kidney.[58,82] Although a recent study on dual-time-point ^{68}Ga-exendin-4 PET/CT showed no increase of tumor-to-background ratio in late scan,[83] considering the longer effective half-life of exendin-4 in the tumor than that in the kidneys,[36] detection of tumors in the tail of the pancreas may benefit from late scans. It was also reported that in some cases, demarcation between tumors in the tail of pancreas and kidney was possible only at late scans[36,58,60] (see **Fig. 5**). Megalin-mediated reabsorption in the proximal tubules after glomerular filtration is responsible for renal retention of radiolabeled peptides, including exendin-4.[84–86] To reduce the reabsorption of the tracer, infusion of succinylated gelatin, a plasma expander to induce low-molecular weight pseudoproteinuria,[87] before tracer injection has been suggested, and the reduced kidney uptake resulted in clearer discrimination of the pancreatic tail from the

kidney signal.[77,82] Different members of radiolabeled exendin-4 have also been developed to reduce the renal uptake. For instance, ^{18}F-labeled derivatives like ^{18}F-TTCOCys40-exendin-4, ^{18}F-(Nle^{14},Lys^{40})exendin-4 showed lower kidney uptake, faster clearance rate, and thus favorable tumor-to-kidney ratio compared with radiometal-labeled exendin derivatives[50,88]; radiolabeled exendin-4 derivatives with addition of an albumin-binding moiety, using antagonistic tracers, using chelator desferrioxamine, or through brush border membrane enzyme-mediated degradation with cleavable linkers results in a significant reduction of kidney uptake and therefore an improved target-to-kidney ratio.[89–93]

Third, as exendin-4 is a biologically active peptide primarily established for the treatment of type 2 diabetes mellitus by targeting GLP-1 receptor, there is a decrease of blood glucose level after injection of radiolabeled exendin-4.[36] Thus, it was suggested that all patients receive an exogenous glucose infusion during the PET/CT examination.[37,63] Furthermore, nausea and sporadic vomiting are the known side effects of radiolabeled exendin-4.[36,60,63]

PERSPECTIVE OF GLUCAGONLIKE PEPTIDE-1 RECEPTOR IMAGING

Overexpression of GLP-1 receptor not only on insulinoma cells but also on native pancreatic β cells provides further applications of GLP-1 receptor imaging. It has been applied for preoperative distinction between insulinoma and nesidioblastosis, a term that refers to neogenesis of islets of Langerhans cells from pancreatic duct epithelium with primary islet-cell hypertrophy. Christ and colleagues[94] reported a case that ^{68}Ga-DOTA-exendin-4 accurately localized a focal type of nesidioblastosis, which was confirmed by histology, with markedly increased diffuse uptake from the tail of the pancreas to the pancreatic corpus. The autoradiography demonstrated more than 3 times higher density of GLP-1 receptor in the islets of this patient with nesidioblastosis when compared with islets of a normal pancreas. Similarly, in our previously reported prospective cohort study, we noted 4 patients clinically diagnosed as nesidioblastosis showed a mild to moderate increase of ^{68}Ga-NOTA-exendin-4 uptake in certain segments or the whole pancreas.[60] In congenital hyperinsulinism of infancy, ^{18}F-fluoro-L-dihydroxyphenylalanine (^{18}F-DOPA) PET is a well-established accurate technique to distinguish between focal and diffuse types of nesidioblastosis and thus to guide surgical resection.[95–97] L-DOPA is a precursor of catecholamines that is converted to dopamine by the aromatic amino acid decarboxylase (AADC), and pancreatic islets take up L-DOPA and convert it to dopamine through the AADC. In contrast to infancy hyperinsulinism, ^{18}F-DOPA PET has very limited value in locating insulinoma or nesidioblastosis in adults with hyperinsulinemic hypoglycemia, because of the intense physiologic uptake in the normal pancreas possibly caused by a strong expression of AADC in the normal adult exocrine pancreas.[98] Therefore, because there is no established imaging modality for assessment and localizing nesidioblatosis in adult patients with hyperinsulinemic hypoglycemia, it is worth further investigating the diagnostic value and clinical relevance of GLP-1 receptor imaging in this field.

Islet transplantation is an effective β-cell replacement therapy and has become an option to treat selected patients with insulin-dependent diabetic mellitus. Clinical attempts to assess the viability of transplanted islets are not reliable without β cell markers. Pattou and colleagues[99] reported GLP-1 receptor imaging with ^{111}In-DTPA-exendin-4 to visualize the transplanted islets in a patient who underwent the resection of greater than 80% of the pancreas for an insulinoma and subsequent healthy islet reimplantation. Focal accumulation of ^{111}In-DTPA-exendin-4 was visible at the site of islet transplantation, and the function of these reimplanted islets and their contribution to the overall insulin secretion was also confirmed. In addition to this clinical case report, several preclinical studies on GLP-1 receptor imaging in determination of viable islet graft volume have also been reported.[50,52,100,101] These results have provided evidence that transplanted functional islets can be imaged with a GLP-1 receptor targeted agent, and this approach may have potential for noninvasive monitoring of islet-cell graft survival after transplantation.

GLP-1 receptor imaging has also been applied to assess pancreatic β cell mass, which is a key issue in diabetes mellitus. Brom and colleagues[102] found a marked reduction in pancreatic uptake of ^{111}In-labeled exendin in 5 patients with type 1 diabetes compared with matching healthy individuals. However, a contradictory result reported by Nalin and colleagues[103] showed that the pancreatic uptake of ^{68}Ga-exendin-4 was not reduced by destruction of β cells in streptozotocin-induced diabetic pigs. Considering imaging of β cell mass is challenging due to the low concentration of β cells in the pancreas, which account for only 1% to 2% of the total pancreatic mass, the high retention of radiolabeled exendin-4 in the kidneys is complicating β cell mass quantification by SPECT and PET imaging. The spill-in and spill-out signal from the highly radioactive kidneys may significantly bias the quantification of the radioactivity levels in the adjacent markedly less radioactive pancreas.[104,105] Thus, approaches to reduce retention of radiolabeled exendin-4 in the kidneys and image corrections are essential to improve β cell mass quantification in future application of GLP-1 receptor imaging in the assessment of diabetes mellitus.

From the perspective of intraoperative imaging-guided surgery, it is interesting to notice the development of fluorescent probes to improve intraoperative delineation and complete resection of insulinoma. Reiner and colleagues[106,107] developed the first and second generation of near-infrared fluorescent probes targeting the GLP-1 receptor, and confirmed the close correspondence between fluorescence signals and β cell mass. Brand and colleagues[108] reported successful synthesis of a bimodal imaging probe with PET and fluorescence (^{64}Cu-E4-Fl) with good radiochemical yield and specific activity. ^{64}Cu-E4-Fl showed good performance in visualizing small xenografts (<2 mm) with PET and pancreatic β cell mass by phosphor autoradiography. Recently, Boss and colleagues[109] studied the GLP-1 receptor targeted optical imaging agent, exendin-4-IRDye 800CW. The probe accumulation in xenografts and the subcutaneous xenografts were clearly visualized. This study provides the first in vivo evidence of the feasibility of GLP-1 receptor targeted fluorescence imaging using exendin-4-IRDye 800CW to guide intraoperative lesion delineation and removal of insulinomas.

SUMMARY

The diagnosis and surgical treatment of insulinoma is dependent on accurate localization with imaging modalities. GLP-1 receptor imaging that targets pancreatic β cells has been highlighted for detecting insulinomas in recent years. Based on the high sensitivity and specificity of GLP-1 receptor imaging in localizing insulinoma, it is recommended to be introduced to clinical practice.

CLINICS CARE POINT

For insulinoma, particularly the benign variant with often low somatostatin receptor expression, GLP-1 receptor imaging is highly sensitive and specific for the preoperative localization.

REFERENCES

1. Grant CS. Insulinoma. Best Pract Res Clin Gastroenterol 2005;19(5):783–98.
2. Wilder RM, Allan FN, Power MH, et al. Carcinoma of the islands of the pancreas. JAMA 1927;89(5):348.
3. Howland G, Campbell WR, Malthby EJ, et al. Dysinsulinism: convulsions and coma due to islet cell tumor of pancreas, with operation and cure. JAMA 1929;93:674.
4. Fidler JL, Fletcher JG, Reading CC, et al. Preoperative detection of pancreatic insulinomas on multiphasic helical CT. AJR Am J Roentgenol 2003; 181(3):775–80.
5. McAuley G, Delaney H, Colville J, et al. Multimodality preoperative imaging of pancreatic insulinomas. Clin Radiol 2005;60(10):1039–50.
6. Rostambeigi N, Thompson GB. What should be done in an operating room when an insulinoma cannot be found? Clin Endocrinol (Oxf) 2009; 70(4):512–5.
7. Sotoudehmanesh R, Hedayat A, Shirazian N, et al. Endoscopic ultrasonography (EUS) in the localization of insulinoma. Endocrine 2007;31(3):238–41.
8. Placzkowski KA, Vella A, Thompson GB, et al. Secular trends in the presentation and

management of functioning insulinoma at the Mayo Clinic, 1987-2007. J Clin Endocrinol Metab 2009;94(4):1069–73.
9. Reubi JC. Peptide receptors as molecular targets for cancer diagnosis and therapy. Endocr Rev 2003;24(4):389–427.
10. Krenning EP, Kwekkeboom DJ, Reubi JC, et al. 111In-octreotide scintigraphy in oncology. Metab Clin Exp 1992;41(9 Suppl 2):83–6.
11. Krenning EP, Kwekkeboom DJ, Bakker WH, et al. Somatostatin receptor scintigraphy with [111In-DTPA-D-Phe1]- and [123I-Tyr3]-octreotide: the Rotterdam experience with more than 1000 patients. Eur J Nucl Med 1993;20(8):716–31.
12. Zimmer T, Stölzel U, Bäder M, et al. Endoscopic ultrasonography and somatostatin receptor scintigraphy in the preoperative localisation of insulinomas and gastrinomas. Gut 1996;39(4): 562–8.
13. Sundin A, Arnold R, Baudin E, et al. ENETS consensus guidelines for the standards of care in neuroendocrine tumors: radiological, nuclear medicine & hybrid imaging. Neuroendocrinology 2017; 105(3):212–44.
14. Reubi JC, Waser B. Concomitant expression of several peptide receptors in neuroendocrine tumours: molecular basis for in vivo multireceptor tumour targeting. Eur J Nucl Med Mol Imaging 2003;30(5):781–93.
15. Korner M, Christ E, Wild D, et al. Glucagon-like peptide-1 receptor overexpression in cancer and its impact on clinical applications. Front Endocrinol (Lausanne) 2012;3:158.
16. Korner M, Stöckli M, Waser B, et al. GLP-1 receptor expression in human tumors and human normal tissues: potential for in vivo targeting. J Nucl Med 2007;48(5):736–43.
17. Heller RS, Aponte GW. Intra-islet regulation of hormone secretion by glucagon-like peptide-1-(7–36) amide. Am J Physiol 1995;269(6 Pt 1):G852–60.
18. Heller RS, Kieffer TJ, Habener JF. Insulinotropic glucagon-like peptide I receptor expression in glucagon-producing alpha-cells of the rat endocrine pancreas. Diabetes 1997;46(5):785–91.
19. Tornehave D, Kristensen P, Rømer J, et al. Expression of the GLP-1 receptor in mouse, rat, and human pancreas. J Histochem Cytochem 2008; 56(9):841–51.
20. Drucker DJ. The biology of incretin hormones. Cell Metab 2006;3(3):153–65.
21. Doyle ME, Egan JM. Mechanisms of action of glucagon-like peptide 1 in the pancreas. Pharmacol Ther 2007;113(3):546–93.
22. Pauly RP, Demuth HU, Rosche F, et al. Improved glucose tolerance in rats treated with the dipeptidyl peptidase IV (CD26) inhibitor Ile-thiazolidide. Metab Clin Exp 1999;48(3):385–9.

23. Eng J, Kleinman WA, Singh L, et al. Isolation and characterization of exendin-4, an exendin-3 analogue, from Heloderma suspectum venom. Further evidence for an exendin receptor on dispersed acini from Guinea pig pancreas. J Biol Chem 1992;267(11):7402–5.

24. Goke R, Fehmann HC, Linn T, et al. Exendin-4 is a high potency agonist and truncated exendin-(9-39)-amide an antagonist at the glucagon-like peptide 1-(7-36)-amide receptor of insulin-secreting beta-cells. J Biol Chem 1993;268(26):19650–5.

25. Wild D, Wicki A, Mansi R, et al. Exendin-4-based radiopharmaceuticals for glucagonlike peptide-1 receptor PET/CT and SPECT/CT. J Nucl Med 2010;51(7):1059–67.

26. Brom M, Joosten L, Oyen WJ, et al. Radiolabelled GLP-1 analogues for in vivo targeting of insulinomas. Contrast Media Mol Imaging 2012;7(2):160–6.

27. Gotthardt M, Fischer M, Naeher I, et al. Use of the incretin hormone glucagon-like peptide-1 (GLP-1) for the detection of insulinomas: initial experimental results. Eur J Nucl Med Mol Imaging 2002;29(5):597–606.

28. Wild D, Béhé M, Wicki A, et al. [Lys40(Ahx-DTPA-111In)NH2]exendin-4, a very promising ligand for glucagon-like peptide-1 (GLP-1) receptor targeting. J Nucl Med 2006;47(12):2025–33.

29. Wicki A, Wild D, Storch D, et al. [Lys40(Ahx-DTPA-111In)NH2]-Exendin-4 is a highly efficient radiotherapeutic for glucagon-like peptide-1 receptor-targeted therapy for insulinoma. Clin Cancer Res 2007;13(12):3696–705.

30. Jodal A, Lankat-Buttgereit B, Brom M, et al. A comparison of three (67/68)Ga-labelled exendin-4 derivatives for β-cell imaging on the GLP-1 receptor: the influence of the conjugation site of NODAGA as chelator. EJNMMI Res 2014;4:31.

31. Eng J. Exendin peptides. Mt Sinai J Med 1992;59(2):147–9.

32. Raufman JP, Singh L, Eng J. Exendin-3, a novel peptide from Heloderma horridum venom, interacts with vasoactive intestinal peptide receptors and a newly described receptor on dispersed acini from Guinea pig pancreas. Description of exendin-3(9-39) amide, a specific exendin receptor antagonist. J Biol Chem 1991;266(5):2897–902.

33. Waser B, Reubi JC. Value of the radiolabelled GLP-1 receptor antagonist exendin(9-39) for targeting of GLP-1 receptor-expressing pancreatic tissues in mice and humans. Eur J Nucl Med Mol Imaging 2011;38(6):1054–8.

34. Gotthardt M, Lalyko G, van Eerd-Vismale J, et al. A new technique for in vivo imaging of specific GLP-1 binding sites: first results in small rodents. Regul Pept 2006;137(3):162–7.

35. Wild D, Mäcke H, Christ E, et al. Glucagon-like peptide 1-receptor scans to localize occult insulinomas. N Engl J Med 2008;359(7):766–8.

36. Christ E, Wild D, Forrer F, et al. Glucagon-like peptide-1 receptor imaging for localization of insulinomas. J Clin Endocrinol Metab 2009;94(11):4398–405.

37. Christ E, Wild D, Ederer S, et al. Glucagon-like peptide-1 receptor imaging for the localisation of insulinomas: a prospective multicentre imaging study. Lancet Diabetes Endocrinol 2013;1(2):115–22.

38. Wenning AS, Kirchner P, Antwi K, et al. Preoperative Glucagon-like peptide-1 receptor imaging reduces surgical trauma and pancreatic tissue loss in insulinoma patients: a report of three cases. Patient Saf Surg 2015;9:23.

39. Sowa-Staszczak A, Pach D, Mikołajczak R, et al. Glucagon-like peptide-1 receptor imaging with [Lys40(Ahx-HYNIC- 99mTc/EDDA)NH2]-exendin-4 for the detection of insulinoma. Eur J Nucl Med Mol Imaging 2013;40(4):524–31.

40. Sowa-Staszczak A, Trofimiuk-Müldner M, Stefańska A, et al. 99mTc Labeled Glucagon-Like Peptide-1-Analogue (99mTc-GLP1) scintigraphy in the management of patients with occult insulinoma. PLoS One 2016;11(8):e0160714.

41. Senica K, Tomazic A, Skvarca A, et al. Superior diagnostic performance of the GLP-1 receptor agonist [Lys(40)(AhxHYNIC-[(99m)Tc]/EDDA)NH(2)]-exendin-4 over conventional imaging modalities for localization of insulinoma. Mol Imaging Biol 2020;22(1):165–72.

42. Selvaraju RK, Velikyan I, Asplund V, et al. Pre-clinical evaluation of [(68)Ga]Ga-DO3A-VS-Cys(40)-Exendin-4 for imaging of insulinoma. Nucl Med Biol 2014;41(6):471–6.

43. Mikkola K, Kirsi M, Yim CB, et al. 64Cu- and 68Ga-labelled [Nle(14),Lys(40)(Ahx-NODAGA)NH2]-exendin-4 for pancreatic beta cell imaging in rats. Mol Imaging Biol 2014;16(2):255–63.

44. Selvaraju RK, Velikyan I, Johansson L, et al. In in vivo imaging of the glucagonlike peptide 1 receptor in the pancreas with 68Ga-labeled DO3A-exendin-4. J Nucl Med 2013;54(8):1458–63.

45. Boss M, Buitinga M, Jansen TJP, et al. PET-based dosimetry of [(68)Ga]Ga-NODAGA-exendin-4 in humans, a tracer for beta cell imaging. J Nucl Med 2020;61(1):112–6.

46. Gao H, Niu G, Yang M, et al. PET of insulinoma using (1)(8)F-FBEM-EM3106B, a new GLP-1 analogue. Mol Pharm 2011;8(5):1775–82.

47. Kiesewetter DO, Gao H, Ma Y, et al. 18F-radiolabeled analogs of exendin-4 for PET imaging of GLP-1 in insulinoma. Eur J Nucl Med Mol Imaging 2012;39(3):463–73.

48. Kiesewetter DO, Guo N, Guo J, et al. Evaluation of an [(18)F]AlF-NOTA analog of exendin-4 for

imaging of GLP-1 receptor in insulinoma. Thera-nostics 2012;2(10):999–1009.

49. Wu H, Liang S, Liu S, et al. 18F-radiolabeled GLP-1 analog exendin-4 for PET/CT imaging of insulinoma in small animals. Nucl Med Commun 2013;34(7):701–8.

50. Wu Z, Liu S, Hassink M, et al. Development and evaluation of 18F-TTCO-Cys40-Exendin-4: a PET probe for imaging transplanted islets. J Nucl Med 2013;54(2):244–51.

51. Li J, Peng J, Tang W, et al. Synthesis and evalua-tion of (18)F-PTTCO-Cys(40)-Exendin-4 for PET im-aging of ectopic insulinomas in rodents. Bioorg Chem 2020;98:103718.

52. Wu Z, Todorov I, Li L, et al. In vivo imaging of trans-planted islets with 64Cu-DO3A-VS-Cys40-Exendin-4 by targeting GLP-1 receptor. Bioconjug Chem 2011;22(8):1587–94.

53. Connolly BM, Vanko A, McQuade P, et al. Ex vivo imaging of pancreatic beta cells using a radiola-beled GLP-1 receptor agonist. Mol Imaging Biol 2012;14(1):79–87.

54. Wu Z, Liu S, Nair I, et al. 64Cu labeled sarcopha-gine exendin-4 for microPET imaging of glucagon like peptide-1 receptor expression. Theranostics 2014;4(8):770–7.

55. Bandara N, Zheleznyak A, K Cherukuri, et al. Eval-uation of Cu-64 and Ga-68 radiolabeled glucagon-like peptide-1 receptor agonists as PET tracers for pancreatic beta cell imaging. Mol Imaging Biol 2016;18(1):90–8.

56. Bauman A, Valverde IE, Fischer CA, et al. Develop-ment of 68Ga- and 89Zr-labeled exendin-4 as po-tential radiotracers for the imaging of insulinomas by PET. J Nucl Med 2015;56(10):1569–74.

57. Antwi K, Fani M, Nicolas G, et al. Localization of hidden insulinomas with ^{68}Ga-DOTA-Exendin-4 PET/CT: a pilot study. J Nucl Med 2015;56(7):1075–8.

58. Luo Y, Yu M, Pan Q, et al. 68)Ga-NOTA-exendin-4 PET/CT in detection of occult insulinoma and eval-uation of physiological uptake. Eur J Nucl Med Mol Imaging 2015;42(3):531–2.

59. Luo Y, Li N, Kiesewetter DO, et al. 68Ga-NOTA-Ex-endin-4 PET/CT in localization of an occult insuli-noma and appearance of coexisting esophageal carcinoma. Clin Nucl Med 2016;41(4):341–3.

60. Luo Y, Pan Q, Yao S, et al. Glucagon-like peptide-1 receptor PET/CT with 68Ga-NOTA-Exendin-4 for detecting localized insulinoma: a prospective cohort study. J Nucl Med 2016;57(5):715–20.

61. Cuthbertson DJ, Banks M, Khoo B, et al. Applica-tion of Ga(68) -DOTA-exendin-4 PET/CT to localize an occult insulinoma. Clin Endocrinol (Oxf) 2016;84(5):789–91.

62. Luo YP, Pan QQ, Li F, et al. [(68)Ga-exendin-4 PET-CT for the localization of occult insulinomas: a prospective cohort study]. Zhonghua Wai Ke Za Zhi 2018;56(11):837–42.

63. Antwi K, Fani M, Heye T, et al. Comparison of glucagon-like peptide-1 receptor (GLP-1R) PET/CT, SPECT/CT and 3T MRI for the localisation of occult insulinomas: evaluation of diagnostic accu-racy in a prospective crossover imaging study. Eur J Nucl Med Mol Imaging 2018;45(13):2318–27.

64. Pallavi UN, Malasani V, Sen I, et al. Molecular imag-ing to the surgeons rescue: gallium-68 DOTA-exen-din-4 positron emission tomography-computed tomography in pre-operative localization of insuli-nomas. Indian J Nucl Med 2019;34(1):14–8.

65. Sood A, Basher RK, Kang M, et al. 68Ga-DOTA-Ex-endin PET-MRI fusion imaging in a case of insuli-noma. Clin Nucl Med 2019;44(7):e428–30.

66. Luo Y, Li J, Yang A, et al. 68Ga-Exendin-4 PET/CT in evaluation of endoscopic ultrasound-guided ethanol ablation of an insulinoma. Clin Nucl Med 2017;42(4):310–1.

67. Hausman MS Jr, Thompson NW, Gauger PG, et al. The surgical management of MEN-1 pancreato-duodenal neuroendocrine disease. Surgery 2004;136(6):1205–11.

68. Falconi M, Mantovani W, Crippa S, et al. Pancreatic insufficiency after different resections for benign tu-mours. Br J Surg 2008;95(1):85–91.

69. Triponez F, Goudet P, Dosseh D, et al. Is surgery beneficial for MEN1 patients with small (< or = 2 cm), nonfunctioning pancreaticoduodenal endo-crine tumor? An analysis of 65 patients from the GTE. World J Surg 2006;30(5):654–62 [discussion: 663–4].

70. Partelli S, Tamburrino D, Lopez C, et al. Active sur-veillance versus surgery of nonfunctioning pancre-atic neuroendocrine neoplasms ≤2 cm in MEN1 patients. Neuroendocrinology 2016;103(6):779–86.

71. Falconi M, Eriksson B, Kaltsas G, et al. ENETS consensus guidelines update for the management of patients with functional pancreatic neuroendo-crine tumors and non-functional pancreatic neuro-endocrine tumors. Neuroendocrinology 2016;103(2):153–71.

72. Antwi K, Nicolas G, Fani M, et al. 68Ga-Exendin-4 PET/CT detects insulinomas in patients with endog-enous hyperinsulinemic hypoglycemia in MEN-1. J Clin Endocrinol Metab 2019;104(12):5843–52.

73. Wild D, Christ E, Caplin ME, et al. Glucagon-like peptide-1 versus somatostatin receptor targeting reveals 2 distinct forms of malignant insulinomas. J Nucl Med 2011;52(7):1073–8.

74. Eriksson O, Velikyan I, Selvaraju RK, et al. Detec-tion of metastatic insulinoma by positron emission tomography with [(68)ga]exendin-4-a case report. J Clin Endocrinol Metab 2014;99(5):1519–24.

75. Velikyan I, Bulenga TN, Selvaraju R, et al. Dosim-etry of [(177)Lu]-DO3A-VS-Cys(40)-Exendin-4 -

impact on the feasibility of insulinoma internal radiotherapy. Am J Nucl Med Mol Imaging 2015; 5(2):109–26.

76. Guleria M, Das T, Amirdhanayagam J, et al. Preparation of [(177)Lu]Lu-DOTA-Ahx-Lys40-Exendin-4 for radiotherapy of insulinoma: a detailed insight into the radiochemical intricacies. Nucl Med Biol 2019;78-79:31–40.

77. Buitinga M, Jansen T, van der Kroon I, et al. Succinylated gelatin improves the theranostic potential of radiolabeled exendin-4 in insulinoma patients. J Nucl Med 2019;60(6):812–6.

78. Rolleman EJ, Melis M, Valkema R, et al. Kidney protection during peptide receptor radionuclide therapy with somatostatin analogues. Eur J Nucl Med Mol Imaging 2010;37(5):1018–31.

79. Melis M, Vegt E, Konijnenberg MW, et al. Nephrotoxicity in mice after repeated imaging using 111In-labeled peptides. J Nucl Med 2010;51(6):973–7.

80. Hepprich M, Antwi K, Waser B, et al. Brunner's gland hyperplasia in a patient after Roux-Y gastric bypass: an important pitfall in GLP-1 receptor imaging. Case Rep Endocrinol 2020;2020:4510910.

81. Antwi K, Hepprich M, Müller NA, et al. Pitfalls in the detection of insulinomas with glucagon-like peptide-1 receptor imaging. Clin Nucl Med 2020; 45(9):e386–92.

82. Antwi K, Nicolas G, Fani M, et al. Volume replacement fluid demarks benign insulinoma with 68Ga-DOTA-Exendin-4 PET/CT. Clin Nucl Med 2019; 44(5):e347–8.

83. Michalski K, Laubner K, Stoykow C, et al. Detection of insulinomas using dual-time-point 68Ga-DOTA-Exendin 4 PET/CT. Clin Nucl Med 2020;45(7):519–24.

84. Melis M, Krenning EP, Bernard BF, et al. Localisation and mechanism of renal retention of radiolabelled somatostatin analogues. Eur J Nucl Med Mol Imaging 2005;32(10):1136–43.

85. Gotthardt M, van Eerd-Vismale J, Oyen WJ, et al. Indication for different mechanisms of kidney uptake of radiolabeled peptides. J Nucl Med 2007; 48(4):596–601.

86. Vegt E, Melis M, Eek A, et al. Renal uptake of different radiolabelled peptides is mediated by megalin: SPECT and biodistribution studies in megalin-deficient mice. Eur J Nucl Med Mol Imaging 2011;38(4):623–32.

87. ten Dam MA, Branten AJ, Klasen IS, et al. The gelatin-derived plasma substitute Gelofusine causes low-molecular-weight proteinuria by decreasing tubular protein reabsorption. J Crit Care 2001;16(3):115–20.

88. Mikkola K, Yim C-B, Lehtiniemi P, et al. Low kidney uptake of GLP-1R-targeting, beta cell-specific PET tracer, 18F-labeled [Nle14,Lys40]exendin-4

analog, shows promise for clinical imaging. EJNMMI Res 2016;6(1):91.

89. Jodal A, Pape F, Becker-Pauly C, et al. Evaluation of (1)(1)(1)In-Labelled Exendin-4 Derivatives Containing Different Meprin beta-Specific Cleavable Linkers. PLoS One 2015;10(4):e0123443.

90. Rylova SN, Waser B, Del Pozzo L, et al. Approaches to improve the pharmacokinetics of radiolabeled glucagon-like peptide-1 receptor ligands using antagonistic tracers. J Nucl Med 2016;57(8):1282–8.

91. Kaeppeli SAM, Jodal A, Gotthardt M, et al. Exendin-4 derivatives with an albumin-binding moiety show decreased renal retention and improved GLP-1 receptor targeting. Mol Pharm 2019;16(9):3760–9.

92. Kaeppeli SAM, Schibli R, Mindt TL, et al. Comparison of desferrioxamine and NODAGA for the gallium-68 labeling of exendin-4. EJNMMI Radiopharm Chem 2019;4(1):9.

93. Zhang M, Jacobson O, Kiesewetter DO, et al. Improving the theranostic potential of exendin 4 by reducing the renal radioactivity through brush border membrane enzyme-mediated degradation. Bioconjug Chem 2019;30(6):1745–53.

94. Christ E, Wild D, Antwi K, et al. Preoperative localization of adult nesidioblastosis using 68Ga-DOTA-exendin-4-PET/CT. Endocrine 2015; 50(3):821–3.

95. Ribeiro MJ, De Lonlay P, Delzescaux T, et al. Characterization of hyperinsulinism in infancy assessed with PET and 18F-fluoro-L-DOPA. J Nucl Med 2005; 46(4):560–6.

96. Mohnike K, Blankenstein O, Christesen HT, et al. Proposal for a standardized protocol for 18F-DOPA-PET (PET/CT) in congenital hyperinsulinism. Horm Res 2006;66(1):40–2.

97. Hardy OT, Hernandez-Pampaloni M, Saffer JR, et al. Accuracy of [18F]fluorodopa positron emission tomography for diagnosing and localizing focal congenital hyperinsulinism. J Clin Endocrinol Metab 2007;92(12):4706–11.

98. Tessonnier L, Sebag F, Ghander C, et al. Limited value of 18F-F-DOPA PET to localize pancreatic insulin-secreting tumors in adults with hyperinsulinemic hypoglycemia. J Clin Endocrinol Metab 2010;95(1):303–7.

99. Pattou F, Kerr-Conte J, Wild D. GLP-1-receptor scanning for imaging of human beta cells transplanted in muscle. N Engl J Med 2010;363(13):1289–90.

100. van der Kroon I, Andralojc K, Willekens SM, et al. Noninvasive imaging of islet Transplants with 111In-exendin-3 SPECT/CT. J Nucl Med 2016; 57(5):799–804.

101. Eter WA, Van der Kroon I, Andralojc K, et al. Noninvasive in vivo determination of viable islet graft

volume by (111)In-exendin-3. Sci Rep 2017;7(1): 7232.

102. Brom M, Woliner-van der Weg W, Joosten L, et al. Non-invasive quantification of the beta cell mass by SPECT with (1)(1)(1)In-labelled exendin. Diabetologia 2014;57(5):950–9.

103. Nalin L, Selvaraju RK, Velikyan I, et al. Positron emission tomography imaging of the glucagon-like peptide-1 receptor in healthy and streptozotocin-induced diabetic pigs. Eur J Nucl Med Mol Imaging 2014;41(9):1800–10.

104. Liu Y. Invalidity of SUV measurements of lesions in close proximity to hot sources due to "shine-through" effect on FDG PET-CT interpretation. Radiol Res Pract 2012;2012:867218.

105. Woliner-van der Weg W, Deden LN, Meeuwis AP, et al. A 3D-printed anatomical pancreas and kidney phantom for optimizing SPECT/CT reconstruction

settings in beta cell imaging using 111In-exendin. EJNMMI Phys 2016;3(1):29.

106. Reiner T, Kohler RH, Liew CW, et al. Near-infrared fluorescent probe for imaging of pancreatic beta cells. Bioconjug Chem 2010;21(7):1362–8.

107. Reiner T, Thurber G, Gaglia J, et al. Accurate measurement of pancreatic islet beta-cell mass using a second-generation fluorescent exendin-4 analog. Proc Natl Acad Sci U S A 2011;108(31): 12815–20.

108. Brand C, Abdel-Atti D, Zhang Y, et al. In vivo imaging of GLP-1R with a targeted bimodal PET/fluorescence imaging agent. Bioconjug Chem 2014;25(7): 1323–30.

109. Boss M, Bos D, Frielink C, et al. Targeted optical imaging of the glucagonlike peptide 1 receptor using exendin-4-IRDye 800CW. J Nucl Med 2020; 61(7):1066–71.

A Critical Review of PET Tracers Used for Brain Tumor Imaging

Austin J. Borja, BA[a,b], Emily C. Hancin, MS, BA[a,c], William Y. Raynor, BS[a,d],
Cyrus Ayubcha, MSc[a,e], Donald K. Detchou, BA[a,b], Thomas J. Werner, MSc[a],
Mona-Elisabeth Revheim, MD, PhD, MHA[a,f,g],
Abass Alavi, MD, MD (Hon), PhD (Hon), DSc (Hon)[a,*]

KEYWORDS

• Brain neoplasms • Neuroimaging • PET • ^{18}F-fluorodeoxyglucose

KEY POINTS

- Because enhancement on computed tomography (CT) and MR reflects blood-brain barrier (BBB) changes, molecular imaging with PET-based techniques is needed to assess brain tumor activity, especially in tumors with intact or partially intact BBB.
- ^{18}F-fluorodeoxyglucose (FDG)-PET has been validated in tumor detection/delineation, recurrence, and prognostication.
- Although FDG remains the most widely used PET tracer in the evaluation of brain tumors, various other tracers, including amino acid indicators, have been studied extensively.
- Breakdown of the BBB plays a major role in visualizing brain tumors by radiolabeled amino acid tracers; therefore, this approach is suboptimal for assessing disease activity beyond CT and MR.

INTRODUCTION

Intracranial neoplasms include both primary tumors and metastases, the latter markedly more common.[1,2] A recent study found that brain metastases were present at diagnosis in 12.1% of patients with metastatic disease.[3] Primary malignancies that metastasize most frequently to the brain include melanoma, lung, renal, breast, and colorectal cancer.[1,3] Based on data from 2010 to 2014, the age-adjusted incidence of primary central nervous system (CNS) tumors in the United States has been reported as 22.64 cases per 100,000 population per year, with an age-adjusted mortality rate of 4.33 per 100,000 per year.[4] Aside from those composed of neuroepithelial tissue, primary tumors arising within the CNS also include meningiomas as well as lymphoma.[5] Most CNS tumors are nonmalignant, and approximately half of these are meningiomas.[6] Among malignant CNS tumors, gliomas occur with the greatest frequency.[6]

In the past, the classification of CNS tumors relied on histologic criteria alone.[7] The 2016 World Health Organization (WHO) Classification of Tumors of the Central Nervous System (2016 CNS WHO) was groundbreaking in its inclusion of genetic criteria.[8] Grade determinations according to the 2016 CNS WHO, however, still require

Conflict of Interest: The authors have declared no conflicts of interest.

[a] Department of Radiology, Hospital of the University of Pennsylvania, 3400 Spruce Street, Philadelphia, PA 19104, USA; [b] Perelman School of Medicine at the University of Pennsylvania, 3400 Civic Center Boulevard, Philadelphia, PA 19104, USA; [c] Lewis Katz School of Medicine at Temple University, 3500 North Broad Street, Philadelphia, PA 19140, USA; [d] Drexel University College of Medicine, 2900 West Queen Lane, Philadelphia, PA 19129, USA; [e] Harvard Medical School, 25 Shattuck Street, Boston, MA 02115, USA; [f] Division of Radiology and Nuclear Medicine, Oslo University Hospital, Sognsvannsveien 20, Oslo 0372, Norway; [g] Institute of Clinical Medicine, Faculty of Medicine, University of Oslo, Problemveien 7, Oslo 0315, Norway
* Corresponding author.
E-mail address: abass.alavi@pennmedicine.upenn.edu

histologic studies to assess for malignant features, which pose limitations due to the invasive nature of CNS tumors as well as potential complications of tissue biopsy. Advances in molecular imaging with PET have contributed to the understanding of CNS tumors and eventually may provide a noninvasive method of grading.[9] For decades, MR imaging with gadolinium contrast has played a role in assessing tumor anatomy, determining response to therapy, and prognostication.[10,11] More recently, diffusion-weighted MR, perfusion-weighted MR, and MR spectroscopy have been proposed for assessing brain tumor characteristics.[12] Because PET allows for direct visualization of metabolic activity, interest in ^{18}F-fluorodeoxyglucose (FDG) and other PET tracers has grown steadily. This has led to the development of new PET tracers, including those derived from amino acids, such as ^{18}F-fluoroethyltyrosine (FET), ^{11}C-methionine (MET), and ^{18}F-dihydroxyphenylalanine (FDOPA).[13] Not only do PET-based techniques have the potential to influence tumor diagnosis and grading by providing valuable insight into tumor activity and heterogeneity, but also they may play a vital role in prognostication and assessing individualized patient responses to therapy. These promising applications of PET imaging, as well as the roles of various PET tracers, are discussed in this communication.

TUMOR DELINEATION

Proper delineation of the entire tumor volume is crucial not only for diagnostic purposes but also for the planning of surgical resection and radiotherapy. Poor penetration of the blood-brain barrier (BBB) by contrast agents used in computed tomography (CT) and MR, however, present a challenge in cases where the BBB is intact. For example, low-grade gliomas often do not enhance on CT or MR, whereas enhancement usually is observed in high-grade gliomas due to disruption of the BBB. Still, high-grade tumors may have areas of intact BBB and may not enhance at all.[13] Furthermore, changes in BBB permeability visualized by contrast-enhanced MR are not specific to tumor activity.[14–16]

PET imaging with FDG, which is a substrate of BBB transporters, therefore, can indicate areas of tumor activity that otherwise cannot be visualized by CT or MR. To differentiate between tumor activity and physiologic uptake by gray matter, the coregistration of FDG-PET and MR images as well as delayed PET imaging has been proposed.[17] Combined PET/MR images correlate both MR-specific characterization and precise anatomic localization with PET to confirm the expected metabolic activity of an active tumor.[18,19] Furthermore, by increasing the time between tracer administration and image acquisition to up to 8 hours, relatively higher elimination of FDG from normal tissue has been found to result in increased contrast between the tumor and physiologic activity.[20]

In addition to FDG, other PET tracers targeting amino acid transport, hypoxia, cellular proliferation, and the 18-kDa mitochondrial translocator protein (TSPO) have been proposed for tumor delineation and characterization. The use of radiolabeled amino acids to evaluate non-CNS malignancies, however, has been so far unsuccessful. For example, many unnatural amino acids undergo substantial urinary excretion, which has limited the use of these indicators in kidney, ureter, or bladder cancers, with few exceptions.[21] Furthermore, agents used in breast cancer research, such as ^{11}C-MET, have a short half-life in the body, which prevents extended or delayed time point imaging.[22] Others, such as ^{18}F-fluciclovine, have failed to distinguish between histologic complete and incomplete responses to neoadjuvant therapy followed by surgical management.[22]

Although these tracers have exhibited significant shortcomings in other organ systems, FET-PET and MET-PET have been used widely to determine tumor volumes in nonenhancing gliomas.[23,24] At first glance, tumor activity assessed by amino acid PET may extend beyond MR contrast enhancement.[23,25–27] A study by Grosu and colleagues[28] compared anatomic imaging by CT and MR to functional imaging with MET-PET or single-photon emission CT (SPECT) with ^{123}I-methyl-tyrosine (IMT) in 44 subjects with recurrent high-grade gliomas (**Fig. 1**). Tumor volume delineation was performed for the planning of fractionated stereotactic radiotherapy using either combined functional and anatomic imaging (36 subjects) or anatomic imaging alone (8 subjects). By showing that patients whose treatment planning was informed by MET-PET or IMT-SPECT had longer survival times compared with patients whose planning relied on anatomic imaging alone, the investigators concluded that functional imaging with amino acid tracers may have a greater role to play in radiation treatment planning and, therefore, could warrant further investigation. Venneti and colleagues[29] utilized ^{18}F-glutamine to assess the metabolic activity of gliomas in mice and humans. They observed decreased tracer uptake following chemotherapeutic or radiation intervention, which the investigators associate with reduced metabolic uptake and tumor burden.

Despite these observations, the utility of amino acid PET for assessing brain tumors has been

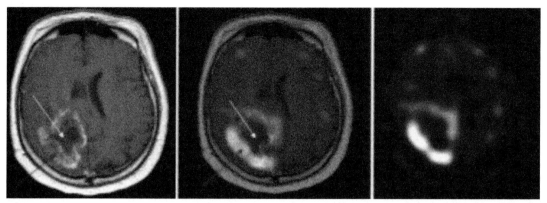

Fig. 1. Recurrent glioblastoma multiforme 6 months after reirradiation (fractionated stereotactic radiotherapy) and temozolomide. The T1 gadolinium(Gd)–MR imaging and ^{123}I-α-methyl-tyrosine (IMT) SPECT show the (tumor) necrosis (*yellow arrows*) in the treated region and the tumor progression on the margin of the irradiated field (*red arrows*). Left panel: T1Gd–MR imaging; Middle panel: ^{123}I-α-methyl-tyrosine (IMT)-SPECT/MR imaging; Right panel: IMT-SPECT imaging. (*From* Grosu AL, Weber WA, Franz M, Stark S, Piert M, Thamm R, et al. Reirradiation of recurrent high-grade gliomas using amino acid PET (SPECT)/CT/MRI image fusion to determine gross tumor volume for stereotactic fractionated radiotherapy. Int J Radiat Oncol Biol Phys. 2005;63(2):511-9; with permission.)

brought into question. As many as 30% of WHO grade II gliomas show no uptake.[16,30–32] By targeting hypoxia rather than amino acid transport, PET imaging with ^{18}F-fluoromisonidazole also shows peripheral uptake beyond MR-enhancing regions that correlate with MET-PET.[16,33] ^{18}F-glutamine is limited as a tracer because, unlike ^{18}F-FDG, it is subject to inactivation by defluorination via enzymes, such as alanine aminotransferase, which renders the tracer unusable in imaging.[34] ^{18}F-fluorothymidine (FLT) targets cellular proliferation but requires a permeable BBB for uptake, a structural change also associated with degenerative processes, such as radiation damage, skewing subsequent imaging observations.[16,35–37] Accordingly, FLT-PET was found to be poor at detecting WHO grade II gliomas.[15,38,39] Glioma tumor delineation also has been proposed using the TSPO ligand ^{18}F-GE-180.[40] Although uptake patterns of both FET and ^{18}F-GE-180 are more extensive than MR enhancement alone, the overlap of spatial distribution between the 2 tracers is only moderate, which places limitations on the potential for the combined effectiveness of these 2 tracers.[41,42] Geisler and colleagues[43] compared FET to MET in evaluating residual tumor following the resection of cerebral gliomas in rats. They found that both FET and MET uptake significantly increased around the area of resection during the first postoperative week, and they suggested that a 14-day delay in imaging to assess the presence of residual tumor is a more appropriate course of action. A delay of this magnitude in imaging is unrealistic in evaluating human subjects, because an initial postoperative MR imaging

may be conducted as early as 72 hours after surgical resection to guide further treatment decisions.[44] In light of the aforementioned limitations and irregularities, the validity of amino acid–based approaches is questionable due to inconsistencies in uptake, limited half-life, susceptibility to degradation, and dependence on BBB abnormalities.

TUMOR GRADING

Management of brain tumors relies heavily on tumor grading, and a noninvasive method of grading that correlates with histologic findings is of great interest.[9,12] In a meta-analysis that considered data from 119 subjects, FDG-PET and FET-PET were shown to facilitate the distinction between high-grade and low-grade gliomas.[45] Accordingly, high FDG uptake in a glioma is consistent with WHO grades III and IV, whereas WHO grade II gliomas are more likely to show less uptake compared with normal cortical activity.[46] Physiologic FDG uptake in cortical and subcortical regions, however, hampers the tumor-to-background ratio and may explain why uptake of MET but not FDG was found to correlate with cellular proliferation in gliomas.[47] Static and kinetic FET-PET parameters were assessed in 162 patients with gliomas by Vomacka and colleagues[48] (**Fig. 2**). By showing that a voxel-based analysis could differentiate among WHO grades and between isocitrate dehydrogenase (IDH) mutation subtypes, the investigators concluded that a rapid and reader-independent technique of quantifying FET-PET with potential for clinical utility is feasible.

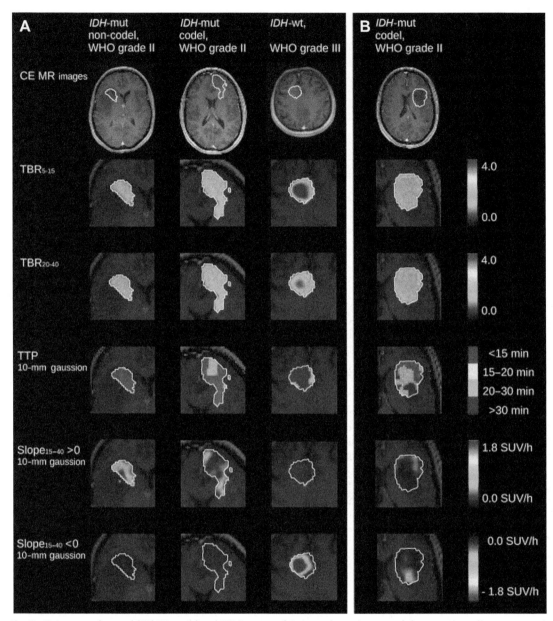

Fig. 2. Contrast-enhanced (CE) T1-weighted MR images of 4 example patients, and the corresponding parametric images of the early and late TBR, the TTP, and the negative and positive slope$_{15-40}$ for the voxels within the BTV (zoom factor 2; BTV marked with white contour; TTP and slope$_{5-15}$ images estimated from dynamic PET data smoothed with a gaussian filter with 10-mm FWHM). (A) Images of 3 example patients with parameter distributions characteristic of 1 *IDH*-mut non-codel WHO grade II glioma, 1 *IDH*-mut codel WHO grade II glioma, and 1 *IDH*-wt WHO grade III glioma. (B) One example patient (*IDH*-mut codel WHO grade II glioma) with a mixed pattern in parametric images, where maximum uptake in TBR images does not colocalize with the hotspot with early TTP and negative slope$_{15-40}$. TBR, tumor-to-brain ratio; TTP, time-to-peak; BTV, biological tumor volume; FWHM, full width half maximum; SUV, standardized uptake value; wt, wildtype; mut, mutant. (*From* Vomacka L, Unterrainer M, Holzgreve A, Mille E, Gosewisch A, Brosch J, et al. Voxel-wise analysis of dynamic (18)F-FET PET: a novel approach for non-invasive glioma characterisation. EJNMMI Res. 2018;8(1):91; with permission.)

FLT-PET also has been proposed to assess tumor grade. Collet and colleagues[49] conducted a study of 39 patients by to differentiate among WHO glioma grades II, III, and IV. Uptake of FLT-PET was found superior to all MR parameters assessed, which included those determined by diffusion-weighted and perfusion-weighted imaging as well as MR spectroscopy.

RESPONSE TO TREATMENT

Treatment options for brain tumors can include surgery, radiotherapy, and chemotherapy, depending on tumor classification and location as well as patient-dependent factors, such as age and other existing health conditions.[50,51] Early response assessment is of vital importance to the management of brain tumors, especially in those that are highly aggressive and heterogeneous. Current practice, however, relying heavily on anatomic modalities, cannot accurately distinguish between true progression and pseudoprogression, which includes treatment-induced changes.[9,12] These limitations may hinder the ability for clinicians to make appropriate treatment decisions, which may have a negative impact on patient outcomes.

FDG-PET has been demonstrated as an excellent modality to determine lesion activity and can accurately identify radiation injuries, which are particularly difficult to identify using conventional modalities.[52] Damage from radiation can present with seizures, changes in personality, and memory deficits in addition to underlying axonal swelling and reactive gliosis. Radiation necrosis describes late-injury lesions where necrosis is present and can be a focal or diffuse process.[53] In cases of diffuse radiation necrosis, periventricular white matter often is involved, whereas focal lesions can be present near or distant to the tumor.[54] Due to BBB disruption present in radiation necrosis, these lesions often exhibit contrast enhancement on CT and MR, thereby appearing similar to tumor regrowth. By using FDG-PET, decreased uptake can be observed in radiation necrosis, whereas tumor recurrence would show increased metabolic activity. Patronas and colleagues[55] were the first to describe this application of FDG-PET in a study of 5 patients. Although the patients had similar clinical presentations with equivocal CT findings, 2 patients were correctly identified as having radiation necrosis confirmed by pathology whereas 3 were found to have tumor recurrence. A later study examined 95 patients with brain metastases or gliomas and showed that FDG-PET could discriminate between radiation necrosis in tumor recurrence with near 100% sensitivity and specificity.[56] Perfect sensitivity and specificity of FDG-PET also were reported in a similar study in 9 patients with high-grade tumors.[57]

Coregistration of FDG-PET with ^{82}Rb(rubidium)-PET images, which show BBB lesions, can help delineate lesions whose boundaries are not clear due to their proximity to the cortex. A study using these modalities to assess for recurrent tumors in 38 cases reported a sensitivity of 81% and a specificity of 88%.[58] In this instance, FDG uptake greater than or equal to normal cortical tissue was considered positive for tumor recurrence. Alternatively, FDG uptake greater than normal white matter was used to evaluate for tumor recurrence in 35 patients who underwent imaging by both FDG-PET and contrast-enhanced MR.[59] False positives were observed by both modalities in the cases of 2 meningiomas and 1 radiation necrosis. In patients who underwent stereotactic radiosurgery, FDG-PET was found to have superior accuracy in evaluating treatment effects on gliomas compared with brain metastases.[60] When PET and contrast-enhanced MR images were coregistered, sensitivity and specificity of 86% and 80% respectively, were obtained. Defining PET-positive findings as any uptake in enhancing regions or uptake greater than adjacent tissue, this study demonstrated high sensitivity without overly compromising specificity.

Compared with the histologic results of 20 patients, FDG-PET findings were found concordant in 15 patients and discordant in 5 patients who had undergone intensive radiotherapy.[61] The investigators concluded that FDG-PET may have less utility depending on the radiotherapy protocol used. PET-positive findings were determined in this study by comparing uptake in the lesion with uptake in the adjacent area or the contralateral hemisphere. A semiquantitative visual score was used by Ricci and colleagues[62] to differentiate radiation necrosis and tumor recurrence in 31 patients by assessing for FDG uptake in lesions greater than or equal to that of the cortex. Compared with histologic diagnoses, FDG-PET was determined to have a sensitivity of 73% and a specificity of 56%. These studies demonstrate the variability in methods used to assess for tumor recurrence, emphasizing the need for widely adopted objective standards in PET image analysis and quantification.

Response assessment has also been proposed with other PET tracers. Although the diagnostic accuracy of FET-PET and FDOPA-PET have been reported to be approximately 80% to 90%,[16,63–68] the accuracy of MET-PET is slightly lower, possibly due to tracer affinity for inflammation.[69–71] Galldiks and colleagues[64] found that FET-PET was able to distinguish pseudoprogression from true progression in 22 patients with treated glioblastoma who presented with concerning MR contrast enhancement (**Fig. 3**). A meta-analysis of 799 patients evaluating the use of FLT-PET in this domain did not demonstrate significant superiority compared with FDG-PET.[72] PET imaging with ^{11}C-choline also has been

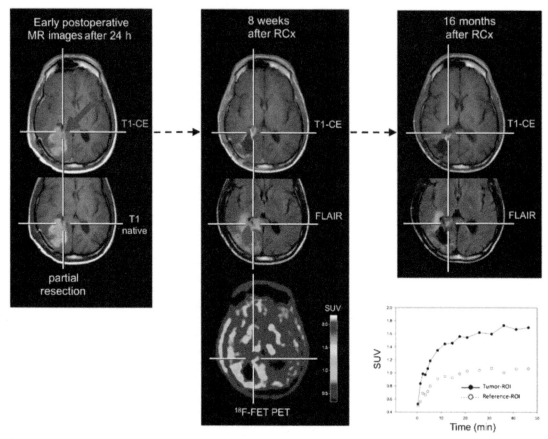

Fig. 3. PET and MR imaging in a 34-year-old glioblastoma patient (patient 7, pseudoprogression group, MGMT promoter methylated) 24 hours after resection and 8 weeks and 16 months after completion of radiochemother-apy (RCx). The early postoperative MR images (*left*) show a small point-shaped residual contrast-enhancing (CE) tumor in the right parietooccipital area (*red arrow* [diameter, 5 mm]). The follow-up MR images 8 weeks after completion of radiochemotherapy suggest tumor progression (*middle, top image*). In contrast, in the area spatially corresponding to the enlarged contrast enhancement, the ^{18}F-FET PET image shows no metabolic active tumor. Dorsolateral to the resection hole, slightly increased metabolic activity (TBR$_{max}$ 1.6) with ^{18}F-FET uptake kinetic pattern I is present. Follow-up MR images after 16 months show a slightly reduced contrast enhancement and FLAIR signal alteration (*right*). After a follow-up of 17 months without any change in treatment, the patient was still alive, clinically stable, and free of tumor progression. MGMT, O^6-methylguanine-DNA methyltransferase; FLAIR, fluid-attenuated inversion recovery. (*From* Galldiks N, Dunkl V, Stoffels G, Hutterer M, Rapp M, Sabel M, et al. Diagnosis of pseudoprogression in patients with glioblastoma using O-(2-[18F]fluoroethyl)-L-tyrosine PET. Eur J Nucl Med Mol Imaging. 2015;42(5):685-95; with permission.)

investigated with a meta-analysis of 118 subjects, which suggests that it is a highly sensitive and spe-cific method of discriminating between true pro-gression and pseudoprogression.[73] These data pose several questions regarding the utility of non-FDG tracers in the identification of these pa-thologies, and further studies are warranted to further elicit their utility in this area.

PROGNOSIS

As discussed previously, conventional modalities, such as CT and MR, suffer from low specificity, which limits their utility in predicting patient sur-vival. Biopsy procedures are hampered by both

their invasiveness and their lack of generalizability as a result of tumor heterogeneity and tumor trans-formation over time. Alternatively, FDG-PET has been established as a powerful predictor of patient outcomes, especially in gliomas.[74,75] The predic-tive power of FDG-PET even has been suggested to be superior to that of pathology according to Di Chiro and Fulham.[76] Several studies have demon-strated that increased FDG uptake in brain tumors after therapy is associated with shorter sur-vival.[77–80] It was found that in 55 high-grade gli-oma patients with MR findings consistent with tumor recurrence, FDG uptake was an indepen-dent predictor of survival.[81] The implications for patient management were investigated in 75 glioma patients.[82] Data acquired from FDG-PET scans contributed to the decision to initiate or withhold treatment in 97% of cases. Furthermore, these decisions were based on PET findings alone in 28% of cases. These results are consistent with another study that showed in 30 patients with suspected tumor progression without surgical confirmation, FDG-PET contributed to the management of 24 patients.[61]

Several known observations must be taken into consideration when interpreting FDG-PET images. For example, edema resulting from radiation injury or BBB breakdown is associated with hypometabolism of the adjacent cortex. This pattern of cortical suppression should not be confused with radiation necrosis, which typically is less extensive.[52] Edema as the etiology for this pattern of hypometabolism has been confirmed by Pourdehnad and colleagues,[83] who correlated FDG-PET with MR in a study of 29 patients. Hypometabolism visualized by PET often can be correlated clinically, such as in visual field defects caused by edema of the visual cortex, and seems to represent a reversible phenomenon.[52] In addition, decreased FDG uptake in the contralateral cerebellum is associated with many supratentorial disorders, such as head injury and stroke, but the implication of this observation is not yet clear.[52]

ALTERNATIVE PET TRACERS

Through its interaction with 5 subtypes of somatostatin receptors (SSTRs), somatostatin plays a role in neurotransmission and cell growth inhibition. SSTR expression can be assessed by PET imaging with ^{68}Ga-DOTA peptides (^{68}Ga-DOTA-TOC, ^{68}Ga-DOTA- NOC, and ^{68}Ga-DOTA-TATE), which have a particular affinity for SSTR2.[9,84] Various CNS tumors, such as gliomas, meningiomas, primitive neuroendocrine tumors, and medulloblastomas, express SSTRs to varying degrees.[85–90] Because SSTR expression is higher in meningiomas compared with normal leptomeningeal tissue, ^{68}Ga-DOTA peptides may have a potential role in the diagnosis and delineation of meningiomas.[91–93] A study of 134 subjects found that PET/CT with ^{68}Ga-DOTA tracers could detect meningiomas that were missed by contrast-enhanced MR (**Fig. 4**).[92] Further investigation into the potential applications of ^{68}Ga-DOTA tracers in determining glioma grade, which is correlated inversely with SSTR expression, and evaluating medulloblastomas, which express high levels of SSTR2 and SSTR3, may be warranted.[86,94–96]

With its primary use in prostate cancer, ^{68}Ga-PSMA (prostate-specific membrane antigen) tracer uptake is not demonstrated in healthy brain tissue. As a result, brain metastases from prostate cancer are easily visualized by ^{68}Ga-PSMA–PET. In addition, it meningiomas, schwannomas, peripheral nerve sheath tumors, and other benign conditions of the nervous system express PSMA and, therefore, may show uptake by ^{68}Ga-PSMA tracers.[97–104] Therefore, activity portrayed by ^{68}Ga-PSMA–PET in the brain may be used to evaluate certain tumors, and incidental uptake should prompt a further work-up for primary causes.

Immuno-PET uses antibody-derived tracers to visualize the expression of tumor-related antigens.[16] In a mouse model of glioblastoma, an ^{89}Zr-labeled monoclonal antibody (^{89}Zr(zirconium)-Df-YY146) was used to evaluate CD146 expression by tumor cells.[105] A strong correlation between uptake of ^{89}Zr-Df-YY146 and CD146 expression caused the authors to conclude that immuno-PET has the potential to guide therapy and assess tumor response. With additional larger prospective studies, these results may have critical consequences in advancing the diagnostic imaging of glioblastoma.

DISCUSSION

The introduction of FDG in August 1976 opened a new era in medical imaging and has had a major impact on the management of many diseases and disorders over the past 4 decades.[106] Although early investigation demonstrated its role in neuropsychiatric disorders, over the years, this tracer has been shown to be effective in detecting a variety of common human diseases, including cancer, inflammation, and metabolic abnormalities.[107–109] Due to the lack of total-body PET imaging capabilities in the 1970s and 1980s, most research studies that were conducted early on in the development of this modality dealt with brain disorders. Although neurology was the main focus of these foundational research studies, efforts were made by investigators at the National Institutes of Health and University of Pennsylvania to examine patients with brain tumors. These early studies clearly demonstrated the potential role of FDG-PET imaging for assessing cancer in general, and particularly in brain tumors, because this malignancy is the most aggressive cancer in human beings.[110] These early investigators were able to show that FDG-PET can differentiate between low-grade and high-grade presentations based on quantitative measurements of glucose metabolism in these tumors. Also, these pioneering studies demonstrated the prognostic importance of FDG in predicting patient outcomes in these serious malignancies. In addition, FDG elucidated the deleterious effects of this cancer in the

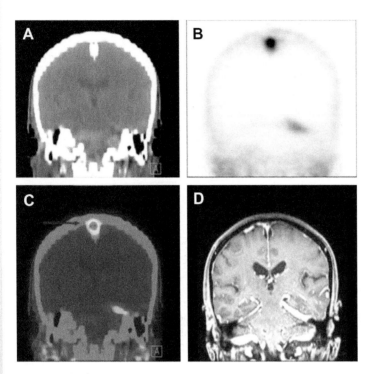

Fig. 4. Detection of a meningioma adjacent to the falx cerebri only by 68Ga-DOTATOC PET/CT: (*A*) *t*he CT image clearly shows a calcified mass; (*B*) PET image; (*C*) the fused PET/CT image shows typical focal radiotracer uptake (*red arrow*); and (*D*) the gadolinium-DTPA enhanced MR image shows a small area of enhancement on the meningeal mass. (*From* Afshar-Oromieh A, Giesel FL, Linhart HG, Haberkorn U, Haufe S, Combs SE, et al. Detection of cranial meningiomas: comparison of (6)(8)Ga-DOTA-TOC PET/CT and contrast-enhanced MRI. Eur J Nucl Med Mol Imaging. 2012;39(9):1409-15; with permission.)

ipsilateral brain hemisphere as well as in the contralateral cerebellum, which was shown to have significantly reduced glucose metabolism.[111]

One of the first attempts made to use a non-FDG tracer with PET was in brain tumors by employing MET for detection and characterization.[112] Over the ensuing 40 years, many similar tracers have been introduced and have been reported to be very effective in characterizing brain tumors.[113,114] Most of such tracers are amino acid derivatives and have been employed for imaging studies elsewhere in the body with minimal success.[115,116] Therefore, assessing brain tumors has become the main applications of these failed tracers in malignances of other organs.

Proponents of such approaches have criticized FDG-PET imaging for having limited value in brain tumors because of its nonspecific uptake in the cortex adjacent to brain tumors located in the white matter.[117,118] This logic would have been acceptable if this phenomenon was a major drawback for FDG as a useful tracer for this purpose. Over the years, the authors and other groups have demonstrated that brain tumors are associated with significant edema in the surrounding white matter, which can be readily visualized by MR.[83,119,120] Such edema frequently is associated with significant suppression of cortical uptake of FDG. Therefore, the validity of the argument by the proponents of non-FDG tracers in examining brain tumors is questionable. Based on numerous published articles on this topic in the literature, tumors with mild to moderate uptake can be distinctly visualized by FDG-PET imaging without interference from the surrounding cortical structures, particularly when fused with MR to correct delineation. Furthermore, the nonspecific uptake of FDG has been used as an argument in the discussion. This nonspecific uptake, however, also is applicable to most of the amino acid tracers.

As in other malignancies, it has been shown that uptake of FDG in brain tumors increases substantially over time and reaches a plateau within several hours. In contrast, FDG uptake in the cortex and other gray matter structures start to decline after 1 hour after the administration of this compound. Therefore, acquiring brain images 2 hours to 3 hours after the injection of FDG substantially enhances the contrast between the tumor and adjacent structures. As such, the performance of FDG-PET in this setting can improve significantly by performing delayed imaging.[17] The recent introduction of PET/MR machines as a practical imaging tool could have a major impact on the role of FDG-PET in assessing brain tumor.[18,121] The high sensitivity and simultaneous acquisition of high-quality images over several hours may have the potential to improve diagnostic efficacy and patient outcomes. In addition, total-body PET instrumentation may additionally serve to improve outcomes, particularly in metastatic disease.[28,122]

BBB breakdown, which is noted in most brain tumors and other cerebral lesions, has been the basis for visualizing such abnormalities by medical imaging techniques. For decades, technetium-based radiotracers were used to detect brain tumors by conventional planar imaging as well as SPECT. Applications of both CT and MR techniques in assessing brain tumors are based heavily on administering contrast agents (iodinated compounds for CT and gadolinium-diethylenetriaminepentaacetic acid for MR) to detect BBB abnormalities.[123,124] Breakdown of the BBB in brain tumors leads to enhanced leakage of these contrast agents in brain tumors. In contrast to FDG, which reveals the true metabolic activity of brain tumors, uptake of most other PET tracers, including radiolabeled amino acids, is associated with the permeable BBB in these lesions, which may be a result of various extraneous processes that do not necessarily reflect the degree or extent of malignancy. Therefore, PET imaging with such tracers mostly leads to visualization of BBB abnormalities that are similarly noted by CT and MR. As such, assessing tumor grade and complications related to radiation therapy with these tracers is somewhat questionable and unjustified at this time.

CLINICS CARE POINTS

- Hybrid modalities involving PET will play a growing role in diagnosing, monitoring, and prognosticating brain tumors.

- By portraying glucose uptake, FDG not only aids in the identification of tumors but can also characterize response to therapy in order to predict patient outcomes. FDG-PET has been extensively validated and confirmed as a suitable modality to evaluate brain tumors.

- Other PET tracers to assess brain tumors are currently under development. However, there is still lack of evidence that many of these experimental tracers, especially amino acid tracers, contribute information beyond what is visible on CT and MR imaging.

DISCLOSURE

The authors have nothing to disclose.

REFERENCES

1. Barnholtz-Sloan JS, Sloan AE, Davis FG, et al. Incidence proportions of brain metastases in patients diagnosed (1973 to 2001) in the Metropolitan Detroit Cancer Surveillance System. J Clin Oncol 2004;22(14):2865–72.
2. Valiente M, Ahluwalia MS, Boire A, et al. The evolving landscape of brain metastasis. Trends Cancer 2018;4(3):176–96.
3. Cagney DN, Martin AM, Catalano PJ, et al. Incidence and prognosis of patients with brain metastases at diagnosis of systemic malignancy: a population-based study. Neuro Oncol 2017; 19(11):1511–21.
4. Ostrom QT, Gittleman H, Liao P, et al. CBTRUS statistical report: primary brain and other central nervous system tumors diagnosed in the United States in 2010-2014. Neuro Oncol 2017;19(suppl_5):v1–88.
5. Wang KY, Chen MM, Malayil Lincoln CM. Adult primary brain neoplasm, including 2016 World Health Organization Classification. Radiol Clin North Am 2019;57(6):1147–62.
6. Barnholtz-Sloan JS, Ostrom QT, Cote D. Epidemiology of brain tumors. Neurol Clin 2018;36(3):395–419.
7. Gupta A, Dwivedi T. A simplified overview of World Health Organization classification update of central nervous system tumors 2016. J Neurosci Rural Pract 2017;8(4):629–41.
8. Louis DN, Perry A, Reifenberger G, et al. The 2016 World Health Organization classification of tumors of the central nervous system: a summary. Acta Neuropathol 2016;131(6):803–20.
9. Shooli H, Dadgar H, Wang YJ, et al. An update on PET-based molecular imaging in neuro-oncology: challenges and implementation for a precision medicine approach in cancer care. Quant Imaging Med Surg 2019;9(9):1597–610.
10. Felix R, Schörner W, Laniado M, et al. Brain tumors: MR imaging with gadolinium-DTPA. Radiology 1985;156(3):681–8.
11. Zhou Z, Lu ZR. Gadolinium-based contrast agents for magnetic resonance cancer imaging. Wiley Interdiscip Rev Nanomed Nanobiotechnol 2013; 5(1):1–18.
12. Nandu H, Wen PY, Huang RY. Imaging in neuro-oncology. Ther Adv Neurol Disord 2018;11. 1756286418759865.
13. Sharma A, McConathy J. Overview of PET tracers for brain tumor imaging. PET Clin 2013;8(2):129–46.
14. Hygino da Cruz LC Jr, Rodriguez I, Domingues RC, et al. Pseudoprogression and pseudoresponse: imaging challenges in the assessment of posttreatment glioma. AJNR Am J Neuroradiol 2011;32(11):1978–85.
15. Dhermain FG, Hau P, Lanfermann H, et al. Advanced MRI and PET imaging for assessment of treatment response in patients with gliomas. Lancet Neurol 2010;9(9):906–20.

16. Werner JM, Lohmann P, Fink GR, et al. Current landscape and emerging fields of PET imaging in patients with brain tumors. Molecules 2020;25(6): 1471.

17. Basu S, Alavi A. Molecular imaging (PET) of brain tumors. Neuroimaging Clin N Am 2009;19(4):625–46.

18. Weber W. Clinical PET/MR. Recent Results Cancer Res 2020;216:747–64.

19. Borja AJ, Hancin EC, Khosravi M, et al. Applications of hybrid PET/magnetic resonance imaging in central nervous system disorders. PET Clin 2020;15(4):497–508.

20. Spence AM, Muzi M, Mankoff DA, et al. 18F-FDG PET of gliomas at delayed intervals: improved distinction between tumor and normal gray matter. J Nucl Med 2004;45(10):1653–9.

21. McConathy J, Yu W, Jarkas N, et al. Radiohalogenated nonnatural amino acids as PET and SPECT tumor imaging agents. Med Res Rev 2012;32(4): 868–905.

22. Ulaner GA, Goldman DA, Corben A, et al. Prospective clinical trial of (18)F-Fluciclovine PET/CT for determining the response to neoadjuvant therapy in invasive ductal and invasive lobular breast cancers. J Nucl Med 2017;58(7):1037–42.

23. Pauleit D, Floeth F, Hamacher K, et al. O-(2-[18F] fluoroethyl)-L-tyrosine PET combined with MRI improves the diagnostic assessment of cerebral gliomas. Brain 2005;128(Pt 3):678–87.

24. Kracht LW, Miletic H, Busch S, et al. Delineation of brain tumor extent with [11C]L-methionine positron emission tomography: local comparison with stereotactic histopathology. Clin Cancer Res 2004; 10(21):7163–70.

25. Galldiks N, Ullrich R, Schroeter M, et al. Volumetry of [(11)C]-methionine PET uptake and MRI contrast enhancement in patients with recurrent glioblastoma multiforme. Eur J Nucl Med Mol Imaging 2010;37(1):84–92.

26. Langen KJ, Galldiks N, Hattingen E, et al. Advances in neuro-oncology imaging. Nat Rev Neurol 2017;13(5):279–89.

27. Lohmann P, Stavrinou P, Lipke K, et al. FET PET reveals considerable spatial differences in tumour burden compared to conventional MRI in newly diagnosed glioblastoma. Eur J Nucl Med Mol Imaging 2019;46(3):591–602.

28. Grosu AL, Weber WA, Franz M, et al. Reirradiation of recurrent high-grade gliomas using amino acid PET (SPECT)/CT/MRI image fusion to determine gross tumor volume for stereotactic fractionated radiotherapy. Int J Radiat Oncol Biol Phys 2005; 63(2):511–9.

29. Venneti S, Dunphy MP, Zhang H, et al. Glutamine-based PET imaging facilitates enhanced metabolic evaluation of gliomas in vivo. Sci Transl Med 2015; 7(274):274ra17.

30. Jansen NL, Graute V, Armbruster L, et al. MRI-suspected low-grade glioma: is there a need to perform dynamic FET PET? Eur J Nucl Med Mol Imaging 2012;39(6):1021–9.

31. Hutterer M, Nowosielski M, Putzer D, et al. [18F]-fluoro-ethyl-L-tyrosine PET: a valuable diagnostic tool in neuro-oncology, but not all that glitters is glioma. Neuro Oncol 2013;15(3):341–51.

32. Pichler R, Dunzinger A, Wurm G, et al. Is there a place for FET PET in the initial evaluation of brain lesions with unknown significance? Eur J Nucl Med Mol Imaging 2010;37(8):1521–8.

33. Kawai N, Maeda Y, Kudomi N, et al. Correlation of biological aggressiveness assessed by 11C-methionine PET and hypoxic burden assessed by 18F-fluoromisonidazole PET in newly diagnosed glioblastoma. Eur J Nucl Med Mol Imaging 2011; 38(3):441–50.

34. Miner MW, Liljenbäck H, Virta J, et al. (2S, 4R)-4-[(18)F]Fluoroglutamine for in vivo PET imaging of glioma xenografts in mice: an evaluation of multiple pharmacokinetic models. Mol Imaging Biol 2020; 22(4):969–78.

35. Montagne A, Toga AW, Zlokovic BV. Blood-brain barrier permeability and gadolinium: benefits and potential pitfalls in research. JAMA Neurol 2016;73(1):13–4.

36. Nowosielski M, DiFranco MD, Putzer D, et al. An intra-individual comparison of MRI, [18F]-FET and [18F]-FLT PET in patients with high-grade gliomas. PLoS One 2014;9(4):e95830.

37. Pöpperl G, Götz C, Rachinger W, et al. Value of O-(2-[18F]fluoroethyl)- L-tyrosine PET for the diagnosis of recurrent glioma. Eur J Nucl Med Mol Imaging 2004;31(11):1464–70.

38. Jacobs AH, Thomas A, Kracht LW, et al. 18F-fluoro-L-thymidine and 11C-methylmethionine as markers of increased transport and proliferation in brain tumors. J Nucl Med 2005;46(12):1948–58.

39. Saga T, Kawashima H, Araki N, et al. Evaluation of primary brain tumors with FLT-PET: usefulness and limitations. Clin Nucl Med 2006;31(12):774–80.

40. Albert NL, Unterrainer M, Fleischmann DF, et al. TSPO PET for glioma imaging using the novel ligand (18)F-GE-180: first results in patients with glioblastoma. Eur J Nucl Med Mol Imaging 2017; 44(13):2230–8.

41. Unterrainer M, Fleischmann DF, Diekmann C, et al. Comparison of (18)F-GE-180 and dynamic (18)F-FET PET in high grade glioma: a double-tracer pilot study. Eur J Nucl Med Mol Imaging 2019;46(3): 580–90.

42. Zanotti-Fregonara P, Pascual B, Rostomily RC, et al. Anatomy of (18)F-GE180, a failed radioligand for the TSPO protein. Eur J Nucl Med Mol Imaging 2020;47(10):2233–6.

43. Geisler S, Stegmayr C, Niemitz N, et al. Treatment-Related Uptake of O-(2-(18)F-Fluoroethyl)-l-

Tyrosine and I-[Methyl-(3)H]-Methionine After Tumor Resection in Rat Glioma Models. J Nucl Med 2019;60(10):1373–9.

44. Lescher S, Schniewindt S, Jurcoane A, et al. Time window for postoperative reactive enhancement after resection of brain tumors: less than 72 hours. Neurosurg Focus 2014;37(6):E3.

45. Dunet V, Pomoni A, Hottinger A, et al. Performance of 18F-FET versus 18F-FDG-PET for the diagnosis and grading of brain tumors: systematic review and meta-analysis. Neuro Oncol 2016;18(3):426–34.

46. Albert NL, Weller M, Suchorska B, et al. Response Assessment in Neuro-Oncology working group and European Association for neuro-Oncology recommendations for the clinical use of PET imaging in gliomas. Neuro Oncol 2016;18(9):1199–208.

47. Kim S, Chung JK, Im SH, et al. 11C-methionine PET as a prognostic marker in patients with glioma: comparison with 18F-FDG PET. Eur J Nucl Med Mol Imaging 2005;32(1):52–9.

48. Vomacka L, Unterrainer M, Holzgreve A, et al. Voxel-wise analysis of dynamic (18)F-FET PET: a novel approach for non-invasive glioma characterisation. EJNMMI Res 2018;8(1):91.

49. Collet S, Valable S, Constans JM, et al. [(18)F]-fluoro-L-thymidine PET and advanced MRI for preoperative grading of gliomas. Neuroimage Clin 2015; 8:448–54.

50. Galldiks N, Lohmann P, Albert NL, et al. Current status of PET imaging in neuro-oncology. Neurooncol Adv 2019;1(1):vdz010.

51. Tan AC, Ashley DM, Lopez GY, et al. Management of glioblastoma: state of the art and future directions. CA Cancer J Clin 2020;70(4):299–312.

52. Hustinx R, Pourdehnad M, Kaschten B, et al. PET imaging for differentiating recurrent brain tumor from radiation necrosis. Radiol Clin North Am 2005;43(1):35–47.

53. Verma N, Cowperthwaite MC, Burnett MG, et al. Differentiating tumor recurrence from treatment necrosis: a review of neuro-oncologic imaging strategies. Neuro Oncol 2013;15(5):515–34.

54. Chen W. Clinical applications of PET in brain tumors. J Nucl Med 2007;48(9):1468–81.

55. Patronas NJ, Di Chiro G, Brooks RA, et al. Work in progress: [18F] fluorodeoxyglucose and positron emission tomography in the evaluation of radiation necrosis of the brain. Radiology 1982;144(4):885–9.

56. Di Chiro G, Oldfield E, Wright DC, et al. Cerebral necrosis after radiotherapy and/or intraarterial chemotherapy for brain tumors: PET and neuropathologic studies. AJR Am J Roentgenol 1988; 150(1):189–97.

57. Doyle WK, Budinger TF, Valk PE, et al. Differentiation of cerebral radiation necrosis from tumor recurrence by [18F]FDG and 82Rb positron emission tomography. J Comput Assist Tomogr 1987;11(4):563–70.

58. Valk PE, Budinger TF, Levin VA, et al. PET of malignant cerebral tumors after interstitial brachytherapy. Demonstration of metabolic activity and correlation with clinical outcome. J Neurosurg 1988;69(6):830–8.

59. Davis WK, Boyko OB, Hoffman JM, et al. [18F]2-fluoro-2-deoxyglucose-positron emission tomography correlation of gadolinium-enhanced MR imaging of central nervous system neoplasia. AJNR Am J Neuroradiol 1993;14(3):515–23.

60. Chao ST, Suh JH, Raja S, et al. The sensitivity and specificity of FDG PET in distinguishing recurrent brain tumor from radionecrosis in patients treated with stereotactic radiosurgery. Int J Cancer 2001; 96(3):191–7.

61. Janus TJ, Kim EE, Tilbury R, et al. Use of [18F]fluorodeoxyglucose positron emission tomography in patients with primary malignant brain tumors. Ann Neurol 1993;33(5):540–8.

62. Ricci PE, Karis JP, Heiserman JE, et al. Differentiating recurrent tumor from radiation necrosis: time for re-evaluation of positron emission tomography? AJNR Am J Neuroradiol 1998;19(3):407–13.

63. Ceccon G, Lohmann P, Stoffels G, et al. Dynamic O-(2-18F-fluoroethyl)-L-tyrosine positron emission tomography differentiates brain metastasis recurrence from radiation injury after radiotherapy. Neuro Oncol 2017;19(2):281–8.

64. Galldiks N, Dunkl V, Stoffels G, et al. Diagnosis of pseudoprogression in patients with glioblastoma using O-(2-[18F]fluoroethyl)-L-tyrosine PET. Eur J Nucl Med Mol Imaging 2015;42(5):685–95.

65. Kebir S, Fimmers R, Galldiks N, et al. Late pseudoprogression in glioblastoma: diagnostic value of dynamic O-(2-[18F]fluoroethyl)-L-Tyrosine PET. Clin Cancer Res 2016;22(9):2190–6.

66. Werner JM, Stoffels G, Lichtenstein T, et al. Differentiation of treatment-related changes from tumour progression: a direct comparison between dynamic FET PET and ADC values obtained from DWI MRI. Eur J Nucl Med Mol Imaging 2019;46(9):1889–901.

67. Cicone F, Minniti G, Romano A, et al. Accuracy of F-DOPA PET and perfusion-MRI for differentiating radionecrotic from progressive brain metastases after radiosurgery. Eur J Nucl Med Mol Imaging 2015;42(1):103–11.

68. Lizarraga KJ, Allen-Auerbach M, Czernin J, et al. 18)F-FDOPA PET for differentiating recurrent or progressive brain metastatic tumors from late or delayed radiation injury after radiation treatment. J Nucl Med 2014;55(1):30–6.

69. Salber D, Stoffels G, Pauleit D, et al. Differential uptake of O-(2-18F-fluoroethyl)-L-tyrosine, L-3H-methionine, and 3H-deoxyglucose in brain abscesses. J Nucl Med 2007;48(12):2056–62.

70. Minamimoto R, Saginoya T, Kondo C, et al. Differentiation of brain tumor recurrence from post-

radiotherapy necrosis with 11C-methionine PET: visual assessment versus quantitative assessment. PLoS One 2015;10(7):e0132515.

71. Nihashi T, Dahabreh IJ, Terasawa T. Diagnostic accuracy of PET for recurrent glioma diagnosis: a meta-analysis. AJNR Am J Neuroradiol 2013; 34(5):944–50. S1-11.

72. Li Z, Yu Y, Zhang H, et al. A meta-analysis comparing 18F-FLT PET with 18F-FDG PET for assessment of brain tumor recurrence. Nucl Med Commun 2015;36(7):695–701.

73. Gao L, Xu W, Li T, et al. Accuracy of 11C-choline positron emission tomography in differentiating glioma recurrence from radiation necrosis: a systematic review and meta-analysis. Medicine (Baltimore) 2018;97(29):e11556.

74. Padma MV, Said S, Jacobs M, et al. Prediction of pathology and survival by FDG PET in gliomas. J Neurooncol 2003;64(3):227–37.

75. Alavi JB, Alavi A, Chawluk J, et al. Positron emission tomography in patients with glioma. A predictor of prognosis. Cancer 1988;62(6):1074–8.

76. Di Chiro G, Fulham MJ. Virchow's shackles: can PET-FDG challenge tumor histology? AJNR Am J Neuroradiol 1993;14(3):524–7.

77. Ericson K, Kihlstrom L, Mogard J, et al. Positron emission tomography using 18F-fluorodeoxyglucose in patients with stereotactically irradiated brain metastases. Stereotact Funct Neurosurg 1996;66(Suppl 1):214–24.

78. Mogard J, Kihlstrom L, Ericson K, et al. Recurrent tumor vs radiation effects after gamma knife radiosurgery of intracerebral metastases: diagnosis with PET-FDG. J Comput Assist Tomogr 1994;18(2): 177–81.

79. Belohlavek O, Simonova G, Kantorova I, et al. Brain metastases after stereotactic radiosurgery using the Leksell gamma knife: can FDG PET help to differentiate radionecrosis from tumour progression? Eur J Nucl Med Mol Imaging 2003;30(1):96–100.

80. Patronas NJ, Di Chiro G, Kufta C, et al. Prediction of survival in glioma patients by means of positron emission tomography. J Neurosurg 1985;62(6): 816–22.

81. Barker FG 2nd, Chang SM, Valk PE, et al. 18-Fluorodeoxyglucose uptake and survival of patients with suspected recurrent malignant glioma. Cancer 1997;79(1):115–26.

82. Deshmukh A, Scott JA, Palmer EL, et al. Impact of fluorodeoxyglucose positron emission tomography on the clinical management of patients with glioma. Clin Nucl Med 1996;21(9):720–5.

83. Pourdehnad M, Basu S, Duarte P, et al. Reduced grey matter metabolism due to white matter edema allows optimal assessment of brain tumors on 18F-FDG-PET. Hell J Nucl Med 2011;14(3): 219–23.

84. Shimon I. Somatostatin receptors in pituitary and development of somatostatin receptor subtype-selective analogs. Endocrine 2003;20(3):265–9.

85. Bashir A, Broholm H, Clasen-Linde E, et al. Pearls and pitfalls in interpretation of 68Ga-DOTATOC PET imaging. Clin Nucl Med 2020;45(6):e279–80.

86. Lee H, Suh M, Choi H, et al. A pan-cancer analysis of the clinical and genetic portraits of somatostatin receptor expressing tumor as a potential target of peptide receptor imaging and therapy. EJNMMI Res 2020;10(1):42.

87. Dutour A, Kumar U, Panetta R, et al. Expression of somatostatin receptor subtypes in human brain tumors. Int J Cancer 1998;76(5):620–7.

88. Fruhwald MC, Rickert CH, O'Dorisio MS, et al. Somatostatin receptor subtype 2 is expressed by supratentorial primitive neuroectodermal tumors of childhood and can be targeted for somatostatin receptor imaging. Clin Cancer Res 2004;10(9): 2997–3006.

89. Fruhwald MC, O'Dorisio MS, Pietsch T, et al. High expression of somatostatin receptor subtype 2 (sst2) in medulloblastoma: implications for diagnosis and therapy. Pediatr Res 1999;45(5 Pt 1):697–708.

90. Ramirez C, Cheng S, Vargas G, et al. Expression of Ki-67, PTTG1, FGFR4, and SSTR 2, 3, and 5 in nonfunctioning pituitary adenomas: a high throughput TMA, immunohistochemical study. J Clin Endocrinol Metab 2012;97(5):1745–51.

91. Gehler B, Paulsen F, Oksuz MO, et al. [68Ga]-DOTATOC-PET/CT for meningioma IMRT treatment planning. Radiat Oncol 2009;4:56.

92. Afshar-Oromieh A, Giesel FL, Linhart HG, et al. Detection of cranial meningiomas: comparison of (6)(8)Ga-DOTATOC PET/CT and contrast-enhanced MRI. Eur J Nucl Med Mol Imaging 2012;39(9):1409–15.

93. Reubi JC, Maurer R, Klijn JG, et al. High incidence of somatostatin receptors in human meningiomas: biochemical characterization. J Clin Endocrinol Metab 1986;63(2):433–8.

94. Kiviniemi A, Gardberg M, Frantzen J, et al. Somatostatin receptor subtype 2 in high-grade gliomas: PET/CT with (68)Ga-DOTA-peptides, correlation to prognostic markers, and implications for targeted radiotherapy. EJNMMI Res 2015;5:25.

95. Kiviniemi A, Gardberg M, Kivinen K, et al. Somatostatin receptor 2A in gliomas: association with oligodendrogliomas and favourable outcome. Oncotarget 2017;8(30):49123–32.

96. Cervera P, Videau C, Viollet C, et al. Comparison of somatostatin receptor expression in human gliomas and medulloblastomas. J Neuroendocrinol 2002;14(6):458–71.

97. Chan M, Hsiao E. Subacute cortical infarct showing uptake on 68Ga-PSMA PET/CT. Clin Nucl Med 2017;42(2):110–1.

98. Vamadevan S, Le K, Shen L, et al. Incidental prostate-specific membrane antigen uptake in a peripheral nerve sheath tumor. Clin Nucl Med 2017;42(7):560–2.

99. Rischpler C, Maurer T, Schwaiger M, et al. Intense PSMA-expression using (68)Ga-PSMA PET/CT in a paravertebral schwannoma mimicking prostate cancer metastasis. Eur J Nucl Med Mol Imaging 2016;43(1):193–4.

100. Kanthan GL, Izard MA, Emmett L, et al. Schwannoma showing avid uptake on 68Ga-PSMA-HBED-CC PET/CT. Clin Nucl Med 2016;41(9):703–4.

101. Jain TK, Jois AG, Kumar VS, et al. Incidental detection of tracer avidity in meningioma in (68)Ga-PSMA PET/CT during initial staging for prostate cancer. Rev Esp Med Nucl Imagen Mol 2017;36(2):133–4.

102. Bilgin R, Ergul N, Cermik TF. Incidental meningioma mimicking metastasis of prostate adenocarcinoma in 68Ga-labeled PSMA ligand PET/CT. Clin Nucl Med 2016;41(12):956–8.

103. Sheikhbahaei S, Afshar-Oromieh A, Eiber M, et al. Pearls and pitfalls in clinical interpretation of prostate-specific membrane antigen (PSMA)-targeted PET imaging. Eur J Nucl Med Mol Imaging 2017;44(12):2117–36.

104. Malik D, Sood A, Mittal BR, et al. Nonspecific uptake of (68)Ga-Prostate-specific membrane antigen in diseases other than prostate malignancy on positron emission tomography/computed tomography imaging: a pictorial assay and review of literature. Indian J Nucl Med 2018;33(4):317–25.

105. Hernandez R, Sun H, England CG, et al. Immuno-PET imaging of CD146 expression in malignant brain tumors. Mol Pharm 2016;13(7):2563–70.

106. Hoilund-Carlsen PF. Abass Alavi: a giant in nuclear medicine turns 80 and is still going strong! Hell J Nucl Med 2018;21(1):85–7.

107. Vaidyanathan S, Patel CN, Scarsbrook AF, et al. FDG PET/CT in infection and inflammation–current and emerging clinical applications. Clin Radiol 2015;70(7):787–800.

108. Borja AJ, Hancin EC, Dreyfuss AD, et al. 18F-FDG-PET/CT in the quantification of photon radiation therapy-induced vasculitis. Am J Nucl Med Mol Imaging 2020;10(1):66.

109. Borja AJ, Hancin EC, Zhang V, Revheim ME, Alavi A. Potential of PET/CT in assessing dementias with emphasis on cerebrovascular disorders. Eur J Nucl Med Mol Imaging 2020;47(11):2493–8.

110. Seymour T, Nowak A, Kakulas F. Targeting aggressive cancer stem cells in glioblastoma. Front Oncol 2015;5:159.

111. Kajimoto K, Oku N, Kimura Y, et al. Crossed cerebellar diaschisis: a positron emission tomography study with l-[methyl-11 C] methionine and 2-deoxy-2-[18 F] fluoro-d-glucose. Ann Nucl Med 2007;21(2):109–13.

112. Bergström M, Collins VP, Ehrin E, et al. Discrepancies in brain tumor extent as shown by computed tomography and positron emission tomography using [68Ga]EDTA, [11C]glucose, and [11C]methionine. J Comput Assist Tomogr 1983;7(6):1062–6.

113. Nariai T, Tanaka Y, Wakimoto H, et al. Usefulness of L-[methyl-11C] methionine-positron emission tomography as a biological monitoring tool in the treatment of glioma. J Neurosurg 2005;103(3):498–507.

114. Ishiwata K, Kubota K, Murakami M, et al. Re-evaluation of amino acid PET studies: can the protein synthesis rates in brain and tumor tissues be measured in vivo? J Nucl Med 1993;34(11):1936–43.

115. Qi Y, Liu X, Li J, et al. Fluorine-18 labeled amino acids for tumor PET/CT imaging. Oncotarget 2017;8(36):60581–8.

116. Zhu A, Lee D, Shim H. Metabolic positron emission tomography imaging in cancer detection and therapy response. Semin Oncol 2011;38(1):55–69.

117. Jung JH, Ahn BC. Current radiopharmaceuticals for positron emission tomography of brain tumors. Brain Tumor Res Treat 2018;6(2):47–53.

118. Jeong YJ, Yoon HJ, Kang DY. Assessment of change in glucose metabolism in white matter of amyloid-positive patients with Alzheimer disease using F-18 FDG PET. Medicine (Baltimore) 2017;96(48):e9042.

119. Schneider T, Kuhne JF, Bittrich P, et al. Edema is not a reliable diagnostic sign to exclude small brain metastases. PLoS One 2017;12(5):e0177217.

120. Kaal EC, Vecht CJ. The management of brain edema in brain tumors. Curr Opin Oncol 2004;16(6):593–600.

121. Hassanzadeh C, Rao YJ, Chundury A, et al. Multiparametric MRI and [(18)F]Fluorodeoxyglucose positron emission tomography imaging is a potential prognostic imaging biomarker in recurrent glioblastoma. Front Oncol 2017;7:178.

122. Vandenberghe S, Moskal P, Karp JS. State of the art in total body PET. EJNMMI Phys 2020;7(1):35.

123. Pasternak JJ, Williamson EE. Clinical pharmacology, uses, and adverse reactions of iodinated contrast agents: a primer for the non-radiologist. Mayo Clin Proc 2012;87(4):390–402.

124. Ibrahim MA, Hazhirkarzar B, Dublin AB. Magnetic resonance imaging (MRI) gadolinium. StatPearls [Internet]. Treasure Island, FL: StatPearls Publishing; 2020.

Preclinical Evaluation of TSPO and MAO-B PET Radiotracers in an LPS Model of Neuroinflammation

Vidya Narayanaswami, PhD[a], Junchao Tong, PhD[b], Christin Schifani, PhD[c], Peter M. Bloomfield, MSc[d], Kenneth Dahl, PhD[e], Neil Vasdev, PhD[f],*

KEYWORDS

- LPS rat model • MAO-B • Neuroinflammation • PET biomarkers • TSPO

KEY POINTS

- A unilateral intrastriatal lipopolysaccharide rat model of neuroinflammation was characterized with the translocator protein 18-kDa (TSPO) tracer, [^{18}F]FEPPA, and the paradigm was extended to monoamine oxidase (MAO)-B PET tracers, [^{11}C]L-deprenyl and [^{11}C]SL25.1188.
- [^{18}F]FEPPA TSPO PET imaging proved to be a robust sensitive biomarker of the early phase of acute neuroinflammation in rats.
- [^{11}C]L-deprenyl detected a later phase of neuroinflammation ascribed to increased MAO-B expression, albeit with suboptimal sensitivity, whereas [^{11}C]SL25.1188 was not suitable for MAO-B PET imaging in rats.

INTRODUCTION

There is emerging interest in understanding the role of the neuroimmune system in the pathophysiology of neurodegenerative and psychiatric diseases.[1,2] Neuroinflammation is a dynamic and complex adaptive immune response triggered by cell damaging processes in the brain, which may include infection, toxins, autoimmunity, trauma, and responses to processes that change neuronal activity.[3,4] Hallmarks of a neuroimmune response involve activation of resident central nervous system (CNS) innate immune glial cells, predominantly microglia and astrocytes, accompanied by a dynamic biochemical cascade of inflammatory factors. This includes but is not limited to the production of cytokines, chemokines, secondary messengers, and reactive oxygen species that modify the CNS microenvironment.[5,6] Microglia and astrocytes function as both the source and target of these inflammatory cytokines and chemokines.[7,8] Acute neuroinflammatory responses are adaptive, promote neuronal survival, and restore homeostasis; however, if the neuroinflammatory response is not transient or tightly controlled within

[a] Azrieli Centre for Neuro-Radiochemistry, Brain Health Imaging Centre, Centre for Addiction and Mental Health, 250 College Street, Room 270, Toronto, Ontario M5T 1R8, Canada; [b] Brain Health Imaging Centre, Centre for Addiction and Mental Health, 250 College Street, Room 339, Toronto, Ontario M5T 1R8, Canada; [c] Brain Health Imaging Centre, Centre for Addiction and Mental Health, 250 College Street, Room 270, Toronto, Ontario M5T 1R8, Canada; [d] Brain Health Imaging Centre, Centre for Addiction and Mental Health, 250 College Street, Room B26A, Toronto, Ontario M5T 1R8, Canada; [e] Azrieli Centre for Neuro-Radiochemistry, Brain Health Imaging Centre, Centre for Addiction and Mental Health, 250 College Street, Room B02, Toronto, Ontario M5T 1R8, Canada; [f] Department of Psychiatry, Brain Health Imaging Centre, Azrieli Centre for Neuro-Radiochemistry, Centre for Addiction and Mental Health, University of Toronto, 250 College Street, Room PET G2, Toronto, Ontario M5T 1R8, Canada
* Corresponding author. 250 College Street, Room PET G2, Toronto, Ontario M5T 1R8, Canada.
E-mail address: neil.vasdev@utoronto.ca

PET Clin 16 (2021) 233–247
https://doi.org/10.1016/j.cpet.2020.12.003
1556-8598/21/© 2020 Elsevier Inc. All rights reserved.

the CNS, then it results in an uncontrolled, chronic neuroinflammatory response.[9] This chronic neuro-inflammatory state is deleterious due to excessive and dysregulated production of proinflammatory factors, resulting in synaptic impairment, oxidative damage, and mitochondrial dysfunction, which can lead to or exacerbate neurodegeneration.[10–13] Chronic neuroinflammatory response also may involve adaptive immunity, indicated by the recruitment and infiltration of peripheral immune cells, via disruption of the blood-brain barrier, which can further initiate neurodegenerative mechanisms.[14,15] Given that neuroinflammation is implicated as an important pathophysiologic mechanism underlying neurologic disorders, in vivo monitoring of neuroinflammation is gaining significant attention in therapeutic areas that include neurodegenerative and psychiatric diseases.

PET imaging biomarkers of neuroinflammation may provide an avenue for early diagnosis and delivery of therapeutics, tracking disease progression, and evaluating response to novel therapeutics in clinical trials.[16] The National Institute on Aging and the Alzheimer's Association created biological diagnostic recommendations for the preclinical, mild cognitive impairment (MCI), and dementia stages of Alzheimer disease (AD). Biomarkers recently have been grouped into (1) β-amyloid deposition; (2) pathologic tau; and (3) neurodegeneration, which collectively are referred to as AT(N).[17] To that end, early integration of quantitative molecular imaging, such as neurodegenerative/neuroinflammatory biomarkers, can be used to confirm drug-target engagement and establish pharmacokinetics of drugs and mechanism of drug action as well as to facilitate patient stratification and trial design.

PET BIOMARKERS OF MICROGLIAL AND ASTROCYTE ACTIVATION: TRANSLOCATOR PROTEIN AND MONOAMINE OXIDASE B

Translocator protein 18-kDa (TSPO), originally named the peripheral benzodiazepine receptor, is an 18-kDa outer mitochondrial membrane protein that is up-regulated in neuroinflammation; hence, it gathered immense clinical research interest as a PET biomarker to target neuroinflammation. Increased TSPO expression, evaluated in vitro using immunohistochemistry and in vivo using TSPO PET imaging, has been reported in clinical research and a wide variety of animal models of neuroinflammatory conditions, including AD, stroke, brain injury, experimental autoimmune encephalitis, and epilepsy.[18–23] Detailed information with regard to development and clinical significance as well as challenges and opportunities associated with clinical research application of TSPO PET radiopharmaceuticals are reviewed elsewhere.[3,4,24,25] Studies that employed the first-generation radioligand [11C]PK11195 reported higher TSPO PET brain signal in patients with amyotrophic lateral sclerosis, AD, and Parkinson disease and in brains of people at risk of Huntington disease compared with controls; however, increases in TSPO PET signal were not found in AD and multiple sclerosis patients in studies that employed second-generation TSPO ligands.[4] Discrepant results in human patient studies were attributed to large interindividual variability in PET signal. Second-generation TSPO ligands, such as [11C]PBR28, [18F]FEPPA, [11C]DAA1106, and [18F]DPA-713, have been subjected to a few limiting factors, including a single-nucleotide polymorphism in the TSPO gene (rs6971 polymorphism), which replaces alanine by threonine (Ala147Thr), subsequently influencing the binding affinity of TSPO ligands according to the exhibited genotype.[24,26] Specifically, second-generation TSPO ligands showed 3 different binding patterns: high-affinity binders (HABs) and low-affinity binders (LABs), that express a single binding site for TSPO with either high affinity or low affinity, respectively, and mixed-affinity binders that express approximately equal numbers of the high-affinity and low-affinity binding sites.[27–29] The impact of the TSPO gene polymorphism on second-generation TSPO tracer binding characteristics initiated a refined approach to clinical research, that is, to incorporate a screening procedure to genotype the participants for TSPO rs6971 polymorphism.[29] Such a revised clinical research protocol has been implemented at the authors' imaging center, where [18F]FEPPA, the fluoroethoxy derivative of PBR28, was developed and successfully translated for human PET imaging studies.[30] Compelling evidence of microglial activation in depression was provided by a human imaging study using [18F]FEPPA PET that demonstrated significant elevation of brain TSPO density in participants with depression compared with healthy controls.[31] Another [18F]FEPPA PET study reported increased TSPO levels in human subjects with cannabis use disorder compared to those in non–cannabis-using controls, prompting further investigation of the role of cannabinoids and -TSPO in neuroimmune signaling.[32]

Development of third-generation TSPO tracers was triggered to improvise the signal-to-noise ratio and overcome the challenge associated with rs6971 polymorphism. To that end, [11C]ER176, a quinazoline analog of PK11195, exhibited little in vitro sensitivity to rs6971; in human brain tissue, the ratio of in vitro binding affinity in HABs to that in LABs was 1.3:1 for ER176, whereas that for PBR28 was 55:1.[27,33] A preliminary first-in-human study revealed that the binding potential (BP) of [^{11}C]ER176 in LABs was one-third lower than in HABs but was comparable to the BP of [^{11}C]PBR28 in HABs,[34] suggesting better sensitivity in detecting abnormalities in patients between participant groups and that LABs may not need to be excluded from studies.[34,35] Further studies employing [^{11}C]ER176 are needed in patient populations displaying neuroinflammation. Although initial clinical studies employing a third-generation TSPO ligand, [^{18}F]GE-180 (flutriciclamide), report insensitivity to the TSPO polymorphism and high lesion-to-background ratio in tumors and multiple sclerosis plaques, further characterization of this tracer is warranted.[36]

Generally, caution must be exercised when interpreting the TSPO PET signal in the context of neuroinflammation. To date, it is not clear whether the presence of the TSPO PET signal indicates either a predominantly pro-inflammatory or anti-inflammatory state; or the presence of destructive or reparative mechanisms. As the knowledge about microglial phenotypes, that is, resting (M0), proinflammatory (M1), and anti-inflammatory (M2), evolves, there is a dire need to examine alterations in TSPO expression relative to phenotypical shift and disease progression. Alongside microglia, astrocytes also play an important role in the neuroinflammatory response. Studies have demonstrated colocalization of TSPO and markers for activated astrocytes, such as glial-fibrillary acidic protein (GFAP), under some conditions, suggesting that TSPO is not specific to microglia but also is expressed in astrocytes.[37,38] Future studies that examine the longitudinal overlap between astrocytic markers and TSPO expression in neuroinflammation models will inform the extent to which astrocytes contribute to the TSPO PET signal.

Astrocytosis, a response to destructive injury, is a complex and highly dynamic process that involves transitioning of astrocytes through sequential protective (A2) and detrimental (A1) stages.[39] There is increasing evidence that morphology and function may be inter-related in astrocyte activation. The initial hypertrophic phase is characterized by overexpression of different markers involving monoamine oxidase (MAO)-B; intermediate filaments, including nestin, vimentin, and GFAP; and followed by an astrodegeneration phase characterized by atrophy and synaptic dysfunction.[40] MAO-B, one of the two subtypes (MAO-A and MAO-B) of the major monoamine metabolizing enzyme, is considered to be localized preferentially (but not exclusively [eg, serotonin neuron cell bodies]) to astrocytes and is up-regulated in activated astrocytes under pathologic conditions.[41] Autoradiography and immunohistochemistry studies have demonstrated that [^{3}H]L-deprenyl (MAO-B ligand) binding partly overlaps with GFAP-positive astrocytes in amyotrophic lateral sclerosis, indicating some specificity of MAO-B to activated astrocytes.[42] Studies also suggest; however, that MAO-B overexpression may be an early event of astrocyte activation and MAO-B may not overlap with other commonly used astroglial markers, including GFAP.[43] Up-regulation of MAO-B in reactive astrocytes activated during neuroinflammatory processes suggests the potential for measuring alterations in MAO-B as a marker of astrogliosis in diseases that include AD and related dementias.[44]

Key advancements in the field of radiochemistry have been instrumental in the development of MAO-B PET radiotracers.[45] To date, limited studies report the use of MAO-B radioligands as imaging tools to assess neuroinflammation. MAO-B PET radiotracers, [^{11}C]L-deprenyl and its deuterated derivative, [^{11}C]L-deprenyl-D$_2$, have been evaluated in vivo in humans.[46,47] [^{11}C]L-deprenyl-D$_2$ was prepared in an attempt to improve the pharmacokinetics by slowing the rate of trapping of the tracer attributed to the kinetic isotope effect.[48,49] A comparison of PET scans between people with MCI and AD employing the PET radiotracer [^{11}C]L-deprenyl-D$_2$ revealed that astrocytosis precedes the development of AD.[44,50] In these studies, PET imaging with [^{11}C]Pittsburgh compound B ([^{11}C]PiB) was used to assess amyloid plaque load in subjects with MCI and AD. Increased [^{11}C]L-deprenyl-D$_2$ binding in the frontal and parietal cortices were found in both the [11C]PiB+ and [11C]PiB− MCI groups as well as the AD cohort, although higher and more widespread [^{11}C]L-deprenyl-D$_2$ binding was found in the [11C]PiB+ MCI group. Follow-up studies conducted by employing the same radioligands reported initially high and then declining astrocytosis in autosomal dominant AD carriers, suggesting astrocyte activation in the early stages of AD pathology to prevent deposition of amyloid.[50]

The irreversible binding of L-deprenyl and its derivatives and presence of radioactive metabolites in the brain prompted development of reversible and selective MAO-B PET radiotracers devoid of brain-penetrant metabolites.[51] To that end, [^{11}C]SL25.1188, a carbamate-based inhibitor of MAO-B with reversible kinetics, was translated successfully for clinical PET research studies and applied to image several human neuropsychiatric populations, including major depressive disorder (MDD) at the authors' center.[52,53] In individuals with MDD, greater

MAO-B levels throughout gray matter regions were associated with longer duration of illness,[54] consistent with a postmortem study that reported similar age-related increases in GFAP levels in the dorsolateral prefrontal cortex of patients with MDD.[54,55] The apparent dissociation, however, between increased [^{11}C]SL25.1188 MAO-B binding[54] and loss of GFAP-immunopositive astrocytes observed in autopsied brain[55,56] in MDD argues for more detailed studies of MAO-B expression at different stages of neuroinflammation and its relationship to other astroglial biomarkers.

To the best of the authors' knowledge, there are no preclinical and clinical in vivo research studies that have investigated TSPO (a primarily microglia marker) and MAO-B (astrocytes preferred) imaging in parallel in the context of neuroinflammation. Complementary to TSPO imaging, PET measurement of MAO-B may allow tracking of different underlying neuroinflammatory states and allow suitable therapeutic intervention.

GOALS

The goal of this study is to characterize and establish a preclinical screening tool for benchmarking new radiotracers targeted toward distinct neuroinflammatory mechanisms that develop at different time points after a damaging stimulus. As a step toward this goal, time-dependent neuroinflammatory responses were evaluated in a central lipopolysaccharide (LPS) rat model of neuroinflammation using PET tracers for TSPO and MAO-B. The well-established TSPO tracer, [^{18}F]FEPPA, was employed to characterize and validate the LPS rat model of neuroinflammation and the paradigm was extended further to characterize alternate PET biomarkers of neuroinflammation, including [^{11}C]L-deprenyl and [^{11}C]SL25.1188, for MAO-B.

EXPERIMENTAL APPROACH

LPS, an endotoxin from the cell wall of gram-negative bacteria, is a known potent immunostimulant that induces inflammatory responses within the brain.[57–59] In the CNS, LPS binds to CD14 receptor, a glycosylphosphatidylinositol-linked membrane protein and, together with the extracellular adaptor protein myeloid differentiation factor-2 (MD-2), binds to the toll-like receptor 4 (TLR4) expressed by microglia causing a direct activation of brain innate immunity.[58] Transduction through TLR4 results in a cascade of intracellular events that leads to the transcription of inflammatory and immune response genes.[60] Animals can respond to LPS stimuli differently, depending on age, species, source of the stimulus, dose, route, and duration of the administration.[59] The authors' approach was to adapt an LPS treatment paradigm that previously has demonstrated immunologic responses to the stimulus[61] with the goal of further characterizing the LPS rat model for PET imaging studies.

Activation of microglia and astrocytes was observed after a single intrastriatal LPS injection in rats, as evidenced by elevations of respective immunohistochemical markers, CD68 and GFAP.[61] Within 1 week post–LPS injection, CD68$^+$ immunoreactive cells were more abundant in the ipsilateral striatum compared with the contralateral striatum and decreased 1 month post–LPS injection; GFAP+ immunoreactive cells were evident 1 week and 1 month post–LPS injection.[61] To that end, the authors hypothesized that a single dose of LPS will activate neuroimmunological responses, thereby serving as a suitable tool to evaluate PET biomarkers of neuroinflammation. Following a single unilateral stereotaxic injection of LPS (50 μg/4 μL of sterile saline) into the striatum, neuroinflammatory responses were evaluated by conducting longitudinal PET/MR imaging studies with multiple tracers ([^{18}F]FEPPA, [^{11}C]L-deprenyl, and [^{11}C]SL25.1188).

Generation of Lipopolysaccharide Rat Model of Neuroinflammation

All animal procedures were carried out in accordance with the Institutional Animal Care and Use Committee ethical guidelines (animal use protocol #783). Adult male Sprague Dawley rats (300–400 g; 2–3 months old) were kept under gas anesthesia (2.5% isoflurane in O_2 at a flow rate of 1 L/min) and positioned in a stereotactic head frame (David Kopf Instruments, Tujunga, California). Coordinates for the right striatum (caudate putamen) to bregma were 0.5-mm anteroposterior, 3-mm lateral, and 5.5/4.5-mm dorsoventral.[62] Stereotaxic coordinates were derived using bregma as reference and thereafter a small hole was drilled in the skull at the appropriate location. Neuroinflammation was induced by a single unilateral stereotaxic injection of LPS into the striatum; 50 μg LPS dissolved in 4 μL of sterile NaCl 0.9% (LPSs from *Escherichia coli* O55:B5, Sigma-Aldrich, St. Louis, Missouri).[61] Animals were housed individually postsurgery, provided free access to food and water, and monitored closely during recovery and PET imaging studies.

In Vivo Small Animal PET/MR Imaging Procedure

Radiosyntheses of PET radiotracers

The syntheses of [^{18}F]FEPPA[30] and [^{11}C]SL25.1188[53] were carried out, as previously described, at the authors' laboratories. [¹¹C]L-deprenyl was synthesized, as previously described, with minor modifications.[63]

Animal preparation

Rats were anesthetized by isoflurane (5% induction; O_2 rate: 2 L/min) and catheterized in the lateral tail vein using a SurFlash Polyurethane IV Catheter 24G × 3/4" (Terumo, Somerset, New Jersey). Following insertion, the catheter was flushed with heparinized saline (30 IU/mL, approximately 200 μL). The animal was transferred to the scanner bed in prone position, the head immobilized in a flat skull position for the duration of the acquisition using built-in ear bars and a bite bar; and the scanner bed temperature initially was set at 40°C but was subject to alteration based on animals' body temperature during the experiment. Anesthesia was maintained throughout the PET/MR scanning procedure (isoflurane: 1.5%–2%; O_2 rate: 1 L/min) and the animals' body temperature and respiration parameters were monitored closely.

PET/MR acquisition

Longitudinal imaging studies were conducted on a nanoScan PET/MR 3T tomograph (Mediso, Budapest, Hungary) with multiple tracers, including [¹⁸F]FEPPA, [¹¹C]L-deprenyl, and [¹¹C]SL25.1188, as outlined in the experimental study design (**Fig. 1**). Longitudinal PET/MR imaging studies were conducted: 1 week and 1 month post–LPS injection to evaluate [¹⁸F]FEPPA uptake (n = 4) and 1 week, 2 weeks, and 1 month post–LPS injection to evaluate [¹¹C]L-deprenyl uptake (n = 3). Preliminary PET/MR imaging studies for [¹¹C]SL25.11885 were conducted 1 day, 1 week, and 1 month post–LPS injection in a separate cohort of animals (n = 2). The PET/MR protocol was based on the authors' previously published procedures, with slight modifications.[64] At first, a scout MR was acquired for subsequent PET field of view positioning. MR images were acquired to define anatomic regions of interest through PET/MR image coregistration. Concomitantly with a

bolus injection of each individual radiotracer (injected radioactivity range: 14–22 MBq), 120-minute, 60-minute, and 90-minute emission list mode scans were acquired for [¹⁸F]FEPPA, [¹¹C]L-deprenyl, and [¹¹C]SL25.11885, respectively.

Blocking of [¹¹C]L-deprenyl uptake by lazabemide (Sigma-Aldrich) was conducted in 2 separate baseline and pretreatment (blocking) experiments at the 1-month time point using a within-subject study design. In the first PET/MR imaging session, brain radiotracer uptake was determined under baseline conditions whereby [¹¹C]L-deprenyl was administered intravenously simultaneously with the start of PET acquisition. The catheter was flushed with heparinized saline (approxiamtely 100 μL) and capped to allow radiotracer injections for the subsequent pretreatment experiment. Before the start of the second PET measurement, the animals were injected with lazabemide (1 mg/kg) intraperitoneally 90 minutes prior to radiotracer injection followed by concomitant PET acquisition.

PET data analyses

The acquired list mode data were sorted either into 39, 3-dimensional (3-D) (for [¹⁸F]FEPPA and [¹¹C]SL25.11885) or into 27, 3-D (for [¹¹C]L-deprenyl) true sinograms. The 3-D sinograms were converted to 2-dimensional (2-D) sinograms using Fourier rebinning (FORE),[65] during which corrections were included for detector geometry and efficiencies, attenuation, and scatter, prior to image reconstruction, using a 2-D–filtered back projection (FBKP) with a Hann filter at a cutoff of 0.50 cm⁻¹. A static image of the complete emission acquisition or after 10 min of acquisition was reconstructed with the manufacturer's proprietary iterative 3-D algorithm (6 subsets and 4 iterations). All image data were corrected for dead time and decay corrected to the start of acquisition. Dynamic PET images were reconstructed using a FORE-FBKP algorithm, and regional brain time activity curves (TACs) were extracted using a stereotaxic MR imaging atlas implemented in PMOD

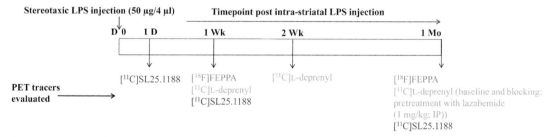

Fig. 1. Experimental study design: longitudinal PET/MR imaging studies were conducted 1 day, 1 week, 2 weeks, and 1 month following intrastriatal LPS injection to characterize TSPO ([¹⁸F]FEPPA) and MAO-B binding ([¹¹C]L-deprenyl and [¹¹C]SL25.1188) in a rat model of neuroinflammation. IP, intraperitoneal.

(v4.004)[66] (PMOD Technologies, Zurich, Switzerland). Standardized uptake values (SUVs) were calculated by normalizing regional radioactivity for injected radioactivity and body weight of the animal. Time-dependent differences in radiotracer uptake was analyzed by Two-way analysis of variance (ANOVA). Tracer binding potential (BP) for the right striatum was estimated using simplified reference tissue model (SRTM) with the left striatum as the reference tissue using the package of Turku PET Centre for PET image analyses (tpcclib 0.7.6, Turku, Finland).[67] Percentages of blocking were calculated by the equation, blocking% = 100 × ($BP_{blocking}$ − $BP_{baseline}$)/ $BP_{baseline}$. Data are presented as mean ±SD. Statistical analyses were performed with paired 2-tailed t-test. Calculations were carried out using Prism v5.0 (GraphPad, San Diego, California) and $P<.05$ was considered statistically significant.

OUTCOMES OF PRECLINICAL STUDIES

All PET radiotracers were produced with high radiochemical purity (>99%) and high molar activity. Rats were injected with 14 MBq to 22 MBq of the respective radiotracer; average molar activities at the time of injection were 201.9 GBq/μmol ± 163.9 GBq/μmol, 181.0 GBq/μmol ± 48.5 GBq/μmol, and 59.0 GBq/μmol ± 27.9 GBq/ μmol; and the injected masses were 0.48 nmol/ kg ± 0.48 nmol/kg, 0.26 nmol/kg ± 0.12 nmol/ kg, and 0.81 ± 0.32 nmol/kg for [18F]FEPPA, [11C]L-deprenyl and [11C]SL25.1188, respectively.

Fig. 2 displays representative static iterative transverse PET images of [18F]FEPPA and [11C]L-deprenyl. [18F]FEPPA uptake expressed in SUV units showed increased tracer retention in the LPS-injected right striatum compared with the left striatum 1 week post–stereotaxic LPS injection (see Fig. 2A) whereas at the 1-month time point [18F]FEPPA binding was attenuated (see Fig. 2B). Fig. 3 demonstrates the TACs of [18F]FEPPA uptake in the left and right striatum 1 week and 1 month post–intrastriatal LPS injection (n = 4). Compared with the left-striatum, washout of [18F]FEPPA was much slower in the LPS-injected striatum 1 week post–LPS injection, suggesting significant [18F] FEPPA retention as a result of LPS injection. Two-way ANOVA analysis of [18F]FEPPA uptake across the time course revealed a significant time × SUV interaction ($F_{38,234}$ = 1.943; $P<.05$ [see Fig. 3A]). Increased [18F]FEPPA binding in the LPS-injected rat striatum was significantly attenuated 1 month post–LPS injection ([see Fig. 3B] time × SUV interaction; $F_{38,234}$ = 0.7675; $P>.05$). As a control, the cerebellum did not show any time-dependent differences of [18F]FEPPA uptake between the left cerebellum and right cerebellum at 1 week and 1 month post-intrastriatal LPS injection ([see Fig. 3D, E] 2-way ANOVA analyses; $P>.05$). The cerebellum exhibited an early peak response and comparable pattern of washout to that of left striatum, confirming that increased [18F]FEPPA binding in the LPS-injected right striatum was local to the neuroinflammatory response induced by LPS. Consistent with results demonstrated in the TACs, the BP of [18F] FEPPA ipsilateral versus contralateral decreased significantly by 63%, from 1.1 ± 0.18 at 1 week to 0.4 ± 0.19 at 1 month post–LPS injection ([Fig. 3C] n = 4; $P<.01$). This early peak and later reduction in [18F]FEPPA response are consistent with previously reported TSPO PET findings using [18F]DPA-714.[61] Taken together, the current results support [18F]FEPPA TSPO PET imaging as a sensitive biomarker of the early phase of acute neuroinflammation in rats.

Alongside establishing a robust [18F]FEPPA response, the LPS rat model of neuroinflammation was extended further to serve as a preliminary screening tool for benchmarking tracers targeted toward alternate neuroinflammatory targets, including MAO-B. Increased concentrations of MAO-B have been proposed as an in vivo marker of neuroinflammation associated with AD.[68] The PET tracer, [11C]L-deprenyl-D_2, binds selectively and irreversibly to MAO-B and has been applied to human studies as an in vivo marker for reactive astrocytosis in neurodegenerative diseases, including AD and amyotrophic lateral sclerosis.[41,50,69,70] To the best of the authors' knowledge, [11C]L-deprenyl-D_2 has not been investigated in rat models of neuroinflammation. As a step toward evaluating [11C]L-deprenyl-D_2 in the LPS rat model of neuroinflammation, the authors conducted a preliminary baseline and blocking study in a control rat to establish the baseline brain uptake of [11C]L-deprenyl-D_2 (data not shown). TACs revealed a fast washout following an early peak SUV of 6 that decreased to less than 1 SUV in 10 minutes and a negligible self-blocking effect with 1 mg/kg of L-deprenyl, suggesting that the deuterated tracer may not be a suitable tool to probe potential up-regulation of MAO-B in the LPS rat model of neuroinflammation. The quick washout of [11C]L-deprenyl-D_2 may be attributed to the kinetic isotope effect of the deuterated analog of [11C]L-deprenyl reported in the humans and nonhuman primates.[47,49] The authors reasoned that, because of lower MAO-B levels in brain along with faster metabolism of the tracer in rats compared with humans and nonhuman primates, [11C]L-deprenyl-D_2 would be less than optimal in MAO-B imaging in rodents. Therefore, [11C]L-deprenyl was considered an

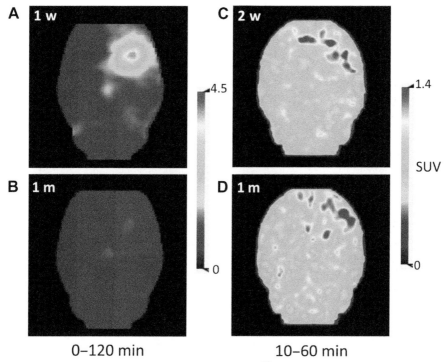

0–120 min   10–60 min

Fig. 2. Representative static iterative transverse PET images of [^{18}F]FEPPA binding (*left*) in LPS-injected rat striatum (*A*) 1 week and (*B*) 1 month post–LPS injection and [^{11}C]L-deprenyl binding (*right*) in LPS-injected rat striatum (*C*) 2 weeks and (*D*) 1 month post–LPS injection.

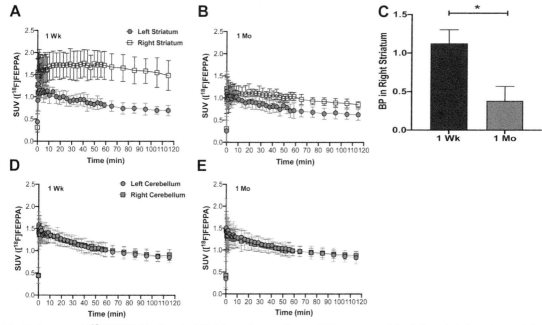

Fig. 3. Increased [^{18}F]FEPPA binding in LPS-injected rat striatum. TACs averaged for left and right striatum (*A*) 1 week and (*B*) 1 month post–LPS injection; TACs averaged for left and right cerebellum (*D*) 1 week and (*E*) 1 month post–LPS injection are shown. (*C*) BP of [^{18}F]FEPPA in right striatum derived by SRTM using left striatum as the reference tissue. Data are presented as mean $\pm$SD; n = 4. *P<0.01, 1 Wk vs. 1 Mo, 2-tailed Student's t-test.

alternate MAO-B tracer in the context of the current study. [^{11}C]L-deprenyl showed relatively slower washout, higher brain retention (average SUV of 0.75 ± 0.06 vs 0.49 ± 0.03; P<.05 in 30–60 min of injection), and larger deprenyl self-blocking effects compared with [^{11}C]L-deprenyl-D$_2$ in rats (data not shown) and, therefore, was used in the LPS model.

In contrast to [^{18}F]FEPPA response, no apparent increase in [^{11}C]L-deprenyl binding was observed in the right striatum 1 week post–LPS injection. Increased [^{11}C]L-deprenyl uptake, however, was observed 2 weeks post–LPS injection, and this signal remained stable up to the 1-month time point, as depicted in the representative static iterative summed (10–60 min) PET images (see **Fig. 2**C, D). TACs of [^{11}C]L-deprenyl uptake at 1 week, 2 weeks, and 1 month post–LPS injection are shown in **Fig. 4** and demonstrate a peak SUV of 4 to 5 approximately 1 minute to 2 minutes post–tracer injection. The magnitude of increases in [^{11}C]L-deprenyl binding in the LPS-injected right striatum compared with the left control site at the 2-week and 1-month time points, albeit small, is depicted in the inserts embedded in the TACs (SUV for [^{11}C]L-deprenyl uptake from 10–60 min time frame). Two-way ANOVA revealed a significant main effect of time and SUV at the 2-week and 1-month time points (P<.05). Importantly, no differences in [^{11}C]L-deprenyl binding were observed in the TACs of [^{11}C]L-deprenyl uptake

between the left cerebellum and right cerebellum at the same time points (see **Fig. 4**E–G) evaluated, suggesting that increased [^{11}C]L-deprenyl binding in the right striatum was specific to MAO-B up-regulation in the LPS-injected site.

Consistent with increased [^{11}C]L-deprenyl uptake observed at the 2-week and 1-month time points post–LPS injection, a trend for increased BP ipsilateral versus contralateral of [^{11}C]L-deprenyl in the LPS-injected right striatum was evident at these time points. The BPs in the right striatum at 1 week, 2 weeks, and 1 month post–LPS injection were 0.05 ± 0.001, 0.10 ± 0.012, and 0.09 ± 0.023, respectively (see **Fig. 4**D), indicating an approximately 2-fold increase in BP 2 weeks and 1 month post–LPS injection. In vivo binding specificity of [^{11}C]L-deprenyl for MAO-B in the LPS rat model was evaluated by pretreatment studies conducted in the presence of lazabemide (n = 2) at the 1-month time point (**Fig. 5**). The representative static iterative summed (10–60 min) PET image (**Fig. 5**A) and comparison of TACs derived from baseline and blocking studies (see **Fig. 5**B) showed that pretreatment with the MAO-B inhibitor not only decreased [^{11}C]L-deprenyl binding throughout the brain but also largely removed the increased binding in the ipsilateral striatum, confirming elevated MAO-B expression induced by LPS. A trend for decreased BP of [^{11}C]L-deprenyl in the LPS-injected right striatum was observed on pretreatment with lazabemide.

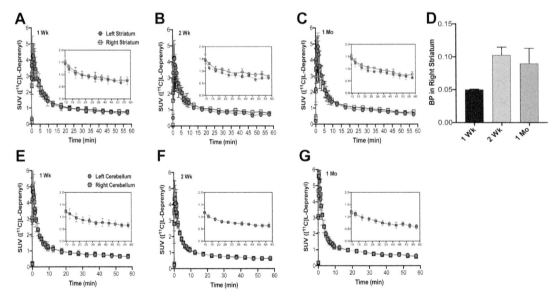

Fig. 4. Moderate increases in [^{11}C]L-deprenyl binding in LPS-injected rat striatum. TACs averaged for left and right striatum (*A*) 1 week, (*B*) 2 weeks, and (*C*) 1 month post–LPS injection; TACs averaged for left and right cerebellum (*E*) 1 week, (*F*) 2 weeks, and (*G*) 1 month post–LPS injection. Inserts show TACs for the 10-minute to 60-minute time frame for the respective brain region and time point. (*D*) BP of [^{11}C]L-deprenyl in right striatum derived by SRTM using left striatum as the reference tissue. Data are presented as mean ±SD; n = 2 to 3.

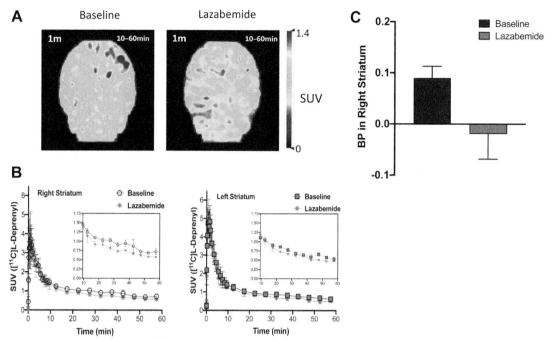

Fig. 5. Moderate increases in [^{11}C]L-deprenyl binding in LPS-injected rat striatum was blocked by pretreatment with lazabemide (1 mg/kg; intraperitoneal). (*A*)Representative static iterative PET images (10–60 min) of [^{11}C]L-deprenyl binding in LPS-injected rat striatum 1 month post–LPS injection at baseline and blocking conditions; (*B*) TACs averaged for right striatum (*left*) and left striatum (*right*) 1 month post–LPS injection under baseline and blocking conditions. (*C*) BP of [^{11}C]L-deprenyl in right striatum derived by SRTM using left striatum as the reference tissue. Data are presented as mean ±SD; n = 2 to 3.

The BPs in the right striatum under baseline and blocking conditions were 0.09 ± 0.02 and −0.02 ± 0.05, respectively, suggesting that the difference in [^{11}C]L-deprenyl binding between ipsilateral and contralateral striatum was eliminated under blocking conditions (see **Fig. 5C**). Taken together, the blocking results suggest the specificity of [^{11}C]L-deprenyl uptake response to MAO-B up-regulation in the LPS-injected site.

MAO-B response in the LPS rat model of neuroinflammation also was probed in preliminary imaging studies using [^{11}C]SL25.1188. In contrast to the response observed with [^{18}F]FEPPA and [^{11}C]L-deprenyl, no increase in [^{11}C]SL25.1188 uptake was observed in the LPS-injected site compared with the contralateral striatum at any time following the surgery (from 1 day up to 4.5 months; for representative average images at 1 day, 1 week, and 1 month postsurgery, see **Fig. 6**). These preliminary results suggest that [^{11}C]SL25.1188 may not be a suitable PET tracer to image MAO-B in a rat model of neuroinflammation.

DISCUSSION

This study characterizes a well-known LPS rat model of neuroinflammation with established tracers for TSPO and MAO-B, which will guide future screening of new PET tracers developed for targets implicated in neuroinflammation. The unilateral intrastriatal LPS rat model has been employed extensively for PET radiotracer development in neuroinflammation, including ligands for TSPO,[61,71–75] although longitudinal studies and this model have not been used for assessment of MAO-B ligands/astrogliosis. Current evidence demonstrates [^{18}F]FEPPA is a sensitive and robust PET biomarker of the early phase of neuroinflammation in rats and suggests that increased TSPO expression precedes the up-regulation of MAO-B in the LPS rat model of neuroinflammation, which is consistent with immunohistochemical evidence in this model of early (hours to 1 week, depending on the biomarker examined) gradually dissipating microglial response and delayed but sustained astrocytes reaction.[76–79] Ory and colleagues[61] showed that although TSPO expression dominated in CD68+ microglia/macrophages at the LPS injection site, it also is expressed, to a much lesser extent, in GFAP+ astrocytes located in the periphery of the injection site. As shown in **Fig. 2**, the highest [^{18}F]FEPPA uptake coincided with the LPS injection site, whereas [^{11}C]L-deprenyl binding appeared to be more distributed at the periphery of [^{18}F]FEPPA hotspot, which agrees with the findings by Ory and colleagues[61] and suggests

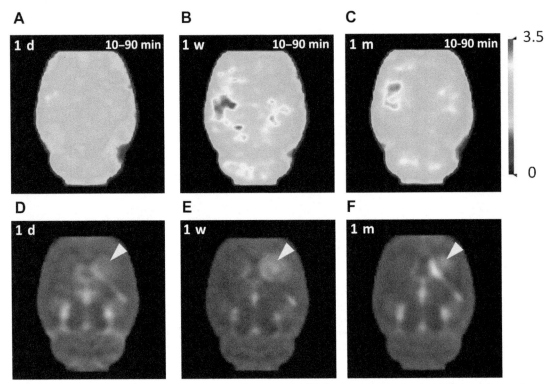

Fig. 6. Representative static iterative transverse PET images of [^{11}C]SL25.1188. Binding in LPS-injected rat striatum (*A*) 1 day, (*B*) 1 week, and (*C*) 1 month post–LPS injection and the corresponding MR (fast spin echo) images (*D*, 1 day; *E*, 1 week; and *F*, 1 month), with injection site (*arrowheads*).

that the late phase of LPS-induced neuroinflammation detected by [^{11}C]L-deprenyl likely was due to increased levels of MAO-B in reactive astrocytes. Detailed histochemical studies will be needed to confirm the PET findings and to pinpoint the role of MAO-B in astrocyte activation. One caveat of this study is the small number of animals examined and the lack of full kinetic analysis with blood sampling of the dynamic PET images, in particular for [^{11}C]L-deprenyl, an irreversible radiotracer, which might have underestimated the binding parameters and reduced the experimental power.

PET imaging of TSPO previously has been investigated in animal models of epileptogenesis to allow visualization of molecular pathways involved in epileptogenesis.[80–82] As part of the neuroinflammatory response, astrogliosis also has been studied in epilepsy.[83,84] Recent studies have reported binding profile of both TSPO and MAO-B PET tracers in acute, latent, and chronic phases of epileptogenesis in a rat pilocarpine model.[85] In vitro autoradiographic studies were conducted on rat brain slices at different time points post–epileptogenic insult to investigate microglial and astrocyte activation, employing [^{18}F]flutriciclamide and [^{18}F]fluorodeprenyl that

target TSPO and MAO-B, respectively.[85,86] Results demonstrated early TSPO up-regulation seen with [^{18}F]flutriciclamide binding. On the other hand, MAO-B autoradiography showed no alterations during the acute phase after the epileptogenic insult but a progressive increase during the latent phase, peaking at the chronic stage, suggesting that astrocyte activation may be triggered by seizures. As a result, TSPO up-regulation was suggested to reflect mainly microglial activation and not astrogliosis given the late activation of astrocytes and the early TSPO peak. Current in vivo results extend previous in vitro findings by demonstrating that increased TSPO expression precedes up-regulation of MAO-B.

It was unexpected that [^{11}C]SL25.1188 failed to detect increased binding in the LPS rat model. Unpublished data from the authors' laboratory suggest that this may be attributed to high nonspecific binding of [^{11}C]SL25.1188 in rat brain in vivo despite successful translation of the new generation reversible PET probe of MAO-B for clinical research.[54] In vitro assay showed that SL25.1188 has approximately 3-fold lower affinity (*Ki*) for rat (8.5-nM) compared with human (2.9-nM) MAO-B,[87] which might have contributed to the authors' failed efforts employing this radiotracer in rats. Thus, [^{11}C]SL25.1188 adds to the list of radiotracers that failed in preclinical studies in rodents but still are useful in higher species[88] and for human clinical research applications, highlighting critical species differences (eg, for MAO-B[89]) and that extra care is needed in preclinical evaluation of MAO-B PET tracers and subsequent clinical translation.

FUTURE DIRECTIONS

There is an urgent need to develop PET tracers for characterizing multiple mechanisms underlying neuroinflammation. By far, TSPO has been the most commonly imaged biomarker of neuroinflammation, although several criticisms surround this target and alternative biomarkers are avidly sought. In order to understand the functional state of the TSPO PET signal in the brain, it is important to determine which microglial phenotypes (M0, M1, or M2) up-regulate TSPO in neuroinflammation. Although mostly considered as a specific marker of microglial activation, TSPO also is overexpressed in activated astrocytes under some conditions.[90–92] To date, astrocytes have been investigated to a lesser extent than microglia for their role in neuroinflammation. Nevertheless, recent studies have emphasized the importance of a bidirectional communication between microglia and astrocytes via physical contacts and secreted molecules. Experimental studies in diverse neurodegenerative diseases imply that microglia define the functions of astrocytes, ranging from neuroprotective to neurotoxic.[93] Conversely, astrocytes appear to regulate microglial phenotypes and functions, including motility and phagocytosis.[94] As a result, caution is advised while interpreting the TSPO PET signal in a clinical research setting and multitracer approaches likely are needed to identify distinct activation states of microglia and astrocytes. Limitations of TSPO have prompted the discovery of alternative biological targets for imaging microglia. The most promising novel tracers are those that target purinergic receptors including P2X$_7$, selective toward the M1 phenotype.[95] In this respect, new tracer development for PET imaging of astrocyte activation has been lagging far behind than that for microglia. Current candidates for MAO-B ([^{11}C]L-deprenyl-D$_2$ and [^{11}C]SL25.1188) suffer from the inherent lack of specificity of MAO-B for astrocytes.[41] The newly developed [^{11}C]BU99008 for the imidazoline 2 binding sites[96] not only has the same limitation as for MAO-B but also has a lack of identity of the so-called I2 receptor.[97] It also is noteworthy that [^{18}F]FEPPA was evaluated in a peripheral LPS-injected mouse model[98]; hence, species differences as well as experimental paradigms should be considered. Consequently, it is essential to develop novel PET tracers that are more specific to either microglia or astrocytes and that can selectively image their distinct inflammatory stages.

SUMMARY

This study characterizes an LPS rat model of neuroinflammation by employing a well-established TSPO tracer and extends this paradigm for evaluation of alternate PET biomarkers of neuroinflammation, including MAO-B. This model may serve as a preliminary screening tool for benchmarking newly developed tracers targeted toward distinct neuroinflammatory mechanisms. Functional interpretation of the TSPO PET signal may be aided with a multitracer approach that uses microglia- and astrocyte-specific PET tracers and/or tracers specific for their respective phenotypes.

CONFLICT OF INTEREST

The authors declare no conflicts of interest.

ACKNOWLEDGMENTS

The authors acknowledge financial support from the National Institute on Aging of the National Institute of Health (R01AG054473), the Canada Foundation for Innovation and the Ontario Research Fund, the Azrieli Foundation, and the Canada Research Chairs Program.

DISCLOSURE

The authors have nothing to disclose.

REFERENCES

1. Lyman M, Lloyd DG, Ji X, et al. Neuroinflammation: the role and consequences. Neurosci Res 2014;79:1–12.
2. Ransohoff RM. How neuroinflammation contributes to neurodegeneration. Science 2016;353(6301): 777–83.
3. Narayanaswami V, Dahl K, Bernard-Gauthier V, et al. Emerging PET radiotracers and targets for imaging of neuroinflammation in neurodegenerative diseases: outlook beyond TSPO. Mol Imaging 2018; 17. 1536012118792317.
4. Werry EL, Bright FM, Piguet O, et al. Recent developments in TSPO PET imaging as a biomarker of neuroinflammation in neurodegenerative disorders. Int J Mol Sci 2019;20(13):3161.
5. Ramesh G, MacLean AG, Philipp MT. Cytokines and chemokines at the crossroads of neuroinflammation, neurodegeneration, and neuropathic pain. Mediators Inflamm 2013;2013:480739.

6. Kempuraj D, Thangavel R, Natteru PA, et al. Neuro-inflammation induces neurodegeneration. J Neurol Neurosurg Spine 2016;1(1):1003.

7. O'Callaghan JP, Sriram K, Miller DB. Defining "neuroinflammation". Ann N Y Acad Sci 2008;1139:318–30.

8. Heneka MT, Kummer MP, Latz E. Innate immune activation in neurodegenerative disease. Nat Rev Immunol 2014;14:463–77.

9. DiSabato DJ, Quan N, Godbout JP. Neuroinflammation: the devil is in the details. J Neurochem 2016;139(Suppl 2):136–53.

10. Glass CK, Saijo K, Winner B, et al. Mechanisms underlying inflammation in neurodegeneration. Cell 2010;140:918–34.

11. Skaper SD, Giusti P, Facci L. Microglia and mast cells: two tracks on the road to neuroinflammation. FASEB J 2012;26:3103–17.

12. González H, Elgueta D, Montoya A, et al. Neuroimmune regulation of microglial activity involved in neuroinflammation and neurodegenerative diseases. J Neuroimmunol 2014;274:1–13.

13. Meeter LH, Kaat LD, Rohrer JD, et al. Imaging and fluid biomarkers in frontotemporal dementia. Nat Rev Neurol 2017;13:406–19.

14. Zlokovic BV. The blood-brain barrier in health and chronic neurodegenerative disorders. Neuron 2008;57:178–201.

15. Sweeney MD, Sagare AP, Zlokovic BV. Blood-brain barrier breakdown in Alzheimer disease and other neurodegenerative disorders. Nat Rev Neurol 2018;14:133–50.

16. Zinnhardt B, Wiesmann M, Honold L, et al. In vivo imaging biomarkers of neuroinflammation in the development and assessment of stroke therapies - towards clinical translation. Theranostics 2018;8(10):2603–20.

17. Jack CR Jr, Bennett DA, Blennow K, et al. NIA-AA research framework: toward a biological definition of Alzheimer's disease. Alzheimers Dement 2018;14:535–62.

18. Mattner F, Katsifis A, Staykova M, et al. Evaluation of a radiolabelled peripheral benzodiazepine receptor ligand in the central nervous system inflammation of experimental autoimmune encephalomyelitis: a possible probe for imaging multiple sclerosis. Eur J Nucl Med Mol Imaging 2005;32:557–63.

19. Martin A, Boisgard R, Theze B, et al. Evaluation of the PBR/TSPO radioligand [18F]DPA-714 in a rat model of focal cerebral ischemia. J Cereb Blood Flow Metab 2010;30:230–41.

20. Dedeurwaerdere S, Callaghan PD, Pham T, et al. PET imaging of brain inflammation during early epileptogenesis in a rat model of temporal lobe epilepsy. EJNMMI Res 2012;2:60.

21. Brendel M, Probst F, Jaworska A, et al. Glial activation and glucose metabolism in a transgenic amyloid

mouse model: a triple-tracer PET study. J Nucl Med 2016;57:954–60.

22. Israel I, Ohsiek A, Al-Momani E, et al. Combined [18F] DPA-714 micro-positron emission tomography and autoradiography imaging of microglia activation after closed head injury in mice. J Neuroinflammation 2016;13:140.

23. Mirzaei N, Tang SP, Ashworth S, et al. In vivo imaging of microglial activation by positron emission tomography with [11C]PBR28 in the 5XFAD model of Alzheimer's disease. Glia 2016;64:993–1006.

24. Cumming P, Burgher B, Patkar O, et al. Sifting through the surfeit of neuroinflammation tracers. J Cereb Blood Flow Metab 2018;38(2):204–24.

25. Tong J, Williams B, Rusjan PM, et al. Concentration, distribution, and influence of aging on the 18 kDa translocator protein in human brain: implications for brain imaging studies. J Cereb Blood Flow Metab 2020;40(5):1061–76.

26. Alam MM, Lee J, Lee SY. Recent progress in the development of TSPO PET ligands for neuroinflammation imaging in neurological diseases. Nucl Med Mol Imaging 2017;51(4):283–96.

27. Owen DR, Howell OW, Tang SP, et al. Two binding sites for [3H]PBR28 in human brain: implications for TSPO PET imaging of neuroinflammation. J Cereb Blood Flow Metab 2010;30:1608–18.

28. Owen DR, Gunn RN, Rabiner EA, et al. Mixed-affinity binding in humans with 18-kDa translocator protein ligands. J Nucl Med 2011;52:24–32.

29. Mizrahi R, Rusjan PM, Kennedy J, et al. Translocator protein (18 kDa) polymorphism (rs6971) explains in-vivo brain binding affinity of the PET radioligand [18F]-FEPPA. J Cereb Blood Flow Metab 2012;32:968–72.

30. Wilson AA, Garcia A, Parkes J, et al. Radiosynthesis and initial evaluation of [18F]-FEPPA for PET imaging of peripheral benzodiazepine receptors. Nucl Med Biol 2008;35:305–14.

31. Setiawan E, Attwells S, Wilson AA, et al. Association of translocator protein total distribution volume with duration of untreated major depressive disorder: a cross-sectional study. Lancet Psychiatry 2018;5:339–47.

32. Da Silva T, Hafizi S, Watts JJ, et al. In vivo imaging of translocator protein in long-term cannabis users. JAMA Psychiatry 2019;76(12):1305–13.

33. Zanotti-Fregonara P, Zhang Y, Jenko KJ, et al. Synthesis and evaluation of translocator 18 kDa protein (TSPO) positron emission tomography (PET) radioligands with low binding sensitivity to human single nucleotide polymorphism rs6971. ACS Chem Neurosci 2014;5(10):963–71.

34. Ikawa M, Lohith TG, Shrestha S, et al. 11C-ER176, a radioligand for 18-kDa translocator protein, has adequate sensitivity to robustly image all three affinity genotypes in human brain. biomarkers

consortium radioligand project team. J Nucl Med 2017;58(2):320–5.

35. Fujita M, Kobayashi M, Ikawa M, et al. Comparison of four 11C-labeled PET ligands to quantify translocator protein 18 kDa (TSPO) in human brain: (R)-PK11195, PBR28, DPA-713, and ER176-based on recent publications that measured specific-to-non-displaceable ratios. EJNMMI Res 2017;7(1):84.

36. Zanotti-Fregonara P, Pascual B, Rostomily RC, et al. Anatomy of 18F-GE180, a failed radioligand for the TSPO protein. Eur J Nucl Med Mol Imaging 2020. https://doi.org/10.1007/s00259-020-04732-y. Online ahead of print.

37. Guilarte TR, Kuhlmann AC, O'Callaghan JP, et al. Enhanced expression of peripheral benzodiazepine receptors in trimethyltin-exposed rat brain: a biomarker of neurotoxicity. Neurotoxicology 1995; 16:441–50.

38. Geloso MC, Corvino V, Marchese E, et al. The dual role of microglia in ALS: mechanisms and therapeutic. Front Aging Neurosci 2017. https://doi.org/10.3389/fnagi.2017.00242.

39. Liddelow SA, Barres BA. Reactive astrocytes: production, function, and therapeutic potential. Immunity 2017;46(6):957–67.

40. Boche D, Gerhard A, Rodriguez-Vieitez E, et al. Prospects and challenges of imaging neuroinflammation beyond TSPO in Alzheimer's disease. Eur J Nucl Med Mol Imaging 2019;46(13):2831–47.

41. Tong J, Rathitharan G, Meyer JH, et al. Brain monoamine oxidase B and A in human parkinsonian dopamine deficiency disorders. Brain 2017;140(9): 2460–74.

42. Ekblom J, Jossan SS, Bergstrom M, et al. Monoamine oxidase-B in astrocytes. Glia 1993;8(2):122–32.

43. Olsen M, Aguilar X, Sehlin D, et al. Astroglial responses to amyloid-beta progression in a mouse model of alzheimer's disease. Mol Imaging Biol 2018;20(4):605–14.

44. Carter SF, Schoell M, Almkvist O, et al. (2012) Evidence for astrocytosis in prodromal Alzheimer disease provided by 11C-deuterium-L-deprenyl: a multitracer PET paradigm combining 11C-Pittsburgh compound B and 18F-FDG. J Nucl Med 2012;53(1): 37–46.

45. Narayanaswami V, Drake LR, Brooks AF, et al. Classics in neuroimaging: development of PET tracers for imaging monoamine oxidases. ACS Chem Neurosci 2019;10:1867–71.

46. Fowler JS, MacGregor RR, Wolf AP, et al. Mapping human brain monoamine oxidase A and B with 11C-labeled suicide inactivators and PET. Science 1987;235(4787):481–5.

47. Fowler JS, Wolf AP, MacGregor RR, et al. Mechanistic positron emission tomography studies: demonstration of a deuterium isotope effect in the monoamine oxidase-catalyzed binding of [11C]L-deprenyl in living baboon brain. J Neurochem 1988;51(5):1524–34.

48. Logan J, Fowler JS, Volkow ND, et al. Reproducibility of repeated measures of deuterium substituted [11C]L-deprenyl ([11C]L-deprenyl-D2) binding in the human brain. Nucl Med Biol 2000; 27(1):43–9.

49. Fowler JS, Wang GJ, Logan J, et al. Selective reduction of radiotracer trapping by deuterium substitution: comparison of carbon-11-L-deprenyl and carbon-11-deprenyl-D2 for MAO B mapping. J Nucl Med 1995;36(7):1255–62.

50. Carter SF, Chiotis K, Nordberg A, et al. Longitudinal association between astrocyte function and glucose metabolism in autosomal dominant Alzheimer's disease. Eur J Nucl Med Mol Imaging 2019;46(2): 348–56.

51. Cumming P, Yokoi F, Chen A, et al. Pharmacokinetics of radiotracers in human plasma during positron emission tomography. Synapse 1999;34:124–34.

52. Rusjan PM, Wilson AA, Miller L, et al. Kinetic modeling of the monoamine oxidase B radioligand [^{11}C]SL25.1188 in human brain with high-resolution positron emission tomography. J Cereb Blood Flow Metab 2014;34:883–9.

53. Vasdev N, Sadovski O, Garcia A, et al. Radiosynthesis of [11C]SL25.1188 via [11C]CO2 fixation for imaging monoamine oxidase B. J Label Compd Radiopharm 2011;54:678–80.

54. Moriguchi S, Wilson AA, Miler L, et al. Monoamine oxidase B total distribution volume in the prefrontal cortex of major depressive disorder: an [11C] SL25.1188 positron emission tomography study. JAMA Psychiatry 2019;76(6):634–41.

55. Si X, Miguel-Hidalgo JJ, O'Dwyer G, et al. Age-dependent reductions in the level of glial fibrillary acidic protein in the prefrontal cortex in major depression. Neuropsychopharmacology 2004; 29(11):2088–96.

56. Rajkowska G, Stockmeier CA. Astrocyte pathology in major depressive disorder: insights from human postmortem brain tissue. Curr Drug Targets 2013; 14(11):1225–36.

57. Ambrosini A, Louin G, Croci N, et al. Characterization of a rat model to study acute neuroinflammation on histopathological, biochemical and functional outcomes. J Neurosci Methods 2005;144:183–91.

58. Russo I, Barlati S, Bosetti F. Effects of neuroinflammation on the regenerative capacity of brain stem cells. J Neurochem 2011;116(6):947–56.

59. Batista CRA, Gomes GF, Candelario-Jalil E, et al. Lipopolysaccharide-induced neuroinflammation as a bridge to understand neurodegeneration. Int J Mol Sci 2019;20(9):2293.

60. Bonow RH, Aid S, Zhang Y, et al. The brain expression of genes involved in inflammatory response, the ribosome, and learning and memory is altered by

centrally injected lipopolysaccharide in mice. Pharmacogenomics J 2009;9:116–26.

61. Ory D, Planas A, Dresselaers T, et al. PET imaging of TSPO in a rat model of local neuroinflammation induced by intracerebral injection of lipopolysaccharide. Nucl Med Biol 2015;42(10):753–61.

62. Paxinos G, Watson C. The rat brain in stereotaxic coordinates. 4th edition. San Diego (CA): Academic Press; 1998.

63. Buccino P, Kreimerman I, Zirbesegger K, et al. Automated radiosynthesis of [(11)C]L-deprenyl-D2 and [(11)C]D-deprenyl using a commercial platform. Appl Radiat Isot 2016;110:47–52.

64. Narayanaswami V, Tong J, Fiorino F, et al. Synthesis, in vitro and in vivo evaluation of 11C-O-methylated arylpiperazines as potential serotonin 1A (5-HT1A) receptor antagonist radiotracers. EJNMMI Radiopharm Chem 2020;5:13.

65. Defrise M, Kinahan PE, Townsend DW, et al. Exact and approximate rebinning algorithms for 3-D PET data. IEEE Trans Med Imaging 1997;16(2):145–58.

66. Schwarz AJ, Danckaert A, Reese T, et al. A stereotaxic MRI template set for the rat brain with tissue class distribution maps and co-registered anatomical atlas: application to pharmacological MRI. Neuroimage 2006;15(32):538–50.

67. Gunn RN, Lammertsma AA, Hume SP, et al. Parametric imaging of ligand-receptor binding in PET using a simplified reference region model. Neuroimage 1997;6(4):279–87.

68. Rodriguez-Vieitez E, Ni R, Gulyás B, et al. Astrocytosis precedes amyloid plaque deposition in Alzheimer APPswe transgenic mouse brain: a correlative positron emission tomography and in vitro imaging study. Eur J Nucl Med Mol Imaging 2015;42(7):1119–32.

69. Johansson A, Engler H, Blomquist G, et al. Evidence for astrocytosis in ALS demonstrated by [11C](L)-deprenyl-D2 PET. J Neurol Sci 2007;255(1–2):17–22.

70. Santillo AF, Gambini JP, Lannfelt L, et al. In vivo imaging of astrocytosis in Alzheimer's disease: an 11C-L-deuteriodeprenyl and PIB PET study. Eur J Nucl Med Mol Imaging 2011;38(12):2202–8.

71. Venneti S, Lopresti BJ, Wang G, et al. A comparison of the high-affinity peripheral benzodiazepine receptor ligands DAA1106 and (R)-PK11195 in rat models of neuroinflammation: implications for PET imaging of microglial activation. J Neurochem 2007;102(6):2118–31.

72. Dickens AM, Vainio S, Marjamäki P, et al. Detection of microglial activation in an acute model of neuroinflammation using PET and radiotracers 11C-(R)-PK11195 and 18F-GE-180. J Nucl Med 2014;55(3):466–72.

73. Perrone M, Moon BS, Park HS, et al. A novel PET imaging probe for the detection and monitoring of

translocator protein 18 kDa expression in pathological disorders. Sci Rep 2016;6:20422.

74. Sridharan S, Lepelletier FX, Trigg W, et al. Comparative evaluation of three TSPO PET radiotracers in a LPS-induced model of mild neuroinflammation in rats. Mol Imaging Biol 2017;19(1):77–89.

75. Moon BS, Jung JH, Park HS, et al. Preclinical comparison study between [18F]fluoromethyl-PBR28 and its deuterated analog in a rat model of neuroinflammation. Bioorg Med Chem Lett 2018;28(17):2925–9.

76. Stern EL, Quan N, Proescholdt MG, et al. Spatiotemporal induction patterns of cytokine and related immune signal molecule mRNAs in response to intrastriatal injection of lipopolysaccharide. J Neuroimmunol 2000;106(1–2):114–29.

77. Herrera AJ, Castaño A, Venero JL, et al. The single intranigral injection of LPS as a new model for studying the selective effects of inflammatory reactions on dopaminergic system. Neurobiol Dis 2000;7(4):429–47.

78. Choi DY, Liu M, Hunter RL, et al. Striatal neuroinflammation promotes Parkinsonism in rats. PLoS One 2009;4(5):e5482.

79. Concannon RM, Okine BN, Finn DP, et al. Differential upregulation of the cannabinoid CB2 receptor in neurotoxic and inflammation-driven rat models of Parkinson's disease. Exp Neurol 2015;269:133–41.

80. Brackhan M, Bascunana P, Postema JM, et al. Serial quantitative TSPO-targeted PET reveals peak microglial activation up to 2 weeks after an epileptogenic brain insult. J Nucl Med 2016;57:1302–8.

81. Yankam Njiwa J, Costes N, Bouillot C, et al. Quantitative longitudinal imaging of activated microglia as a marker of inflammation in the pilocarpine rat model of epilepsy using [11C]-(R)-PK11195 PET and MRI. J Cereb Blood Flow Metab 2016;37:1251–63.

82. Russmann V, Brendel M, Mille E, et al. Identification of brain regions predicting epileptogenesis by serial [(18)F]GE-180 positron emission tomography imaging of neuroinflammation in a rat model of temporal lobe epilepsy. Neuroimage Clin 2017;15:35–44.

83. Bergström M, Kumlien E, Lilja A, et al. Temporal lobe epilepsy visualized with PET with 11C-L-deuterium-deprenyl–analysis of kinetic data. Acta Neurol Scand 1998;98:224–31.

84. Kumlien E, Nilsson A, Hagberg G, et al. PET with 11C-deuterium-deprenyl and 18F-FDG in focal epilepsy. Acta Neurol Scand 2001;103:360–6.

85. Bascuñana P, Gendron T, Sander K, et al. Ex vivo characterization of neuroinflammatory and neuroreceptor changes during epileptogenesis using candidate positron emission tomography biomarkers. Epilepsia 2019;60(11):2325–33.

86. Gendron T, Sander K, Cybulska K, et al. Ring-closing synthesis of dibenzothiophene sulfonium salts and their use as leaving groups for aromatic

(18)F-fluorination. J Am Chem Soc 2018;140: 11125–32.

87. Bramoullé Y, Puech F, Saba W, et al. Radiosynthesis of (S)-5-methoxymethyl-3-[6-(4,4,4-trifluorobutoxy) benzo[d]isoxazol-3-yl] oxazolidin-2-[11C]one ([11C]SL25.1188), a novel radioligand for imaging monoamine oxidase-B with PET. J Label Compd Radiopharm 2008;51(3):153–8.

88. Saba W, Valette H, Peyronneau MA, et al. [(11)C] SL25.1188, a new reversible radioligand to study the monoamine oxidase type B with PET: preclinical characterisation in nonhuman primate. Synapse 2010;64(1):61–9.

89. Novaroli L, Daina A, Favre E, et al. Impact of species-dependent differences on screening, design, and development of MAO B inhibitors. J Med Chem 2006;49(21):6264–72.

90. Lavisse S, Guillermier M, Herard AS, et al. Reactive astrocytes overexpress TSPO and are detected by TSPO positron emission tomography imaging. J Neurosci 2012;32(32):10809–18.

91. Pannell M, Economopoulos V, Wilson TC, et al. Imaging of translocator protein upregulation is selective for pro-inflammatory polarized astrocytes and microglia. Glia 2020;68(2):280–97.

92. Tournier BB, Tsartsalis S, Ceyzériat K, et al. Fluorescence-activated cell sorting to reveal the cell origin of radioligand binding. J Cereb Blood Flow Metab 2020;40(6):1242–55.

93. Liddelow S, Guttenplan K, Clarke L, et al. Neurotoxic reactive astrocytes are induced by activated microglia. Nature 2017;541:481–7.

94. Jha MK, Kim JH, Song GJ, et al. Functional dissection of astrocyte-secreted proteins: implications in brain health and diseases. Prog Neurobiol 2018; 162:37–69.

95. Janssen B, Vugts DJ, Windhorst AD, et al. PET imaging of microglial activation-beyond targeting TSPO. Molecules 2018;23(3):607.

96. Wilson H, Dervenoulas G, Pagano G, et al. Imidazoline 2 binding sites reflecting astroglia pathology in Parkinson's disease: an in vivo ^{11}C-BU99008 PET study. Brain 2019;142(10):3116–28.

97. Keller B, García-Sevilla JA. Immunodetection and subcellular distribution of imidazoline receptor proteins with three antibodies in mouse and human brains: effects of treatments with I1- and I2-imidazoline drugs. J Psychopharmacol 2015;29(9): 996–1012.

98. Vignal N, Cisternino S, Rizzo-Padoin N, et al. [18F] FEPPA a TSPO radioligand: optimized radiosynthesis and evaluation as a PET radiotracer for brain inflammation in a peripheral LPS-injected mouse model. Molecules 2018;23(6):1375.

Tau Imaging in Head Injury

Cyrus Ayubcha, MSc[a], Mateen Moghbel, MD[b], Austin J. Borja, BA[c,d],
Andrew Newberg, MD[e,f], Thomas J. Werner, MSc[c],
Abass Alavi, MD, MD (Hon), PhD (Hon), DSc (Hon)[c], Mona-Elisabeth Revheim, MD, PhD, MHA[g,h,*]

KEYWORDS

- Tau • Chronic traumatic encephalopathy • PET • Neurodegeneration • Imaging • CTE

KEY POINTS

- Misfolded tau proteins underlie chronic traumatic encephalopathy (CTE) related to head trauma.
- Tau-PET radiotracers have shown superior specificity and selectivity.
- Tau-PET imaging of head trauma populations has shown elevated tau uptake related to CTE.

INTRODUCTION

Tau proteins play a significant role in a variety of degenerative neurologic conditions. Postmortem neuropathology studies of victims of repeat and severe head trauma have defined a unique spatial expression of neurologic tauopathies in these individuals known as chronic traumatic encephalopathy (CTE). Established and newly developed radiotracers are now being applied to head injury populations with the intent of diagnosis and disease monitoring. This review assesses the role of tau in head injury, the state of tau radiotracer development, and the potential clinical value of tau-PET as derived from head injury studies.

NEUROPATHOLOGY OF TAU PROTEINS IN HEAD INJURY

Tau protein expression is concentrated in the central nervous system (CNS).[1] Tau in the human brain is mostly contained in neurons, although minor expression has been observed in astrocytes and oligodendrocytes.[2] Tau proteins in intraneuronal regions are concentrated within axons and minimal prevalence has been observed in somatodendritic regions, including the cellular membrane, nuclear membrane, and mitochondrial membrane.[1,3] Although multiple functions of tau proteins have been characterized, the most common functions involve stabilizing microtubule (MT) structures, membrane binding, and axonal transport.[4] Recent findings have also suggested that the interactions between MT and tau proteins are purposed to allow long labile domains so as to allow for dynamic growth and contractions.[5]

Nevertheless, the functions of tau are varied depending on the particular location of the tau proteins. In cytoskeletal regions, the binding of tau proteins to MTs either acts to directly stabilize MTs or create a bridge to link MTs and other cytoskeletal structures.[3] Tau proteins are required for the proper formation of postsynaptic structures, dendritic spines, and terminals where tau proteins act as neurotrophic factors in neurogenesis.[6] Certain domains of the tau protein have the capability of binding to the lipid bilayers in the cellular

[a] Harvard Medical School, 25 Shattuck Street, Boston, MA 02115, USA; [b] Department of Radiology, Massachusetts General Hospital, Boston, MA, USA; [c] Department of Radiology, Hospital of the University of Pennsylvania, 3400 Spruce Street, Philadelphia, PA 19104, USA; [d] Perelman School of Medicine, University of Pennsylvania, 3400 Civic Center Boulevard, Philadelphia, PA 19104, USA; [e] Department of Integrative Medicine and Nutritional Sciences, Marcus Institute of Integrative Health, Thomas Jefferson University, Philadelphia, PA, USA; [f] Department of Radiology, Thomas Jefferson University, Philadelphia, PA, USA; [g] Division of Radiology and Nuclear Medicine, Oslo University Hospital, Sognsvannsveien 20, Oslo 0372, Norway; [h] Institute of Clinical Medicine, Faculty of Medicine, University of Oslo, Problemveien 7, Oslo 0315, Norway
* Corresponding author. Division of Radiology and Nuclear Medicine, Oslo University Hospital, Sognsvannsveien 20, Oslo 0372, Norway.
E-mail address: monar@ous-hf.no

PET Clin 16 (2021) 249–260
https://doi.org/10.1016/j.cpet.2020.12.009
1556-8598/21/© 2020 The Authors. Published by Elsevier Inc. This is an open access article under the CC BY license (http://creativecommons.org/licenses/by/4.0/).

membrane, and although the purpose of such membrane associations is speculated, the prevalence of tau-membrane binding has been correlated with tau aggregation. Tau proteins exhibit similar binding processes, although the most characterized binding interaction has been those involving MTs.[4] Tau proteins are natively unfolded, a paper-clip form of tau is present in the intracellular space as a result of intramolecular binding; otherwise, binding interactions with the MT structure alters the protein to expose the MT binding region of the tau proteins, which allows interactions between MT structures and the tau protein (**Fig. 1**).[3]

Tau proteins exist in 8 different conformations and 6 particular isoforms derived from alternative splicing of the MT-associated protein tau (MAPT) gene.[3,7] Of the 6 isoforms, each is differentiated by the number of N-terminal inserts (0N, 1N, 2N) and the number of MT binding repeats in the C-terminal (3R, 4R).[3] The ratio of isoforms varies over the developmental period and varies between regions of the human brain. For instance, the fetal brain expresses only 1 form of the tau isoform, whereas the fully developed brain confers all 6 isoforms. The 3R and 4R isoforms are equally expressed in the cerebral cortex of healthy adults[8]; otherwise, there is a notable discrepancy in the prevalence of N-terminal variants; for example, 0N, 1N, and 2N tau represent 40%, 50%, and 10% of the total CNS tau, respectively.[9] With respect to the proportions of tau protein isoform,

there are significant differences between humans and other species.[3] Once synthesized, tau proteins may undergo a variety of posttranslational modifications, including phosphorylation, glycation, acetylation, oxidation, polyamination, sumoylation, and ubiquitylation.[3]

Tau proteins are salient to the understanding of head injury. Head injuries, depending on the severity, can produce a series of complex and diverse neurophysiological consequences. The primary injury involves the immediate consequences of the physical insult, whereas secondary injury relates to a pathophysiological cascade. A common category of primary injuries is diffuse axonal injuries, which result from torsion and blunt forces. Specifically, external forces can harm the integrity of axonal structures such that axonal MT structures release previously bounded tau proteins into the parenchymal cerebrospinal fluid (CSF). Secondary injury has been associated with inflammatory pathways activation, neuronal metabolism and perfusion alteration, excitotoxicity, free radical generation, mitochondrial dysfunction, axonal degeneration, and neuronal dysfunction.[10] Of note, secondary injury (eg, axonal degeneration) has been understood as the most contributory to the proliferation of tau proteins in the parenchymal space.

This relationship between free tau proteins as a result of head trauma has been examined by many studies in the context of fluid biomarkers. Following traumatic brain injuries (TBIs),

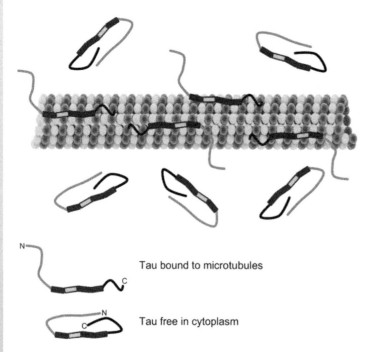

Fig. 1. Binding of tau to MTs. Tau associates with MTs primarily through the MT binding domain, comprising either 3 or 4 repeats. The N and C termini of tau are closely associated when tau is free in the cytoplasm, giving rise to the proposed "paper-clip" model of tau conformation. On binding to MTs, the terminal regions of tau become separated and the N terminus of tau projects away from the MT surface. (*From* Guo, T., W. Noble, and D.P. Hanger, Roles of tau protein in health and disease. Acta neuropathologica, 2017. 133(5): p. 665-704.; with permission.)

Tau bound to microtubules

Tau free in cytoplasm

biomarkers can be assayed primarily in CSF or peripheral blood, although CSF is often preferred.[11] Several studies have thoroughly confirmed the association of several CSF biomarkers with axonal injury after mild (mTBI), moderate, and severe TBI (sTBI). More sensitive assays used by studies on sports-related mTBIs are associated with acute increases of tau in plasma where the concentration of tau correlated with the duration of postconcussive symptoms and the concentrations steadily declined during rehabilitation.[12] sTBI events have correlated with greater concentrations of tau in CSF samples where tau protein levels in ventricular CSF have directly related to TBI severity, lesion size, hypoxia, and clinical outcomes.[13] In those with repeated injury (eg, boxers, contact sport athletes), elevated levels of tau in CSF samples were observed more than a week after the sporting event, where normalization of tau levels occurred 2 to 3 months from incident.[13]

Within the context of head injury, the most serious consequences of the accumulation of tau proteins are seen in unique neurologic tauopathies, namely CTE, in which tau aggregation is linked to subsequent neurodegenerative processes.[14] Epidemiologic studies have linked TBI, single event and repeat, to the development of tauopathies.[10] Although the etiology of tauopathies are somewhat speculative, the pathologic characterization of neurologic tauopathies is generally agreed on.[15] Tauopathies are defined by the intraneuronal presence of tau aggregates termed neurofibrillary tangles (NFT), which are composed of multiple units of hyperphosphorylated MT-associated tau isoforms. The particular form of neurodegeneration leads to a unique distribution and identity of prions[15] (**Figs. 2** and **3**, **Table 1**[16]).[17]

In most tauopathy cases, tau proteins are hyperphosphorylated to become unbounded from MT

Stage I

Stage II

Stage III

Stage IV

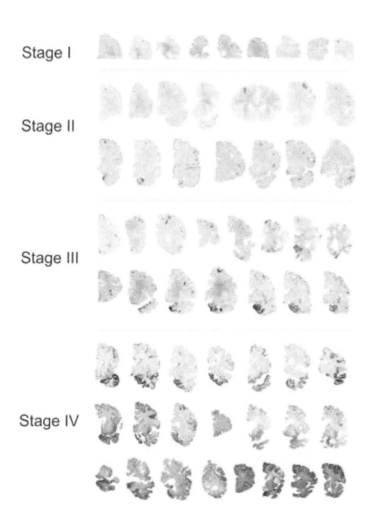

Fig. 2. Stages of CTE. In stage I CTE, p-tau pathology is found in discrete foci in the cerebral cortex, most commonly in the superior or lateral frontal cortices, typically around small vessels at the depths of sulci. In stage II CTE, there are multiple foci of p-tau at the depths of the cerebral sulci and there is localized spread of neurofibrillary pathology from these epicenters to the superficial layers of adjacent cortex. The medial temporal lobe is spared neurofibrillary p-tau pathology. In stage III CTE, p-tau pathology is widespread; the frontal, insular, temporal and parietal cortices show widespread neurofibrillary degeneration with greatest severity in the frontal and temporal lobes, concentrated at the depths of the sulci. Also, in stage III CTE, the amygdala, hippocampus, and entorhinal cortex show substantial neurofibrillary pathology that is found in earlier CTE stages. In stage IV CTE, there is widespread severe p-tau pathology affecting most regions of the cerebral cortex and the medial temporal lobe, sparing calcarine cortex in all but the most severe cases. All images, CP-13 immunostained 50 μ tissue sections. (*From* McKee, A.C., et al., The neuropathology of chronic traumatic encephalopathy. Brain pathology, 2015. 25(3): p. 350-364; with permission.)

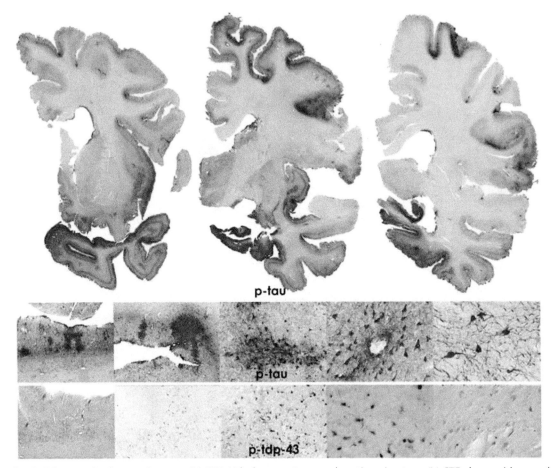

Fig. 3. Microscopic changes in stage IV CTE. Whole-mount coronal sections in stage IV CTE show widespread p-tau pathology affecting most regions of the cerebral cortex and medial temporal lobe. Astrocytic tangles are prominent and there is marked neuronal loss in the cortex, amygdala, and hippocampus. There are also widespread pTDP-43 abnormalities. All images: 50 μ tissue sections, CP-13, or p-TDP-43 immunostain. (*From* McKee, A.C., et al., The neuropathology of chronic traumatic encephalopathy. Brain pathology, 2015. 25(3): p. 350-364; with permission.)

structures; these hyperphosphorylated proteins then accumulate within cells with MAPT mutations. However, changes in isoforms or phosphorylation patterns as a result of such mutations result in tau aggregation that is insoluble and harmful to neuronal function and axonal transport.[18] Tau aggregates retain prion properties by way of seeding and spreading.[19] Minimal exposure to tau seeds can further lead to misfolding and aggregation. This phenomenon is observed when tau proteins mislocalized into the soma and dendrites are transferred between the neurons.[10] It has been observed that tau proteins can spread using the connectome network pattern and either spread preformed NFT or seed subsequent tau accumulation.[10] Sparse tau aggregation generally develops naturally with age, however, and increased density and unique distributions of tau and other abnormal

protein aggregates (eg, beta-amyloid plaques) in the context of clinical dementia become indicative of neurodegenerative disease.[15]

Concerning TBI, NFTs can be observed within 6 hours of the event, and postmortem studies of those with single-event moderate to sTBI have shown higher levels of NFTs than in controls.[10] It is further understood that the risk of CTE is directly related to the number and severity of TBI events.[10] Interestingly, although the distribution of tau aggregates and, to a lesser extent, beta-amyloid plaques, is unique in CTE, there is not unique phosphorylation or a specific isoform that differentiates CTE from other neurodegenerative conditions.[20] Further, the ratio of tau proteins to beta-amyloid plaques is particularly elevated in CTE and is a unique characteristic of this neurodegenerative condition.

Table 1
Pathologic classification of chronic traumatic encephalopathy

Stage	Macroscopic Observations	Microscopic Observations
I	• Unremarkable	• *Principal Characteristic*: One to 2 isolated perivascular focal epicenters of immunoreactive p-tau neurofibrillary tangles (NFT) and neurites (lesions) at the depths of the cerebral sulci in the parietal, frontal and temporal cortices • Beta-amyloid plaques are absent in subjects younger than 50 y • P-tau reactive microglia may exist
II	• Mild enlargement of lateral ventricles • Varying enlargement of the third ventricle • Pallor of the locus coeruleus and substantia nigra	• *Principal Characteristic*: Multiple perivascular foci consisting of p-tau NFT, pre-tangles, and neurites are found in multiple cortices and the superficial cortical layers of surrounding regions such as the gyral crests and sulcal walls • Active microglia exist in the subcortical white matter with surrounding axonal swelling • Beta-amyloid plaques are absent in subjects younger than 50 y
III	• Decreased brain weight • Mild atrophy in the frontal and temporal lobes • Enlargement of the lateral and third ventricles • Potential cavum septum pellucidum, septal fenestration or perforation in some patients	• *Principal Characteristic*: Multiple perivascular neurites, p-tau NFT, pre-tangles, and neurofibrillary lesions of degeneration in the amygdala, hippocampus, entorhinal cortex, and perirhinal cortex • Diminished myelinated nerve fibers, axonal dystrophy and axonal loss can be observed • Beta-amyloid plaques are rarely observed • TAR DNA-binding protein 43 (TDP-43) immunopositive neurites may exist in some cases
IV	• Deceased brain weight • Cerebral atrophy within the temporal, frontal, medial frontal lobes along with the anterior thalamus • Diffuse white matter and corpus callosum atrophy • Cavum septum, perforations, fenestration or absence of posterior septum in most patients	• *Principal Characteristic*: Dense p-tau foci ubiquitously distributed in the cerebrum, diencephalon, and brainstem • Neuronal degeneration of the cortex, astrocytosis in the white matter, gliosis, loss of myelinated nerve fibers, axonal dystrophy, and TDP-43 immunopositive neurites are observed in most cases • Beta-amyloid plaques may be observed

From Ayubcha, C., et al., A critical review of radiotracers in the positron emission tomography imaging of traumatic brain injury: FDG, tau, and amyloid imaging in mild traumatic brain injury and chronic traumatic encephalopathy. European Journal of Nuclear Medicine and Molecular Imaging, 2020; with permission.

TAU RADIOTRACERS IN HEAD INJURY

The strong link between the presence of NFT and neurocognitive decline has strongly motivated the development of tau radiotracers that can assess the magnitude and localization of abnormal protein aggregates (**Table 2**).[7] In the context of most tauopathies, tau radiotracers are required to cross plasma cell membranes and the blood-brain barrier to reach intracellular tau proteins; tau NFT radiotracers must provide high selectivity given similar structures between NFT and β-amyloid aggregates; radiotracers must further account for the variation in NFT with respect to tertiary structures, posttranslational modifications, and isoforms.[7] As such, there is a need for specificity and breadth when developing tau radiotracers.

Table 2
Tau radiotracers

Radiotracer	Description
[18F]FDDNP	Although one of the first radioligands developed for tau, this radioligand has low selectivity for tau. Uptake most often reflects amyloid and tau aggregates.
[18F]THK523	As a result of in vitro, ex vivo, and in vivo studies, this radiotracer has proven more selective for phosphorylated tau rather than β-amyloid. [18F]THK253 is mostly retention by white matter, which harms quantification. Imaging in non-Alzheimer's Disease (non-AD) tauopathies has not shown expected uptake patterns. Other THK compounds have presented a higher binding affinity for tau.
[18F]THK5351	[18F]THK5351 has faster kinetics and lower white matter binding compared with other [18F]THK derivatives. Off-target binding of all THK radiotracers was observed in the striatal regions and MAO-B sites. [18F]THK5351 has proven to have a lower binding affinity and higher increased off-target binding as compared with [18F]AV1451.
[18F]AV1451	[18F]AV1451, also known as [18F]T807 and flortaucipir, confers significantly lower white matter retention while indicating a higher binding affinity for tau as compared with beta-amyloid and other aggregates. Notable off-target binding of [18F]AV1451, likely due to iron and, in the basal ganglia, the substantia nigra, and the choroid plexus is observed.
[11C]PBB3	[11C]PBB3 has one of the highest affinities for neurofibrillary tangles (NFTs) as compared with other prions. Efficient blood-brain barrier penetration and minimal washout were noted. Limited white matter binding but retention in the venous sinuses were observed. This radiotracer can bind 3R and 4R tau isoforms in non-AD tauopathies. Nevertheless, the metabolite character and low half-life of the radiotracer can limit quantification.
Analogues of [11C]PBB3	New fluorinated PBB3 derivatives have attempted to overcome limitations in [11C] half-life, off-target binding in striatal regions, and limited dynamic range. Preliminary investigations have shown success in addressing these limiting characteristics.
[18F] Genentech tau probe 1	Preliminary research has shown that the Genentech tau probe 1 (GTP-1) has advantageous kinetics. Uptake has correlated with disease progression, severity, and differentiation between diseased patients and healthy controls.
[18F]RO6958948	[18F]RO6958948 is high-affinity tau with desirable kinetic characteristics (eg, rapid blood-brain barrier passage and minimal washout). Exploratory studies have shown tau accumulation in Braak-stage regions. [18F]RO6958948, [18F]AV1451, and [18F] THK535 demonstrated similar binding patterns for tau aggregates in AD, but none of the findings were remarkable in the context of non-AD tauopathies.
[18F]MK-6240	[18F]MK-6240 presents high specificity and selectivity for NFT along with sufficient pharmacokinetic properties. As of yet, no significant off-target binding has been observed but rapid washout has been noted.

Data from Hall, B., et al., In vivo tau PET imaging in dementia: pathophysiology, radiotracer quantification, and a systematic review of clinical findings. Ageing research reviews, 2017. 36: p. 50-63.

Interestingly, these challenges are less significant to the application of tau imaging in the context of head injury. Limitations in the concentration of tau proteins as compared with beta-amyloid plaques have posed a significant challenge to tau imaging in dementias, but this is not the case in CTE. In CTE, the prevalence of tau is significantly greater than that of beta-amyloid. As such, highly specific tau radiotracers can excel in binding to tau aggregates with less risk of off-site binding. In addition, there are higher concentrations of tau aggregates in perivascular space, which allows easier access of radiotracers to tau aggregates. As such, tau radiotracers in the context of CTE, as compared with other tauopathy dementias, are likely to perform well.

TAU PET IMAGING STUDIES IN HEAD INJURY

Using many of the noted radiotracers, many studies have applied tau PET to TBI populations. Most tau-PET imaging of individuals with single-event TBIs takes place long after the original insult, whereas most studies use patients with years of mTBI experiences through sports or military combat. Takahata and colleagues[21] used [11C]PBB3-PET to assess tau patterns in 27 individuals with either repeat mTBI or sTBI as compared with 15 healthy control subjects. Increased uptake in the cerebrum and white matter correlated to psychosis and other neuropsychiatric symptoms.[21] Gorgraptis and colleagues[22] applied [18F]AV145-PET in 21 subjects with moderate to sTBI and 11 healthy control subjects; elevated whole brain and right occipital lobe uptake of [18F]AV145 were observed in the TBI group. Robinson and colleagues[23] observed increased white matter uptake of [18F]AV145 and notable uptake in the cerebellum, occipital lobe, inferior temporal lobe, and frontal lobe across 16 military veterans with a history of blast neurotrauma. However, no controls were used in this study as comparators.

Several studies have used National Football League (NFL) players as their study population, whereas most studies have aligned well with non-NFL populations with a few notable

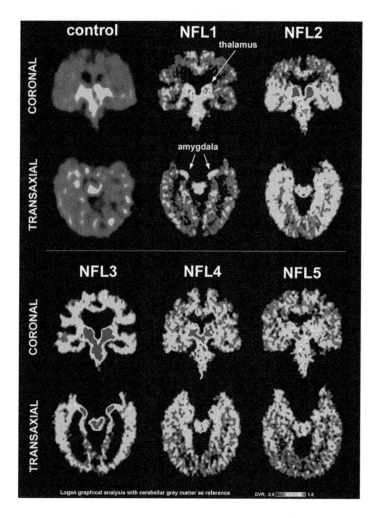

Fig. 4. [18F]FDDNP-PET results for NFL players and a control. Coronal and transaxial [18F]FDDNP-PET scans of the retired NFL players include the following: NFL1: 59-year-old linebacker with mild cognitive impairment (MCI), who experienced momentary loss of consciousness after each of 2 concussions; NFL2: 64-year-old quarterback with age-consistent memory impairment, who experienced momentary loss of consciousness and 24-hour amnesia following 1 concussion; NFL3: 73-year-old guard with dementia and depression, who suffered brief loss of consciousness after 20 concussions, and a 12-hour coma following 1 concussion; NFL4: 50-year-old defensive lineman with MCI and depression, who suffered 2 concussions and loss consciousness for 10 minutes following one of them; NFL5: 45-year-old center with MCI, who suffered 10 concussions and complained of light sensitivity, irritability, and decreased concentration after the last two. The players' scans show consistently high signals in the amygdala and subcortical regions and a range of cortical binding from extensive to limited, whereas the control subject shows limited binding in these regions. Red and yellow areas indicate high [18F]FDDNP binding signals. (*From* Small, G.W., et al., PET scanning of brain tau in retired national football league players: preliminary findings. The American Journal of Geriatric Psychiatry, 2013. 21(2): p. 138–144; with permission.)

exceptions. Dickstein and colleagues[24] examined one player with [18F]AV145-PET and found increased uptake in the gray matter–white junction along with the bilateral cingulate, occipital lobe, and orbitofrontal cortices, and temporal lobes. Mitsis and colleagues[25] observed increased [18F]AV1451 uptake in the 1 NFL player and 1 patient with sTBI in whom differential uptake patterns were observed. The NFL subject conferred higher uptake in the nigral and striatal regions, whereas the subcortical and hippocampal regions were more avid in the scans of the subject with sTBI.[25] Okonkwo and colleagues[26] also observed elevated [18F]AV1451 uptake in 2 patients with TBI as compared with age-sex matched controls. Wooten and colleagues[27] assessed the [18F] AV1451-PET scans of 5 athletes, 2 veterans, and 1 vehicular accident patient as compared with 11 healthy subjects; regions with higher uptake in the TBI group were correlated with poor white matter function.

Larger studies with NFL players were performed by Barrio and colleagues[28] and Stern and colleagues[29] applied [18F] AV1451 to 16 NFL players and 31 healthy controls to find elevated uptake in the bilateral superior frontal,

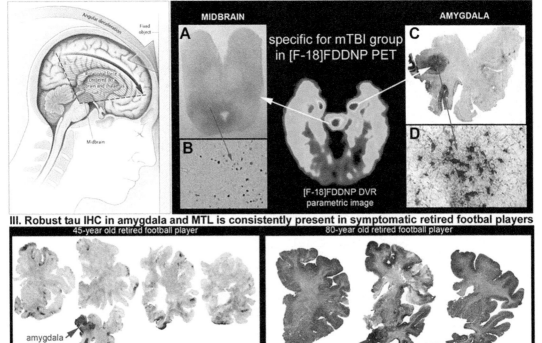

Fig. 5. Involvement of amygdala and midbrain areas in concussion-based mTBI is supported by both mechanistic concept of injury (*I*) and by the results of neuropathological examinations in deceased retired American football players with premortem complaints of functional impairments (*II* and *III*). (*I*) Rotation of the brain in the sagittal plane during a concussion, associated with significant accelerations and deceleration, will have significant negative effect on the brain tissue in the midbrain and thalamus (*green shaded area*) and on the affected cortical areas (*red area*). Stretching, compression, and shearing of axons during such sudden brain movements are hypothesized to be the cause of axonal injury. Similarly, rotation in the coronal plane has been shown to lead to consistent damage to midbrain region tracts (27). (*II*) (*A–D*) show results of tau immunohistochemistry (IHC) and demonstrate that in the mTBI group areas of increased [18F]FDDNP signal in amygdala and dorsal midbrain coincide with presence of dense tau deposits in periaqueductal gray in dorsal midbrain (*A, B*) and in amygdala (*C, D*). (*III*) Amygdala and medial temporal lobe (MTL) areas are affected in the brains of retired professional American football players who died due to suicide (*left*; 45-year-old retired player) or due to natural causes (*right*; 80-year-old retired NFL player). Amygdala and MTL areas are the first areas with high density of tau deposits in the neocortex and remain one of the most affected cortical regions in most retired professional American football player cases. (*From* Barrio, J.R., et al., In vivo characterization of chronic traumatic encephalopathy using [F-18] FDDNP PET brain imaging. Proceedings of the National Academy of Sciences, 2015. 112(16): p. E2039-E2047; with permission.)

bilateral medial temporal, and left parietal regions. Barrio and colleagues[28] used [18F] FDDNP-PET to study uptake patterns among 14 NFL players and 28 healthy controls. Although [18F]FDDNP is bound to beta-amyloid and tau aggregates, the limited prevalence of beta-amyloid in CTE implies that much of the unique uptake in these populations as compared with the control are likely driven my tau aggregate accumulation and not beta-amyloid deposition.[28]

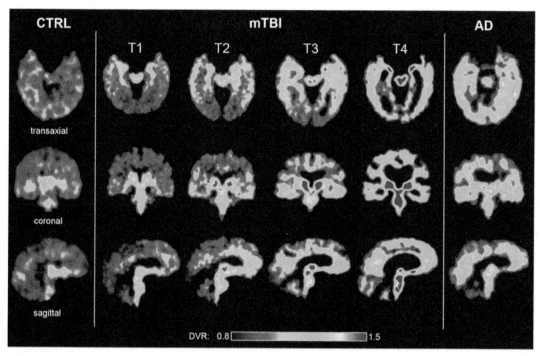

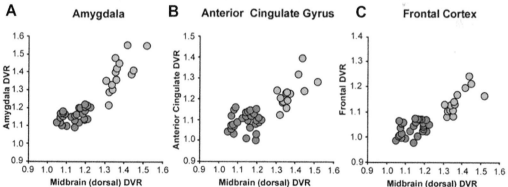

Fig. 6. [18F]FDDNP distribution volume ratios (DVR) parametric images showing patterns T1 to T4 of increased [18F]FDDNP signal observed in the mTBI group compared with cognitive control subjects (*left*). The T1 pattern shows involvement of 2 core areas that have consistently increased [18F]FDDNP signal in all 4 patterns: amygdala (limbic) and dorsal midbrain (subcortical). Patterns T2 to T4 are marked by increase of [18F]FDDNP signal in these 2 core regions and progressively larger number of subcortical, limbic, and cortical areas. Although more complex patterns (eg, T4) overlap with AD in the cortex, midbrain and amygdala signals are elevated above the levels in AD. An AD case is shown in the right column for comparison. (*Lower*) (*A*) is a 2-dimensional scatter plot showing [18F]FDDNP DVR values in 2 core areas consistently involved in CTE (subcortical structures [dorsal midbrain] and limbic structures [amygdala]), clearly demonstrating separation of mTBI and control (CTRL) groups. (*B, C*) demonstrate similar separation effect when dorsal midbrain is compared with cortical areas typically associated with CTE and its mood disorders, namely anterior cingulate gyrus (ACG) (*B*) and frontal lobe (*C*). Subjects with mTBI are represented by green circles, and CTRL subjects are represented by blue circles. (*From* Barrio, J.R., et al., In vivo characterization of chronic traumatic encephalopathy using [F-18] FDDNP PET brain imaging. Proceedings of the National Academy of Sciences, 2015. 112(16): p. E2039-E2047; with permission.)

Nevertheless, Barrio and colleagues[28] noted increased uptake in the amygdala, anterior cingulate gyrus, and frontal cortex in the NFL players. Chen and colleagues[30] used [18F]FDDN-PET in a study population of 7 military veterans, 15 retired players with mTBI histories, and 28 healthy controls; findings were consistent with Barrio and colleagues,[28] but it was noted that military personnel had limited uptake in the amygdala and striatum relative to the player population. Vasilevskaya and colleagues[31] applied [18F] AV1451-PET to 38 former contact sport athletes. In this study, the presence of APOE4 alleles aligned with high cortical gray matter PET tau uptake such that the presence of APOE4 may incline individuals to accumulate tau aggregates more so than others[31] (**Fig. 4**,[32] **Figs. 5** and **6**,[28] **Fig. 7**[33]).

Given that the present diagnosis of CTE is contingent on postmortem neuropathological examination, some of the most convincing tau-PET studies have attempted to confirm their imaging with postmortem analysis of the brain. Mantyh and colleagues[34] studied 1 former NFL player with [18F] AV1451-PET with subsequent postmortem analysis of the individual who was subsequently diagnosed with stage IV CTE, TDP 43 encephalopathy, and stage 3 Braak NFT. Uptake was most avid in degenerated and hypometabolic

regions in the frontotemporal region; this overlapped postmortem tau aggregates in the left fusiform, inferior temporal gyri, and juxtacortical frontal white matter. High uptake with minimal tau deposition was noted in the basal ganglia, thalamus, motor cortex, and calcarine cortex.[34] Omalu and colleagues[33] assessed the [18F] FDDNP-PET scan of 1 former NFL player and respective postmortem analysis to find that [18F] FDDNP-PET uptake correlated with tau deposition, most notably in the parasagittal and paraventricular regions of the brain and the brain stem. No correlation with amyloid or TDP-43 deposition was observed such that regions of the brain most involved in shearing and rotational forces were most linked to tau deposition; such deposition patterns would align with the unique patterns found in CTE.[33]

Marquié and colleagues[35] did not perform any in vivo imaging, rather autoradiographic binding patterns of [18F]AV1451 were observed in 5 postmortem brains diagnosed with stage II through stage IV CTE. [18F]AV1451 binding observed in all NFT regions as confirmed by immunostaining and a limited signal was observed in white matter and other non–tangle-containing regions. Quantification of tau burden and tracer uptake was correlated.[35] Previously mentioned in vivo studies have

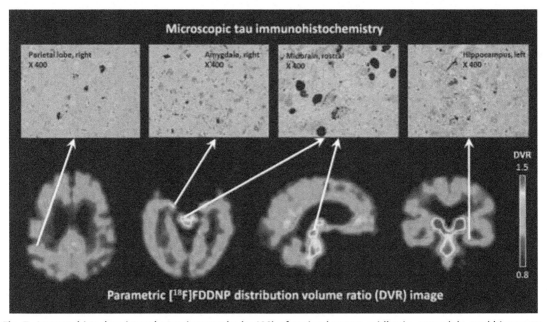

Fig. 7. Immunohistochemistry photomicrographs (× 400) of parietal cortex, midbrain, amygdala, and hippocampus show the presence of tau neuropathological deposits in these regions. (*Lower*) Representative transaxial (2 sections), sagittal (*middle*), and coronal sections (*right*) of [18F]FDDNP-PET images with high signals in the periventricular subcortical regions, amygdala, and midbrain. Warmer colors (*red and yellow*) show areas with higher [18F]FDDNP binding signals. (*From* Omalu, B., et al., Postmortem autopsy-confirmation of antemortem [F-18] FDDNP-PET scans in a football player with chronic traumatic encephalopathy. Neurosurgery, 2018. 82(2): p. 237–246; with permission.)

not found such consistent binding patterns and strong correlations, which may be indicative of a difference between the ex vivo and in vivo environments.

SUMMARY

In reviewing this literature, there are several apparent takeaways. There are variations in the binding patterns between different tau radiotracers. Nevertheless, there is consistently uptake in certain regions across studies; aberrant binding is expected given the variation in small studies and potential off-site radiotracer binding. However, the literature suggests that larger studies may be more consistent in finding uptake in regions where tau aggregates are normally observed in CTE populations. Overall, the evidence suggests that tau-PET imaging will continue to play a significant role in TBI and CTE. These studies have shown considerable promise in the imaging of tau and prospective larger studies may substantiate the use of a particular radiotracer in the assessment of long-term TBI ramifications and the diagnosis of CTE. In particular, there is a notable need for future studies that incorporate in vivo imaging and postmortem pathologic study.

CLINICS CARE POINTS

- Patients with a history of head trauma should be assessed for long-term sequalae associated with head injury.
- Tau deposition is associated with chronic ramifications of head trauma.
- Tau-PET has shown promise in assessing the progression of chronic symptoms and degenerative conditions associated with head trauma.

CONFLICT OF INTEREST

The authors have declared no conflicts of interest.

DISCLOSURE

The authors have nothing to disclose.

REFERENCES

1. Melková K, Vojtěch Z, Subhash N, et al. Structure and functions of microtubule associated proteins tau and MAP2c: similarities and differences. Biomolecules 2019;9(3):105.
2. Müller R, Heinrich M, Heck S, et al. Expression of microtubule-associated proteins MAP2 and tau in cultured rat brain oligodendrocytes. Cell Tissue Res 1997;288(2):239–49.
3. Guo T, Noble W, Hanger DP. Roles of tau protein in health and disease. Acta neuropathol 2017;133(5):665–704.
4. Zhang B, Arpita M, Sharon S, et al. Microtubule-binding drugs offset tau sequestration by stabilizing microtubules and reversing fast axonal transport deficits in a tauopathy model. Proc Natl Acad Sci U S A 2005;102(1):227–31.
5. Qiang L, Xiaohuan S, Timothy OA, et al. Tau does not stabilize axonal microtubules but rather enables them to have long labile domains. Curr Biol 2018;28(13):2181–9.e4.
6. Ittner LM, Thomas F, Yazi DK, et al. Parkinsonism and impaired axonal transport in a mouse model of frontotemporal dementia. Proc Natl Acad Sci U S A 2008;105(41):15997–6002.
7. Hall B, Elijah M, Simon C, et al. In vivo tau PET imaging in dementia: pathophysiology, radiotracer quantification, and a systematic review of clinical findings. Ageing Res Rev 2017;36:50–63.
8. Goedert M, Spillantini MG, Jakes R, et al. Multiple isoforms of human microtubule-associated protein tau: sequences and localization in neurofibrillary tangles of Alzheimer's disease. Neuron 1989;3(4):519–26.
9. Goedert M, Jakes R. Expression of separate isoforms of human tau protein: correlation with the tau pattern in brain and effects on tubulin polymerization. EMBO J 1990;9(13):4225–30.
10. Edwards G III, Jing Z, Pramod KD, et al. Traumatic brain injury induces tau aggregation and spreading. J Neurotrauma 2020;37(1):80–92.
11. Strathmann FG, Stefanie S, Kyle G, et al. Blood-based biomarkers for traumatic brain injury: evaluation of research approaches, available methods and potential utility from the clinician and clinical laboratory perspectives. Clin Biochem 2014;47(10–11):876–88.
12. Bogoslovsky T, Jessica G, Andreas J, et al. Fluid biomarkers of traumatic brain injury and intended context of use. Diagnostics (Basel) 2016;6(4):37.
13. Zetterberg H, Smith DH, Blennow K. Biomarkers of mild traumatic brain injury in cerebrospinal fluid and blood. Nat Rev Neurol 2013;9(4):201.
14. Irwin DJ. Tauopathies as clinicopathological entities. Parkinsonism Relat Disord 2016;22:S29–33.
15. Spillantini MG, Goedert M. Tau pathology and neurodegeneration. Lancet Neurol 2013;12(6):609–22.
16. Ayubcha C, Mona-Elisabeth R, Andrew N, et al. A critical review of radiotracers in the positron emission tomography imaging of traumatic brain injury:

FDG, tau, and amyloid imaging in mild traumatic brain injury and chronic traumatic encephalopathy. Eur J Nucl Med Mol Imaging 2020. https://doi.org/10.1007/s00259-020-04926-4.

17. McKee AC, Bobak A, Thor DS, et al. The neuropathology of chronic traumatic encephalopathy. Brain Pathol 2015;25(3):350–64.

18. Soto C, Pritzkow S. Protein misfolding, aggregation, and conformational strains in neurodegenerative diseases. Nat Neurosci 2018;21(10):1332–40.

19. Holmes BB, Jennifer LF, Thomas EM, et al. Proteopathic tau seeding predicts tauopathy in vivo. Proc Natl Acad Sci U S A 2014;111(41):E4376–85.

20. Puvenna V, Madeline E, Manoj B, et al. Is phosphorylated tau unique to chronic traumatic encephalopathy? Phosphorylated tau in epileptic brain and chronic traumatic encephalopathy. Brain Res 2016; 1630:225–40.

21. Takahata K, Yasuyuki K, Naruhiko S, et al. PET-detectable tau pathology correlates with long-term neuropsychiatric outcomes in patients with traumatic brain injury. Brain 2019;142(10):3265–79.

22. Gorgoraptis N, Lucia ML, Alex W, et al. In vivo detection of cerebral tau pathology in long-term survivors of traumatic brain injury. Sci Transl Med 2019; 11(508):eaaw1993.

23. Robinson ME, Ann CM, David HS, et al. Positron emission tomography of tau in Iraq and Afghanistan Veterans with blast neurotrauma. Neuroimage Clin 2019;21:101651.

24. Dickstein D, Pullman MY, Fernandez C, et al. Cerebral [18 F] T807/AV1451 retention pattern in clinically probable CTE resembles pathognomonic distribution of CTE tauopathy. Transl Psychiatry 2016;6(9):e900.

25. Mitsis E, Riggio S, Kostakoglu L, et al. Tauopathy PET and amyloid PET in the diagnosis of chronic traumatic encephalopathies: studies of a retired NFL player and of a man with FTD and a severe head injury. Transl Psychiatry 2014;4(9):e441.

26. Okonkwo DO, Ross CP, Davneet SM, et al. [18F] FDG,[11C] PiB, and [18F] AV-1451 PET imaging of neurodegeneration in two subjects with a history of repetitive trauma and cognitive decline. Front Neurol 2019;10:831.

27. Wooten DW, Ortiz-Terán L, Zubcevik N, et al. Multi-modal signatures of tau pathology, neuronal fiber integrity, and functional connectivity in traumatic brain injury. J Neurotrauma 2019;36(23): 3233–43.

28. Barrio JR, Gary WS, Koon-Pong W, et al. In vivo characterization of chronic traumatic encephalopathy using [F-18] FDDNP PET brain imaging. Proc Natl Acad Sci U S A 2015;112(16):E2039–47.

29. Stern RA, Adler CH, Chen K, et al. Tau positron-emission tomography in former national football league players. New England journal of medicine 2019;380(18):1716–25.

30. Chen ST, Prabha S, David AM, et al. FDDNP-PET Tau brain protein binding patterns in military personnel with suspected chronic traumatic encephalopathy. J Alzheimers Dis 2018;65(1):79–88.

31. Vasilevskaya A, Foad T, Charles B, et al. Interaction of APOE4 alleles and PET tau imaging in former contact sport athletes. Neuroimage Clin 2020;26: 102212.

32. Small GW, Vladimir K, Prabha S, et al. PET scanning of brain tau in retired national football league players: preliminary findings. Am J Geriatr Psychiatry 2013;21(2):138–44.

33. Omalu B, Gary WS, Julian B, et al. Postmortem autopsy-confirmation of antemortem [F-18] FDDNP-PET scans in a football player with chronic traumatic encephalopathy. Neurosurgery 2018; 82(2):237–46.

34. Mantyh WG, Salvatore S, Alex L, et al. Tau positron emission tomographic findings in a former US football player with pathologically confirmed chronic traumatic encephalopathy. JAMA Neurol 2020; 77(4):517–21.

35. Marquié M, Cinthya A, Ana CA, et al. [18 F]-AV-1451 binding profile in chronic traumatic encephalopathy: a postmortem case series. Acta neuropathol Commun 2019;7(1):164.

Molecular Imaging of Neurodegenerative Parkinsonism

Kirk A. Frey, MD, PhD[a,b,*], Nicolaas I.L.J. Bohnen, MD, PhD[c,d,e]

KEYWORDS

- Parkinson disease • Progressive supranuclear palsy • Multiple system atrophy
- Corticobasal degeneration • Positron tomography

KEY POINTS

- Accurate clinical diagnosis of parkinsonian neurodegenerative conditions remains difficult, particularly for the atypical parkinsonisms.
- Imaging biomarkers can define pathologic changes in vulnerable neuronal populations in neurodegenerative parkinsonism.
- Distinct types and patterns of misfolded protein aggregate deposits in pathologic assessments distinguish among neurodegenerative parkinsonisms.
- Molecular imaging tracers targeting distinct protein aggregates in parkinsonisms are not yet available, and are under development.

INTRODUCTION

Neurodegenerative Movement Disorders with Parkinsonism

There are several neurodegenerative disorders associated with clinical signs and symptoms of parkinsonism. The core features are slowness of voluntary movements (bradykinesia) together with muscle stiffness at rest (rigidity), with variable anatomic distribution. There ae additional clinical features that may be present that can assist in classification of the underlying neurologic disorder as Parkinson disease (PD; idiopathic PD), multiple system atrophy (MSA), progressive supranuclear palsy (PSP), or corticobasal degeneration (CBD). Together, MSA, PSP, and CBD are often referred to as Parkinson-plus or as atypical parkinsonism (atypical PD [aPD]) syndromes. Distinction of the diagnoses at symptomatic onset is often difficult, because typifying signs and symptoms may require subsequent disease progression to manifest. Compared with autopsy pathologic diagnoses, the accuracy of clinical diagnoses may be no greater than 75%.[1,2] With longitudinal evaluations in specialty neurology movement disorder clinics, the differential diagnosis of aPD remains challenging.[3] Thus, specific clinical tests and reliable distinctive biomarkers would have significant impact on diagnosis accuracy and on selection of patients for future trials of novel therapeutics.

[a] Department of Radiology (Nuclear Medicine and Molecular Imaging), University of Michigan, 1500 East Medical Center Drive, Room B1-G505 UH, Ann Arbor, MI 48109-5028, USA; [b] Department of Neurology, University of Michigan, 1500 East Medical Center Drive, Room B1-G505 UH, Ann Arbor, MI 48109-5028, USA; [c] Department of Radiology (Nuclear Medicine and Molecular Imaging), University of Michigan, 24 Frank Lloyd Wright Drive, Box 362, Ann Arbor, MI 48105, USA; [d] Department of Neurology, University of Michigan, 24 Frank Lloyd Wright Drive, Box 362, Ann Arbor, MI 48105, USA; [e] Ann Arbor Veterans Administration Medical Center, Ann Arbor, MI, USA
* Corresponding author. Department of Radiology (Nuclear Medicine and Molecular Imaging), University of Michigan, 1500 East Medical Center Drive, Room B1-G505 UH, Ann Arbor, MI 48109-5028.
E-mail address: kfrey@umich.edu

PET Clin 16 (2021) 261–272
https://doi.org/10.1016/j.cpet.2020.12.002

Parkinson Disease

PD was described initially by James Parkinson[4] in 1817 in a collection of patients from his practice with progressive movement difficulties (see Ref.[5] for recent review). Bradykinesia and rigidity, with predominant onset asymmetrically in an upper extremity, together with a characteristic rest tremor are signs supporting clinical diagnosis of PD.[3,6] Patients may perceive weakness in the involved limb, but objective examination reveals no significant loss of strength, weakness being related to loss of dexterity and voluntary movement attributable to underlying bradykinesia and rigidity. The most reliable clinical confirmation of the PD diagnosis is a dramatic and sustained (over years) symptomatic response to dopamine (DA)-replacement and augmentation pharmacotherapy.

The neuropathologic changes in PD are widely distributed in the nervous system. Initially, it was appreciated that degeneration of dopaminergic neurons in the substantia nigra and adjacent ventral tegmental area, associated with prominent eosinophilic cytoplasmic inclusions, Lewy bodies, were omnipresent and diagnostic of PD.[7] More recently, it is appreciated that neurodegeneration associated with Lewy bodies or with Lewy neurites together with neuronal losses are seen also in the peripheral autonomic nervous system, the medullary autonomic motor nuclei, the pontine locus coeruleus, serotonergic nuclei throughout the brain stem, basal forebrain cholinergic nuclei, and in cerebral limbic and neocortices.[8] This widespread distribution has been detected most readily by immunochemistry targeting the presence of the protein alpha-synuclein (αS) as a major constituent of Lewy bodies[9] and also of Lewy neurites, the latter often difficult to recognize in basic histopathologic tissue stains. The involvement of multiple sites of neurodegeneration is associated with the evolution of theoretic models proposing a progressive spread of αS disorder from peripheral organs (intestinal tract or nasal mucosa) centrally to the involved brain stem and cerebral sites.[10] A multitude of clinical symptoms, including constipation, anosmia, rapid eye movement (REM) behavioral sleep disorder, affective dysregulation (depression and anxiety), as well as cognitive impairment and dementia are now recognized in addition to the parkinsonian movement abnormalities considered classic in the diagnosis of PD.[11]

Multiple System Atrophy

MSA is a condition with variable clinical presentation, most often dichotomized as cerebellar, characterized by predominance of dystaxic control of voluntary limb movements, speech, and posture (MSAc), or as parkinsonian, characterized by rigidity and bradykinesia as seen in PD (MSAp).[12,13] In some patients, clinical features of both MSAc and MSAp are present, referred to as mixed MSA (MSAm). MSAp is often difficult to distinguish from PD at symptom onset. A differentiating MSA feature is the presence of prominent autonomic deficits, including orthostatic hypotension, bowel and urinary bladder dysfunction, and erectile dysfunction.[13]

Current pathologic diagnosis of MSA relies on the immunologic detection of abnormal protein aggregates in numerous characteristic anatomic loci.[14–16] Like PD, the protein accumulations contain αS; however, there are prominent cytoplasmic deposits in glial cells (glial cytoplasmic inclusions [GCIs]) not seen in PD.[17–20] The anatomic distribution of GCI does not differ significantly between MSAc and MSAp, including spinal cord autonomic tracts, cerebellar white matter, medulla, pons and cerebral peduncle, the substantia nigra, striatum, and the globus pallidus.[21] The findings suggest that the 2 clinical phenotypes MSAc and MSAp may represent differential initial involvement of the cerebellar versus basal ganglia sites of disorder, but that, over time, the distributions of pathologic changes may become less distinct. Recent analyses indicate presence of inclusions also in neurons of some loci; however, these are less numerous and of less certain clinical salience than the GCI.[14,22]

Progressive Supranuclear Palsy

PSP, also known as the Steele-Richardson-Olszewski syndrome, is yet another condition that may resemble PD at symptom onset.[23,24] Distinguishing features of PSP are a relative symmetry of parkinsonian limb involvement and more proximal/axial distribution of rigidity than the more distal limb predominance typical of early PD. There is often loss of postural reflexes and stability at presentation of PSP. The rest tremor seen often in PD is typically absent. Many patients with PSP develop abnormal eye movements with prominent inability to redirect gaze in the vertical plane, but with maintained oculovestibular reflex eye movements (Richardson syndrome). However, the characteristic ocular palsy may be a feature of advanced disease progression in many patients with PSP and is not always seen.

Neuropathologic changes in PSP consist of cytoplasmic protein deposits containing amorphous and filamentous microtubule-associated tau protein.[25–28] The cellular distribution typically involves astrocytes, termed tufted astrocytes, for PSP diagnosis. Inclusions are seen also in neurons (ballooned neurons) and in oligodendroglia. The distribution of pathology in PSP typically involves neuronal losses and astrocytic changes in the frontal cerebral cortices, the basal ganglia (particularly affecting the globus pallidus), and midbrain (affecting the substantia nigra, subthalamic nucleus, and superior colliculus). Cerebellar dentate nucleus and the superior cerebellar peduncle are also atrophic and show neuronal and axonal loss.

Corticobasal Degeneration

Of the atypical Parkinson syndromes, CBD may have least overlap with PD but can be a diagnostic confound in some cases. Typical signs of CBD, often termed corticobasal syndrome (CBS), are an asymmetrical limb-predominant rigidity associated with severe impairment of voluntary movement and adoption of a dystonic posture (most commonly a flexed upper extremity posture).[29,30] Examination often reveals somatosensory abnormality in the involved limb, attributable to primary sensory cortical dysfunction. Highly supportive features, although not always present, include sensory stimulus–induced myoclonus in the involved limb and/or the so-called alien limb phenomenon, where the involved extremity appears to intentionally (but involuntarily) interfere with task-related use of the uninvolved contralateral extremity.

Pathologic changes in CBD are closely related to those of PSP, and there is pathologic diagnosis overlap in series of clinically diagnosed CBS and PSP. Changes in glia and neurons involve cytoplasmic inclusions of tau protein aggregates as well as neuronal losses.[31,32] Distinctive changes in CBD are presence of astrocytic plaques, oligodendroglial inclusions termed coiled bodies, and neuronal deposits termed corticobasal inclusions. Typically, pathologic changes are seen in the pericentral cerebral cortices, striatum, thalamus, and substantia nigra.

Differential Diagnoses of Parkinson Syndromes

The parkinsonian syndromes may be distinguished clinically from differential symptomatic features in some cases. As noted earlier, each syndrome may have specific diagnostic features (**Table 1** for summary), increasing classification accuracy. However, despite these clinical clues, many patients are incorrectly diagnosed in life, and many patients lack expression of defining characteristics. Perhaps the most reliable clinical biomarker is the response of rigidity and bradykinesia to administration of DA-augmenting therapy (levodopa) or DA receptor agonists. These dihydroxyphenylalanine (DOPA)-mimetic treatments offer substantial, often dramatic, relief of symptoms in PD. In MSA and PSP, there can be apparent medication benefit; however, it is usually incomplete and poorly maintained over time with disease progression. There is usually no convincing effect of DOPA-mimetic intervention in CBD. A degree of placebo effect may account for the small and poorly sustained initial benefits of therapy seen in some patients with aPD.

However, there are no effective symptomatic therapies for MSA, PSP, or CBD, and no protective or disease-modifying therapies for any of the neurodegenerative parkinsonian disorders. Accurate and early diagnosis will be necessary to develop new and effective therapies, and sensitive fluid (blood and cerebrospinal fluid) and molecular imaging biomarkers are currently under investigation for this purpose.

MOLECULAR IMAGING OF PARKINSONIAN NEURODEGENERATIONS

Functional neuroimaging, most commonly using [^{18}F]fluorodeoxyglucose (FDG) PET, may distinguish patients with PD and patients with aPD[33,34]; however, in the United States, this application of FDG-PET is not routinely covered by medical insurance providers. Univariate patterns of metabolic abnormality distinguish MSA and CBD most clearly, with prominent bilateral cerebellar and striatal hypometabolism in MSA[35] and prominent interhemispheric asymmetrical precentral and postcentral cerebral cortical, thalamic, and striatal hypometabolism in CBD.[36] Unmedicated patients with PD may have conspicuous increased striatal FDG metabolism. Patients with PSP can show mild-intensity prefrontal cerebral cortical and striatal hypometabolism. Elegant multivariate image analysis approaches identify robust principal component metabolic patterns that accurately classify all of the PD and aPD conditions.[33,37,38] However, these image processing tools are not yet routinely available in the clinical setting. Statistically based comparisons of individual patient FDG patterns can also be of diagnostic value in parkinsonian disorders.[39,40]

Neuropharmacologic Imaging Targets

Dopamine synapses

Most molecular imaging studies in PD and aPD have focused on characterizations of vulnerable neuronal populations known to undergo degenerative changes (see Ref.[41] for recent summary). Foremost among these are targeted studies of DA neurons and synapses using several specific neurochemical characteristics of these neurons

Table 1
Differential diagnoses of Parkinson syndromes

Parkinsonian Disorder	Distinctive Supporting Clinical Features
PD	• Asymmetric limb brady-kinesia/rigidity onset • Rest tremor • Significant, sustained response to DOPA-mimetic therapy
MSA	• Autonomic dysfunction • Cerebellar dysfunction • Poor or no response to DOPA-mimetic therapy
PSP	• Supranuclear ocular palsy • Symmetric, proximal limb and axial rigidity • Postural instability at onset • Poor or no response to DOPA-mimetic therapy
Corticobasal degeneration	• Prominent asymmetric limb dystonia at onset • Primary somatosensory cortical deficits • Stimulus-sensitive myoclonus • Alien limb phenomenon • Poor or no response to DOPA-mimetic therapy

Abbreviation: DOPA, dihydroxyphenylalanine.

(**Fig. 1**). Initial studies showing specific visualization of striatal DA terminals and their degeneration in PD were conducted with the false neurotransmitter precursor, [18F]fluorodopa (FDOPA). Subsequent investigations showed similar imaging depictions of DA terminals on the bases of monoaminergic synaptic vesicle transporters (VMAT2 imaging with [11C]dihydrotetrabenazine) and of the presynaptic DA reuptake transporter (DAT) with a variety of cocaine-analog radiotracers.[42] Recent DAT imaging studies suggest very early changes in the nigral synapses detected with [11C]PE2I[43,44] or [18F]FA-PE2I.[45] There is differential loss of DAT compared with FDOPA over time with progression of PD, indicating differential compensation or regulation of the imaging targets.[44] The DAT targeted imaging approach has led to clinical availability and use of the single-photon emission computed tomography (SPECT) radiotracer [123I]ioflupane (see Ref.[46] for review). Reduced DAT tracer binding is observed in the striatum of all of the neurodegenerative parkinsonian syndromes,[42,47,48] with some distinction

between MSAc and MSAp subtypes; reductions are of greater intensity and more asymmetric in MSAp.[49,50] Thus, reduced striatal DAT imaging is a clinical biomarker of nigrostriatal projection disorder, but does not provide specific differential information on PD versus an aPD disorder.

Recent studies probing DA synaptic integrity and function in PD have focused on additional pathologic aspects. There are interesting findings of synaptic DA levels involving changes in DA-D2 receptor availability depicted with the D2 antagonist [11C]raclopride, and, more selectively, with the agonist [11C]PHNO[51] (see Ref.[52] for mechanistic review). Studies in PD have revealed unique insights into the pharmacodynamics of levodopa responses in PD. Symptomatic progression of disease severity, the development of shortened therapeutic response duration, and the subsequent onset of levodopa-induced dyskinesia are predicted by the intensity and duration of DA receptor occupancy after levodopa challenge.[53] Of great interest also is the presence of apparent placebo-related DA release because of altered D2 receptor availability (see Ref.[54] for review).

Serotonin and norepinephrine synapses

Recent studies depict the distribution of presynaptic serotonergic lesions in PD from the serotonin reuptake transporter (SERT) images with [11C] DASB. Decreases are observed widely among the structures innervated by the brain stem raphe nuclei, including the midbrain, thalamus, hypothalamus, and striatum.[55–58] Correlations of reduction in the anterior cingulate cortex with symptoms of anxiety and depression and reductions in the caudate nucleus and orbitofrontal cortex with apathy have been identified.[59]

Additional studies targeting imaging of the presynaptic noradrenergic terminals from the presynaptic norepinephrine transporter (NET) with the radioligand [11C]MeNER have revealed neurodegeneration of the locus coeruleus projections in PD.[60,61] Widespread reductions throughout the brain stem and cerebrum are seen, with the most significant reductions in the midbrain and thalamus. More intense reductions are observed in patients with PD expressing polysomnographic evidence of RBD.[60] Progressively reduced tracer binding in the primary motor cortex is seen with advanced clinical stages of PD.[62]

In addition, peripheral neuroimaging of sympathetic cardiac innervation from the NET ligand [11C]HED reveals characteristic patterns of denervation in PD.[63] The pattern of loss differs from that seen in diabetic autonomic neuropathy, suggesting primary PD disorder affecting the sympathetic ganglion rather than sympathetic axons. The

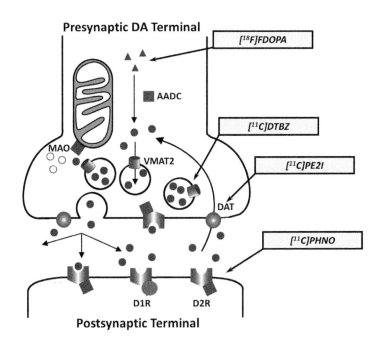

Presynaptic DA Terminal

[18F]FDOPA

AADC

[11C]DTBZ

MAO

VMAT2

[11C]PE2I

DAT

[11C]PHNO

D1R   D2R

Postsynaptic Terminal

Fig. 1. Neurochemical attributes of a nigrostriatal DA synapse with identification of neuroimaging targets and representative PET radioligands (*yellow boxes*). Human brain DA terminal imaging is reported on the bases of [18F]fluorodopa imaging synthesis of DA, [11C]dihydrotetrabenazine (DTBZ) binding to the vesicular monoamine transporter, [11C]PE2I binding to the presynaptic plasmalemmal DA transporter, and [11C]PHNO binding to DA D2 (molecular d2 and d3) receptors. Levodopa, solid triangles (▲); DA, solid circles (●); metabolites, empty circles (○).AADC, aromatic amino acid decarboxylase; D1R, DA D1 subtype receptor; D2R, DA D2 subtype receptor; DAT, presynaptic plasmalemmal DA reuptake transporter; MAO, monoamine oxidase; VMAT2-type-2 vesicular monoamine transporter.

distribution and severity of these defects increases over time in longitudinal studies.

Cholinergic synapses

Prior molecular imaging studies implicate a role of cholinergic systems changes in motor and nonmotor symptoms of PD, including postural instability and gait difficulties (PIGD), sensory processing during postural control, dyskinesias, cognitive impairment, REM sleep behavioral disorder, and impaired sense of smell (see Ref.[64] for review). These studies were mainly performed using acetylcholinesterase PET or nicotinic receptor PET or SPECT ligands. More recently, the human use introduction of an [18F]-labeled vesicular acetylcholine transporter (VAChT) ligand, [18F]fluoroethoxybenzovesamicol ([18F]FEOBV) offers advantages of a higher spatial resolution PET ligand compared with prior VAChT SPECT studies and also allows more robust equilibrium imaging at delayed postinjection times.[65] Importantly, [18F]FEOBV PET shows more distinct binding in the primary sensorimotor cortex, anterior cingulum, limbic system, and cerebellar vermis.[66] A novel observation is evidence of more heterogeneous binding within the thalamic complex, including visualization of the lateral geniculate nucleus, and vestibular cerebellar nuclei (flocculus and nodulus) that may be unique to humans.[66] These anatomically focal areas remain largely underexamined in the available literature and present novel opportunities for cholinergic imaging–clinical phenotyping studies in PD.

Regional cholinergic system changes were reported recently on [18F]FEOBV PET associated with PIGD motor features of freezing of gait and falls in PD.[67] Distinct topographic patterns were observed with evidence of lower cholinergic integrity in striatal, limbic, and mesofrontal regions in patients with freezing of gait. In contrast, distinct cholinergic transporter changes were seen in the lateral geniculate nucleus, caudate nucleus, and prefrontal cortices. Involvement of the lateral geniculate nucleus implicates a role of decreased visual attention in the pathophysiology of falls in PD. More diffuse striatal involvement in freezing of gait may point to an important role of cholinergic interneurons in this episodic mobility disturbance in PD.

There is accumulating evidence for a role of nicotinic receptors underlying levodopa-induced dyskinesias in PD.[68] For example, a recent [123I] 5-IA brain nicotinic acetylcholine receptor SPECT study showed evidence of higher binding in the caudate nucleus in patients with PD with dyskinesias versus without dyskinesias.[69] This finding was observed in the absence of significant differences in striatal DAT binding between dyskinetic versus nondyskinetic patients.

Recent trends in cholinergic ligand imaging studies of PD include the exploration of extracerebral regions. For example, a [11C]donepezil study found evidence of lower intestinal binding in patients with PD compared with controls, suggesting that parasympathetic denervation is present early in the disease course in PD.[70] However, [11C] donepezil binding may lack specificity in part because of binding to sigma receptors. Nevertheless, decreased intestinal [¹¹C]donepezil binding has also been observed in vagotomized patients, supporting that [¹¹C]donepezil PET may have at least partial validity as a measure of intestinal parasympathetic denervation.[71] Therefore, cholinergic imaging of peripheral autonomic organs may have the potential to identify patients in whom PD may begin as a spreading αS disorder (or other disease-triggering mechanism) in the gut.

Patients who are nonmanifesting carriers of mutations in the leucine-rich repeat kinase 2 (LRRK2) gene may provide a different opportunity to study cholinergic system changes in prodromal PD. Liu and colleagues[72] investigated [¹¹C]PMP acetylcholinesterase brain PET changes in LRRK2 carriers and found evidence of significantly increased cortical hydrolysis rates in nonmanifesting carriers compared with control subjects, and higher cortical and higher thalamic rates in symptomatic carriers compared with patients with idiopathic PD. Although these findings may suggest a possible compensatory role of the cholinergic system in early neurodegeneration, these preliminary observations need to be confirmed in independent studies.

Imaging Pathologic Proteinopathies

Definite diagnoses of neurodegenerative conditions rest on confirmatory changes in postmortem pathology. Neurodegenerative parkinsonism syndromes are characterized by pathologic accumulations of abnormal posttranslational processing and misfolding of characteristic proteins associated with aggregate deposits. Recent advances in molecular imaging permit the in vivo imaging of some proteinopathies. Best recognized is the ability of radioligands to depict the deposition of fibrillary beta-amyloid (Aβ) in Alzheimer disease (AD) using [¹¹C]Pittsburgh compound-B (PiB) (see review in Ref.[73]), which was followed by the development of several ¹⁸F-labeled tracers for clinical studies. Parkinsonian neurodegenerations are associated diagnostically with accumulations of αS or tau aggregates. These imaging targets are under investigation for potential in vivo molecular classification of parkinsonism and are reviewed later.

In general, there are important similarities, but critical distinctions, in the evolution of new molecular proteinopathy probes compared with the neuropharmacologic markers discussed previously. The neurochemical neuropharmacologic imaging targets are generally known from prior preclinical pharmacotherapeutic research, and are associated with multiple pharmacophore examples conferring specificity and confirmation of targeting in molecular biochemical and binding assays. In contrast, the proteinopathy deposits are characterized pathologically by special histologic tissue stains and by binding of specific antibodies in immunohistochemistry. The concepts of binding specificity and the details of small-molecule interactions with the deposits are limited. In the case of PiB, chemical ligand similarity to the pathologic Aβ staining reagent thioflavin-T was critical. However, radioligand evaluations and development depend on human pathologic tissue sources of binding targets, and preclinical assays often critically depend on tissue sampling and processing approaches. More recent investigations are targeting the potential ultrastructural identification of unique proteinopathy epitopes that may be disease specific and may serve as molecular interaction targets for new ligands (see Ref.[74] for summary and review).

Aβ amyloid imaging

Aβ deposition does not define the diagnoses of neurodegenerative parkinsonism conditions; however, its accumulation depicted in PET imaging has been investigated as an additional characteristic, particularly in PD. Increased PET imaging of Aβ deposition, in the intensity range of patients with AD, is detected with increasing prevalence from approximately 20% at age 60 years to more than 40% at age 80 years in cognitively normal patients.[75] Patients with mild cognitive impairment (MCI) have substantially higher prevalence of positive AB PET. It is suggested that the signs of cognitive impairment do not strongly parallel Aβ deposition, and that neurofibrillary tangle (NFT) accumulation and neurodegeneration more closely relate to MCI and dementia signs.[76] The prevalence of increased Aβ deposition in cognitively normal patients with PD may differ from neurologically normal persons. It seems in several studies that the prevalence of positive Aβ PET is much lower than that in normal aging.[77,78] Furthermore, it seems that Aβ levels below the typical AD intensity range may be associated with cognitive deficits in patients with PD with MCI.[79–83] In particular, apathy in patients with PD correlates strongly with Aβ deposition in cingulate cortex and anterior striatum.[84] A relationship between integrity of serotonergic cortical terminals and intensity of PET Aβ deposition suggests a possible interaction of αS disorder with the process of amyloidosis.[85]

Tau aggregate imaging

Following development of Aβ PET imaging ligands, attention turned to possible imaging of the second proteinopathy required for diagnosis of AD, the NFT. Detailed molecular and structural analyses of NFT reveal that the deposits in AD consist of hyperphosphorylated and misfolded tau protein.[86] Tau, a microtubule-associated protein, plays a physiologic role by binding interaction and stabilization of polymerized tubulin in microtubules. Subsequent directed studies of tau expression and distribution revealed several isoforms of primary structure, depending on the number of domains interacting with microtubules per molecule. Tau with 3 interacting domains is termed 3R and that with 4 domains 4R tau isoforms. The NFT deposits in AD comprise 3R and 4R tau isoforms. Protein deposits in other neurodegenerations are also comprised of tau, including the presence of more amorphous and straight filamentous deposits of 4R tau in PSP and CBD.[86–88] Targeted imaging of these deposits is then of great interest in potential classification of aPD.

Initial PET imaging of tau deposits targeted NFT depositions in AD and was pursued with a variety of distinct ligands.[88] Most frequently used thus far is the tracer [^{18}F]AV-1451 ([^{18}F]fluortaucipir; previously designated [^{18}F]T807). Studies reveal AV-1451 depiction of cerebrocortical NFT in AD, progressively expanding in distribution with worsening of dementia.[88] It was hoped that the tracer might additionally recognize 4R tau fibrils in PSP or CBD. Many investigations have explored this possibility, with controversial and mixed results. Studies report increased AV-1451 activity in the basal ganglia and midbrain of subjects with PSP, as would be anticipated by the known distribution of neuropathology,[89–91] and also in CBD.[92] However, other investigators do not report significant increases in PSP attributable to tau binding.[93–95] Additional investigations of AV-1451 in postmortem human brain tissues reveal a complex pattern of interactions. It is clear that the tracer has high-affinity binding to NFT in the AD cortex.[96–98] There is additionally evidence that off-target tracer binding is seen corresponding with the distribution of neuromelanin,[96] and perhaps also to monoamine oxidases,[99] potentially accounting for basal ganglia signal in PET images. It is reported that ventral midbrain AV-1451 PET signal may be reduced in patients with PD compared with normal persons,[100,101] potentially reflecting the losses of melanized substantia nigra neurons.

An additional tau PET ligand, designated [^{11}C] PBB3 has been evaluated because of apparent higher affinity for 4R tau fibrils.[102–105] Several investigators report increased tracer accumulation in patients with PSP; however, the tracer also depicts the NFT deposits in AD. This lack of specificity as well as technical constraints related to tracer synthesis and handling limits is widespread use. Nevertheless, PBB3 indicates the possibility of distinct sites for tracer interaction with 4R tau fibrils, leading to current investigation to identify potential 4R-specific high-affinity radiotracers. The possibility of PBB3 interaction with other proteinopathies, including αS in PD, has been explored in vitro and seems to be of sufficiently low intensity that it is not likely to contribute to PET imaging signal[106]

αS aggregate imaging

The remaining proteinopathy characteristic of parkinsonism conditions consists of aggregated αS, as characterized in PD and MSA. As mentioned earlier, the αS deposits in these conditions are distinct from one another both in ultrastructure and in the typical cellular types and locations of accumulation. There is intense interest in the development of radioligands depicting αS deposits; however, there is limited evidence of successful human imaging translation as yet. Several investigators are actively pursuing αS-targeting imaging ligands[74,107–109] and exploring strategies using molecular modeling together with αS samples derived from tissue samples.[74,107] Interim results suggest the possibility of sites that could serve as ligand binding domains; however, there has not yet been successful translation to a PET ligand with positive results in PD or MSA imaging. A difficulty encountered, and not unique to αS ligand development, is the potential for overlap of binding with other proteinopathy deposits present at higher abundance in some patients, such as Aβ.[109] As mentioned previously, the lack of well-characterized and selective small molecules interacting with specific proteinopathy deposits is a significant obstacle to discovery of novel central nervous system–active PET ligands.

DISCUSSION

Recent PET imaging research in PD and related aPD disorders has advanced the initial focus on imaging losses of nigrostriatal AD terminals achieved over the prior 30 years. Studies now depict subtle differences between differing presynaptic DA imaging targets that may suggest altered regulatory changes, ligand specificities, or other neuropathologic features. Studies also inform on the changes and treatment-related synaptic DA levels in PD, providing explanations for altered duration of therapeutic responses, development of therapeutic complications, and also the substrate underlying placebo responses. Presynaptic DA imaging has now led to the achievement of clinical translation of DAT imaging, used for investigation of atypical parkinsonism or tremor, unresponsive to appropriate treatment.

PD is not an isolated degeneration of DA neurons, as confirmed by detailed neuropathologic and neurochemical studies. Imaging research has achieved substantial progress in detecting pathologic changes in nondopaminergic vulnerable neuronal populations in PD, including losses of noradrenergic, serotonergic, and cholinergic projections. These aspects may relate to the frequently observed clinical symptoms and signs in patients with PD that are unresponsive to DA replacement therapy, and suggest opportunities for new symptomatic therapy approaches.

Most new imaging research approaches in parkinsonism do not permit diagnostic distinction among PD and aPD syndromes; however, this is a major unmet need for advancement in the development of new and potentially neuroprotective therapy. An underused and underappreciated tool that may afford good diagnostic potential is the use of FDG-PET imaging in parkinsonism. Several investigators report the ability of FDG to accurately distinguish and classify PD, PSP, MSA, and CBD. In some instances, particularly MSA and CBD, the FDG imaging features may be identified in routine qualitative image review. In studies showing the ability to make optimized distinctions among all of the parkinsonism conditions, advanced computational image analyses are needed to augment qualitative image review. These clinical image analytical tools are not yet widely used or available but could be distributed in future imaging clinics. An important additional current limitation is lack of routine insurance coverage for FDG-PET imaging of parkinsonism in the United States.

New molecular PET imaging approaches in neurodegenerations involve the targeting of pathologic proteinopathy deposits, often constituting and defining autopsy diagnoses. Progress in imaging AD from Aβ amyloid plaque and NFT tau accumulations suggests the feasibility of developing PET ligands selectively targeting the 4R tau deposits characteristic of PSP and CBD and of the αS deposits defining PD and MSA. Although there is not yet translational availability of selective ligands for these targets, they may constitute the most selective approaches to diagnostic imaging biomarkers. To the extent that the protein depositions may represent the primary neurodegeneration mechanisms in these disorders, selective PET imaging tracers could serve additionally as staging/severity markers and perhaps even as markers of engagement and effect of new targeted therapeutics.

FUTURE DIRECTIONS

As discussed earlier, the most promising potential new PET ligands in neurodegenerative parkinsonisms target the pathologic depositions of αS and of 4R tau fibrils. The development of new proteinopathy ligands is challenged by a lack of small-molecule pharmacologic tools to aid in the identification of selective brain-penetrating ligands. An evolving focus on high-resolution molecular imaging of the protein deposits, including use of samples derived from postmortem sources, may permit in silico molecular modeling and identification of unique prototypic imaging ligands.

SUMMARY

Recent PET molecular imaging of PD and related aPD disorders increasingly emphasizes non-DA terminal degeneration processes. Studies include advanced investigations of DA terminal function and regulation as well as non-DA neuronal changes. A major unmet clinical and research need is the development of a reliable and routinely available diagnostic biomarker able to accurately distinguish PD and aPD conditions. FDG-PET imaging together with advanced computational analyses could serve this purpose if the needed imaging processing tools can be clinically distributed. Promising, highly specific biomarker imaging on the basis of distinct pathologic protein depositions of 4R tau or of αS may soon be available to fill both diagnostic classification and potential disease staging, progression, and therapeutic response assessments.

CLINICS CARE POINTS

- Imaging referrals are most commonly encountered in patients with medication-unresponsive parkinsonism. In these potential patients with aPD, clinical diagnosis is unreliable.

- Molecular imaging of striatal DA terminals in suspected aPD does not distinguish between PD, MSA, PSP, or CBD.

- FDG-PET imaging in suspected aPD can accurately distinguish among the conditions, but may require use of ancillary statistical image analysis approaches. FDG is not routinely approved for diagnosis of parkinsonism in the United States.

ACKNOWLEDGMENTS

The authors were supported by a grant designated U01 NS100611 from the US National Institutes of Health during preparation of this article.

DISCLOSURE

The authors have nothing to disclose.

REFERENCES

1. Joutsa J, Gardberg M, Röyttä M, et al. Diagnostic accuracy of parkinsonism syndromes by general neurologists. Parkinsonism Relat Disord+ 2014; 20:840–4.
2. Tolosa E, Wenning G, Poewe W. The diagnosis of Parkinson's disease. Lancet Neurol 2006;5:75–86.
3. Hughes AJ, Daniel SE, Ben-Shlomo Y, et al. The accuracy of diagnosis of parkinsonian syndromes in a specialist movement disorder service. Brain 2002; 125:861–70.
4. Parkinson, J. An essay on the shaking palsy. London, Sherwood, Neely and Jones, 1817. Hovever, this is pretty difficult to locate in most library resources. The monograph was re-printed verbatum on pages 145-218 of the book: Critchley M, James Parkinson, London. MacMillan & Co, LTD, 1955.
5. Obeso JA, Stamelou M, Goetz CG, et al. Past, present, and future of Parkinson's disease: a special essay on the 200th Anniversary of the Shaking Palsy. [Review]. Mov Disord 2017;32:1264–310.
6. Gelb DJ, Oliver E, Gilman S. Diagnostic criteria for Parkinson's disease. Arch Neurol 1999;56:33–9.
7. Dickson DW, Braak H, Duda JE, et al. Neuropathological assessment of Parkinson's disease: refining the diagnostic criteria. Lancet Neurol 2009;8:1150–7.
8. Braak H, Del Tredici K, Rüb U, et al. Staging of brain pathology related to sporadic Parkinson's disease. Neurobiol Aging 2003;24:197–211.
9. Spillantini MG, Schmidt ML, Lee VM-Y, et al. α-Synuclein in Lewy bodies. Nature 1997;388:839–40.
10. Beach TG, Adler CH, Lue L, et al. Unified staging system for Lewy body disorders: correlation with nigrostriatal degeneration, cognitive impairment and motor dysfunction. Acta Neuropathol 2009;117: 613–34.
11. Langston JW. The Parkinson's complex: parkinsonism is just the tip of the iceberg. Ann Neurol 2006;59:591–6.
12. Ozawa T, Paviour D, Quinn NP, et al. The spectrum of pathological involvement of the striatonigral and olivopontocerebellar systems in multiple system atrophy: clinicopathological correlations. Brain 2004; 127:2657–71.
13. Gilman S, Wenning GK, Low PA, et al. Second consensus statement on the diagnosis of multiple system atrophy. Neurology 2008;71:670–6.
14. Koga S, Dickson DW. Recent advances in neuropathology, biomarkers and therapeutic approach of multiple system atrophy. [Review]. J Neurol Neurosurg Psychiatr 2018;89:175–84.
15. Papp MI, Kahn JE, Lantos PL. Glial cytoplasmic inclusions in the CNS of patients with multiple system atrophy (striatonigral degeneration, olivopontocerebellar atrophy and Shy–Drager syndrome). J Neurol Sci 1989;94:79–100.
16. Inoue M, Yagishita S, Ryo M, et al. The distribution and dynamic density of oligodendroglial cytoplasmic inclusions (GCIs) in multiple system atrophy: a correlation between the density of GCIs and the degree of involvement of striatonigral and olivopontocerebellar systems. Acta Neuropathol 1997;93:585–91.
17. Wakabayashi K, Yoshimoto M, Tsuji S, et al. Alpha-synuclein immunoreactivity in glial cytoplasmic inclusions in multiple system atrophy. Neurosci Lett 1998;249:180–2.
18. Spillantini MG, Crowther RA, Jakes R, et al. Filamentous alpha-synuclein inclusions link multiple system atrophy with Parkinson's disease and dementia with Lewy bodies. Neurosci Lett 1998;251: 205–8.
19. Dickson DW, Lin W, Liu WK, et al. Multiple system atrophy: a sporadic synucleinopathy. Brain Pathol 1999;9:721–32.
20. Dickson DW, Liu W, Hardy J, et al. Widespread alterations of alpha-synuclein in multiple system atrophy. Am J Pathol 1999;155:1241–51.
21. Halliday GM, Holton JL, Revesz T, et al. Neuropathology underlying clinical variability in patients with synucleinopathies. Acta Neuropathol 2011; 122:187–204.
22. Cykowski MD, Coon EA, Powell SZ, et al. Expanding the spectrum of neuronal pathology in multiple system atrophy. Brain 2015;138:2293–309.
23. Litvan I, Agid Y, Calne D, et al. Clinical research criteria for the diagnosis of progressive supranuclear palsy (Steele-Richardson-Olszewski syndrome): report of the NINDS-SPSP international workshop. Neurology 1996;47:1–9.
24. Boxer AL, Yu JT, Golbe LI, et al. Advances in progressive supranuclear palsy: new diagnostic criteria, biomarkers, and therapeutic approaches. [Review]. Lancet Neurol 2017;16:552–63.
25. Dickson DW, Ahmed Z, Algom AA, et al. Neuropathology of variants of progressive supranuclear palsy. [Review]. Curr Opin Neurol 2010;23: 394–400.
26. Dickson DW, Kouri N, Murray ME, et al. Neuropathology of frontotemporal lobar degeneration-tau (FTLD-tau). [Review]. J Mol Neurosci 2011;45:384–9.
27. Dickson DW. Parkinson's disease and parkinsonism: neuropathology. Cold Spring Harb Perspect Med 2012;2(8):a009258.

28. Koga S, Parks A, Kasanuki K, et al. Cognitive impairment in progressive supranuclear palsy is associated with tau burden. Mov Disord 2017;32: 1772–9.

29. Mathew R, Bak TH, Hodges JR. Diagnostic criteria for corticobasal syndrome: a comparative study. J Neurol Neurosurg Psychiatr 2012;83:405–10.

30. Alexander SK, Rittman T, Xuereb JH, et al. Validation of the new consensus criteria for the diagnosis of corticobasal degeneration. J Neurol Neurosurg Psychiatr 2014;85:925–9.

31. Komori T, Arai N, Oda M, et al. Astrocytic plaques and tufts of abnormal fibers do not coexist in corticobasal degeneration and progressive supranuclear palsy. Acta Neuropathol 1998;96:401–8.

32. Kouri N, Whitwell JL, Josephs KA, et al. Corticobasal degeneration: a pathologically distinct 4R tauopathy. Nat Rev Neurol 2011;7:263–72.

33. Eckert T, Barnes A, Dhawan V, et al. FDG PET in the differential diagnosis of parkinsonian disorders. Neuroimage 2005;26:912–21.

34. Peralta C, Biafore F, Depetris TS, et al. Recent advancement and clinical implications of [18]FDG-PET in Parkinson's disease, atypical parkinsonisms, and other movement disorders. [Review]. Curr Neurol Neurosci Rep 2019;19(56):06.

35. Gilman S. Functional imaging with positron emission tomography in multiple system atrophy. J Neural Transm (Vienna) 2005;112:1647–55.

36. Pardini M, Huey ED, Spina S, et al. FDG-PET patterns associated with underlying pathology in corticobasal syndrome. Neurology 2019;92:e1121–35.

37. Teune LK, Renken RJ, Mudali D, et al. Validation of parkinsonian disease-related metabolic brain patterns. Mov Disord 2013;28:547–51.

38. Tripathi M, Tang CC, Feigin A, et al. Automated differential diagnosis of early parkinsonism using metabolic brain networks: a validation study. J Nucl Med 2016;57:60–6.

39. Caminiti SP, Alongi P, Majno L, et al. Evaluation of an optimized [18 F]fluoro-deoxy-glucose positron emission tomography voxel-wise method to early support differential diagnosis in atypical Parkinsonian disorders. Eur J Neurol 2017;24:687-e26.

40. Brajkovic L, Kostic V, Sobic-Saranovic D, et al. The utility of FDG-PET in the differential diagnosis of Parkinsonism. Neurol Res 2017;39(8):675–84.

41. Maiti B, Perlmutter JS. PET imaging in movement disorders. [Review]. Semin Nucl Med 2018;48: 513–24.

42. Brooks DJ. Molecular imaging of dopamine transporters. [Review]. Ageing Res Rev 2016;30: 114–21.

43. Pagano G, Niccolini F, Wilson H, et al. Comparison of phosphodiesterase 10A and dopamine transporter levels as markers of disease burden in early Parkinson's disease. Mov Disord 2019;34:1505–15.

44. Li W, Lao-Kaim NP, Roussakis AA, et al. [11] C-PE2I and [18] F-Dopa PET for assessing progression rate in Parkinson's: a longitudinal study. Mov Disord 2018;33:117–27.

45. Fazio P, Svenningsson P, Cselenyi Z, et al. Nigrostriatal dopamine transporter availability in early Parkinson's disease. Mov Disord 2018;33:592–9.

46. Tatsch K, Poepper G. Nigrostriatal dopamine terminal imaging with dopamine transporter SPECT: an update. [Review]. J Nucl Med 2013;54:1331–8.

47. Antonini A, Benti R, De Notaris R, et al. 123I-Ioflupane/SPECT binding to striatal dopamine transporter (DAT) uptake in patients with Parkinson's disease, multiple system atrophy, and progressive supranuclear palsy. Neurol Sci 2003;24(3):149–50.

48. Hammesfahr S, Antke C, Mamlins E, et al. FP-CIT and IBZM-SPECT in corticobasal syndrome: results from a clinical follow-up study. Neurodegener Dis 2016;16:342–7.

49. Kim HWm, Kim JS, Oh M, et al. Different loss of dopamine transporter according to subtype of multiple system atrophy. Eur J Nucl Med Mol Imaging 2016;43:517–25.

50. Bu LL, Liu FT, Jiang CF, et al. Patterns of dopamine transporter imaging in subtypes of multiple system atrophy. Acta Neurol Scand 2018;138:170–6.

51. Payer DE, Guttman M, Kish SJ, et al. D3 dopamine receptor-preferring [11C]PHNO PET imaging in Parkinson patients with dyskinesia. Neurology 2016; 86:224–30.

52. Laruelle M. Imaging synaptic neurotransmission with in vivo binding competition techniques: a critical review. J Cereb Blood Flow Metab 2000;20: 423–51.

53. Stoessl AJ. Central pharmacokinetics of levodopa: lessons from imaging studies. [Review]. Mov Disord 2015;30:73–9.

54. Quattrone A, Barbagallo G, Cerasa A, et al. Neurobiology of placebo effect in Parkinson's disease: what we have learned and where we are going. [Review]. Mov Disord 2018;33:1213–27.

55. Albin RL, Koeppe RA, Bohnen NI, et al. Spared caudal brainstem SERT binding in early Parkinson's disease. J Cereb Blood Flow Metab 2008; 28:441–4.

56. Roussakis AA, Politis M, Towey D, et al. Serotonin-to-dopamine transporter ratios in Parkinson disease: relevance for dyskinesias. Neurology 2016; 86:1152–8.

57. Pagano G, Niccolini F, Fusar-Poli P, et al. Serotonin transporter in Parkinson's disease: a meta-analysis of positron emission tomography studies. [Review]. Ann Neurol 2017;81:171–80.

58. Fu JF, Klyuzhin I, Liu S, et al. Investigation of serotonergic Parkinson's disease-related covariance pattern using [11C]-DASB/PET. NeuroImage Clin 2018;19:652–60.

59. Maillet A, Krack P, Lhommee E, et al. The prominent role of serotonergic degeneration in apathy, anxiety and depression in de novo Parkinson's disease. Brain 2016;139:2486–502.

60. Sommerauer M, Fedorova TD, Hansen AK, et al. Evaluation of the noradrenergic system in Parkinson's disease: an ^{11}C-MeNER PET and neuromelanin MRI study. Brain 2018;141:496–504.

61. Nahimi A, Sommerauer M, Kinnerup MB, et al. Noradrenergic deficits in Parkinson disease imaged with ^{11}C-MeNER. J Nucl Med 2018;59:659–64.

62. Sommerauer M, Hansen AK, Parbo P, et al. Decreased noradrenaline transporter density in the motor cortex of Parkinson's disease patients. Mov Disord 2018;33:1006–10.

63. Wong KK, Raffel DM, Bohnen NI, et al. 2-Year natural decline of cardiac sympathetic innervation in idiopathic Parkinson disease studied with ^{11}C-Hydroxyephedrine PET. J Nucl Med 2017;58:326–31.

64. Bohnen NI, Kanel P, Muller M. Molecular imaging of the cholinergic system in Parkinson's disease. Int Rev Neurobiol 2018;141:211–50.

65. Petrou M, Frey KA, Kilbourn MR, et al. In vivo imaging of human cholinergic nerve terminals with (-)-5-^{18}F-fluoroethoxybenzovesamicol: biodistribution, dosimetry, and tracer kinetic analyses. J Nucl Med 2014;55:396–404.

66. Albin RL, Bohnen NI, Muller MLTM, et al. Regional vesicular acetylcholine transporter distribution in human brain: a [^{18}F]fluoroethoxybenzovesamicol positron emission tomography study. J Comp Neurol 2018;526:2884–97.

67. Bohnen NI, Kanel P, Zhou Z, et al. Cholinergic system changes of falls and freezing of gait in Parkinson's disease. Ann Neurol 2019;85:538–49.

68. Quik M, Bordia T, Zhang D, et al. Nicotine and nicotinic receptor drugs: potential for Parkinson's disease and drug-induced movement disorders. Int Rev Neurobiol 2015;124:247–71.

69. Brumberg J, Kusters S, Al-Momani E, et al. Cholinergic activity and levodopa-induced dyskinesia: a multitracer molecular imaging study. Ann Clin Transl Neurol 2017;4:632–9.

70. Fedorova TD, Seidelin LB, Knudsen K, et al. Decreased intestinal acetylcholinesterase in early Parkinson disease: an ^{11}C-donepezil PET study. Neurology 2017;88:775–81.

71. Fedorova TD, Knudsen K, Hartmann B, et al. In vivo positron emission tomography imaging of decreased parasympathetic innervation in the gut of vagotomized patients. Neurogastroenterol Motil 2020;32:e13759.

72. Liu SY, Wile DJ, Fu JF, et al. The effect of LRRK2 mutations on the cholinergic system in manifest and premanifest stages of Parkinson's disease: a cross-sectional PET study. Lancet Neurol 2018;17:309–16.

73. Rowe CC, Villemagne VL. Brain amyloid imaging. J Nucl Med 2011;52:1733–40.

74. Mathis CA, Lopresti BJ, Ikonomovic MD, et al. Small-molecule PET tracers for imaging proteinopathies. [Review]. Semin Nucl Med 2017;47:553–75.

75. Jansen WJ, Ossenkoppele R, Knol DL, et al. Prevalence of cerebral amyloid pathology in persons without dementia: a meta-analysis. JAMA 2015;313:1924–38.

76. Jack CR Jr, Holtzman DM. Biomarker modeling of Alzheimer's disease. Neuron 2013;80:1347–58.

77. Petrou M, Dwamena BA, Foerster BR, et al. Amyloid deposition in Parkinson's disease and cognitive impairment: a systematic review. Mov Disord 2015;30:928–35.

78. Mashima K, Ito D, Kameyama M, et al. Extremely low prevalence of amyloid positron emission tomography positivity in Parkinson's disease without dementia. Eur Neurol 2017;77:231–7.

79. Petrou M, Bohnen NI, Muller ML, et al. Abeta-amyloid deposition in patients with Parkinson disease at risk for development of dementia. Neurology 2012;79:1161–7.

80. Shah N, Frey KA, Muller ML, et al. Striatal and cortical beta-amyloidopathy and cognition in Parkinson's disease. Mov Disord 2016;31:111–7.

81. Akhtar RS, Xie SX, Chen YJ, et al. Regional brain amyloid-beta accumulation associates with domain-specific cognitive performance in Parkinson disease without dementia. PLoS ONE 2017;12:e0177924 [Electronic Resource].

82. Fiorenzato E, Biundo R, Cecchin D, et al. Brain amyloid contribution to cognitive dysfunction in early-stage Parkinson's disease: the PPMI dataset. J Alzheimers Dis 2018;66:229–37.

83. Kim J, Ghadery C, Cho SS, et al. Network patterns of beta-amyloid deposition in Parkinson's disease. Mol Neurobiol 2019;56:7731–40.

84. Zhou Z, Muller MLTM, Kanel P, et al. Apathy rating scores and beta-amyloidopathy in patients with Parkinson disease at risk for cognitive decline. Neurology 2020;94:e376–83.

85. Kotagal V, Spino C, Bohnen NI, et al. Serotonin, beta-amyloid, and cognition in Parkinson disease. Ann Neurol 2018;83:994–1002.

86. Buée L, Bussière T, Buée-Scherrer V, et al. Tau protein isoforms, phosphorylation and role in neurodegenerative disorders. Brain Res Brain Res Rev 2000;33:95–130.

87. Villemagne VL, Furumoto S, Fodero-Tavoletti M, et al. The challenges of tau imaging. Future Neurol 2012;7:409–21.

88. Villemagne VL, Fodero-Tavoletti MT, Masters CL, et al. Tau imaging: early progress and future directions. Lancet Neurol 2015;14:114–24.

89. Schonhaut DR, McMillan CT, Spina S, et al. [18] F-flortaucipir tau positron emission tomography distinguishes established progressive supranuclear palsy from controls and Parkinson disease: a multicenter study. Ann Neurol 2017;82:622–34.

90. Whitwell JL, Lowe VJ, Tosakulwong N, et al. [18 F] AV-1451 tau positron emission tomography in progressive supranuclear palsy. Mov Disord 2017;32: 124–33.

91. Smith R, Schain M, Nilsson C, et al. Increased basal ganglia binding of [18] F-AV-1451 in patients with progressive supranuclear palsy. Mov Disord 2017;32:108–14.

92. Smith R, Scholl M, Widner H, et al. In vivo retention of ^{18}F-AV-1451 in corticobasal syndrome. Neurology 2017;89:845–53.

93. Coakeley S, Cho SS, Koshimori Y, et al. Positron emission tomography imaging of tau pathology in progressive supranuclear palsy. J Cereb Blood Flow Metab 2017;37:3150–60.

94. Passamonti L, Vazquez Rodriguez P, Hong YT, et al. ^{18}F-AV-1451 positron emission tomography in Alzheimer's disease and progressive supranuclear palsy. Brain 2017;140:781–91.

95. Marquie M, Normandin MD, Meltzer AC, et al. Pathological correlations of [F-18]-AV-1451 imaging in non-alzheimer tauopathies. Ann Neurol 2017;81:117–28.

96. Marquie M, Normandin MD, Vanderburg CR, et al. Validating novel tau positron emission tomography tracer [F-18]-AV-1451 (T807) on postmortem brain tissue. Ann Neurol 2015;78(5):787–800.

97. Lowe VJ, Curran G, Fang P, et al. An autoradiographic evaluation of AV-1451 Tau PET in dementia. Acta Neuropathol Commun 2016;4:58.

98. Sander K, Lashley T, Gami P, et al. Characterization of tau positron emission tomography tracer [18F] AV-1451 binding to postmortem tissue in Alzheimer's disease, primary tauopathies, and other dementias. Alzheimers Demen 2016;12:1116–24.

99. Vermeiren C, Motte P, Viot D, et al. The tau positron-emission tomography tracer AV-1451 binds with similar affinities to tau fibrils and monoamine oxidases. Mov Disord 2018;33:273–81.

100. Hansen AK, Knudsen K, Lillethorup TP, et al. In vivo imaging of neuromelanin in Parkinson's disease using ^{18}F-AV-1451 PET. Brain 2016;139: 2039–49.

101. Coakeley S, Cho SS, Koshimori Y, et al. [18F]AV-1451 binding to neuromelanin in the substantia nigra in PD and PSP. Brain Struct Funct 2018;223: 589–95.

102. Maruyama M, Shimada H, Suhara T, et al. Imaging of tau pathology in a tauopathy mouse model and in Alzheimer patients compared to normal controls. Neuron 2013;79:1094–108.

103. Perez-Soriano A, Arena JE, Dinelle K, et al. PBB3 imaging in Parkinsonian disorders: evidence for binding to tau and other proteins. Mov Disord 2017;32:1016–24.

104. Endo H, Shimada H, Sahara N, et al. In vivo binding of a tau imaging probe, [11 C]PBB3, in patients with progressive supranuclear palsy. Mov Disord 2019;34:744–54.

105. Ono M, Sahara N, Kumata K, et al. Distinct binding of PET ligands PBB3 and AV-1451 to tau fibril strains in neurodegenerative tauopathies. Brain 2017;140:764–80.

106. Koga S, Ono M, Sahara N, et al. Fluorescence and autoradiographic evaluation of tau PET ligand PBB3 to alpha-synuclein pathology. Mov Disord 2017;32:884–92.

107. Hsieh CJ, Ferrie JJ, Xu K, et al. Alpha synuclein fibrils contain multiple binding sites for small molecules. ACS Chem Neurosci 2018;9:2521–7.

108. Verdurand M, Levigoureux E, Zeinyeh W, et al. In silico, in vitro, and in vivo evaluation of new candidates for alpha-synuclein PET imaging. Mol Pharm 2018;15:3153–66.

109. Josephson L, Stratman N, Liu Y, et al. The binding of BF-227-like benzoxazoles to human α-synuclein and amyloid β peptide fibrils. Mol Imaging 2018; 17. 1536012118796297.

Non-^{18}F-FDG/^{18}F-NaF Radiotracers Proposed for the Diagnosis and Management of Diseases of the Heart and Vasculature

Emily C. Hancin, MS, BA[a,b], William Y. Raynor, BS[a,c], Austin J. Borja, BA[a,d],
Thomas J. Werner, MSc[a], Mona-Elisabeth Revheim, MD, PhD, MHA[e,f],
Abass Alavi, MD, MD (Hon), PhD (Hon), DSc (Hon)[a,*]

KEYWORDS

- Atherosclerosis • PET/CT • Radiotracers • Cardiopathology • Inflammation • Infection

KEY POINTS

- 18F-FDG and 18F-NaF have been used extensively in the identification of various cardiovascular diseases, but not without limitations.
- Several other PET radiotracers have been identified as possible markers for cardiovascular-associated inflammation and infection.
- Non-18F-FDG/18F-NaF molecules may have utility as alternative radiotracers in the detection and management of cardiovascular diseases, but few have demonstrated clinical value.

INTRODUCTION

Cardiovascular disease (CVD) encompasses a myriad of pathologic developments in the heart and peripheral vasculature.[1] These pathologies collectively represent the leading cause of death globally as of 2016, and mortality is projected to increase by approximately 6 million by 2030, an alarming statistic especially in the face of substantially increasing health care costs.[2] Therefore, it is imperative to take measures to improve patient outcomes for individuals with CVD, an effort that is bolstered by advances in imaging used for diagnosis and treatment. A multitude of techniques have been used to visualize cardiac pathologies, such as MR imaging, computed tomography (CT), and ultrasound.[3–8] However, PET, which uses positron-emitting radiotracers for structural and functional visualization, has demonstrated several advantages in the identification of cardiac disease.[9–12]

^{18}F-fluorodeoxyglucose (^{18}F-FDG), the analogue of glucose used to proxy glycolytic activity, is especially useful in diseases where increased cell metabolism is a hallmark, as in neurodegenerative disease, inflammation, and neoplasia.[13–16] Another well-known radiotracer used in PET, ^{18}F-sodium fluoride (^{18}F-NaF), has

[a] Department of Radiology, Hospital of the University of Pennsylvania, 3400 Spruce Street, Philadelphia, PA 19104, USA; [b] Lewis Katz School of Medicine at Temple University, 3500 North Broad Street, Philadelphia, PA 19104, USA; [c] Drexel University College of Medicine, 2900 Queen Lane, Philadelphia, PA 19129, USA; [d] Perelman School of Medicine at the University of Pennsylvania, 3400 Civic Center Boulevard, Philadelphia, PA 19104, USA; [e] Division of Radiology and Nuclear Medicine, Oslo University Hospital, Sognsvannsveien 20, Oslo 0372, Norway; [f] Institute of Clinical Medicine, Faculty of Medicine, University of Oslo, Problemveien 7, Oslo 0315, Norway

* Corresponding author. Department of Radiology, Hospital of the University of Pennsylvania, 3400 Spruce Street, Philadelphia, PA 19104, USA
E-mail address: abass.alavi@pennmedicine.upenn.edu

PET Clin 16 (2021) 273–284
https://doi.org/10.1016/j.cpet.2020.12.005
1556-8598/21/© 2020 Elsevier Inc. All rights reserved.

been particularly powerful in identifying plaque burden associated with arterial calcifications.[17–19] Because of their efficacy in the imaging of arterial inflammation and molecular calcification, ^{18}F-FDG and ^{18}F-NaF, respectively, are currently front-runners in the imaging of cardiac pathologies using PET, and global assessment of CVD using these tracers has been proposed as a powerful alternative to localized tracer detection.[20] However, both of these tracers have limitations that set boundaries on the types and degrees of pathologic developments they can identify. For example, patients undergoing ^{18}F-FDG-PET are required to follow a high-fat, low-carbohydrate diet, along with a period of prolonged fasting and unfractionated heparin administration.[21–23] Because ^{18}F-NaF has high affinity for bone, quantification of uptake in the heart and adjacent vessels is influenced by spillover, which has been reported to cause overestimation of blood pool activity in the internal jugular vein.[24] The solution to this limitation was to measure blood pool activity in the lumen of the superior vena cava, which is less susceptible to spillover.

Recently, there has been a growing number of studies that have presented other radiotracers that may have the potential to improve the diagnostic accuracy of PET, to the equivalence of or even more so than these two traditional tracers. This comprehensive review examines recent developments with non-^{18}F-FDG and non-^{18}F-NaF radiotracers in the detection of inflammatory and infectious CVD. We assert that, although alternative radiotracers provide new avenues of investigation into cardiac disease identification and treatment, a global approach to diagnostic imaging is optimal.

ATHEROSCLEROSIS

One of the most notorious and ubiquitous CVDs is atherosclerosis, a chronic inflammatory disease that is typically most notable at arterial branch points, which are characterized by nonlaminar blood flow.[25] The progression of atherosclerosis is characterized first by chronic endothelial damage induced by such conditions as hyperlipidemia or hypertension, followed by the formation of a fatty streak in the intimal layer of the vessel wall.[26] Once the low-density lipoproteins have been oxidized, they serve as chemoattractants for monocytes, which migrate to the lesion and are activated to foamy macrophages.[27] Together with smooth muscle cells, these macrophages aggregate into the fibrous cap that becomes the atherosclerotic plaque.[28] Unstable or high-risk plaques are characterized by plaques with a necrotic core, infiltration with monocytes/macrophages, increased density of vasa vasorum, and microcalcifications.[29–31] Proinflammatory cytokines are secreted by macrophages (ie, interleukin-1, -6, and -8), and the oxidation of lipoproteins in the atheromatous plaque triggers the production of bone-associated proteins in the areas of cell death and ischemia.[29–31] The stimulated osteogenesis and formation of hydroxyapatite crystals increase the vulnerability of the plaque to further damage and possible rupture, causing a stroke or myocardial infarction.[32]

The alpha-V-beta-3 integrin pathway has been shown to play a part in the pathogenesis of atherosclerosis, because it is associated with endothelial cell inflammation, activated macrophages, and increased nuclear factor-κB-dependent cytokine production.[33,34] Jenkins and colleagues[35] used PET/CT with ^{18}F-fluciclatide as a radiotracer in 46 patients with atherosclerotic disease as a measurement of plaque burden. They identified significantly increased tracer uptake in regions of increased alpha-V-beta-3 integrin receptors, which reflects the degree of angiogenesis and inflammation consistent with plaque burden (**Fig. 1**). Guibbal and colleagues[36] synthesized and tested the efficacy of ^{18}F-darapladib, a radiolabeled lipoprotein-associated phospholipase A$_2$ ligand, as a tracer in mouse models of atherosclerosis. They found that, compared with ^{18}F-FDG, ^{18}F-darapladib accumulated in higher amounts in atherosclerotic carotid samples, and they concluded that these data may present a potential future avenue of detecting atherosclerosis by way of lipid-laden macrophages or lipoproteins. Senders and coworkers[37] used PET/MR imaging in rabbits, using [89]Zr-labeled human antibody Fab fragment LA25 ([89]Zr-LA25) as a tracer to image oxidation-specific epitopes, such as oxidized phospholipids and malondialdehyde, which are indicative of proinflammatory response in patients with atherosclerotic diseases. The authors determined that the [89]Zr-LA25 tracer identified malondialdehyde-acetaldehyde epitopes in the abdominal aorta of atherosclerotic rabbits, which may reflect the presence of plaques in that region.

Li and coworkers[38] used ^{68}Ga-fucoidan, a ligand of P-selectin, which is highly expressed in the endothelium components of active atherosclerotic plaques, to investigate whether it could be used as a tracer in PET detection of plaque formation. Using a mouse model of atherosclerosis, they observed increased tracer uptake through autoradiography and PET, which demonstrates the potential for this tracer in detecting plaque formation.[38] Derlin and colleagues[39] took advantage of the important role of chemokines in

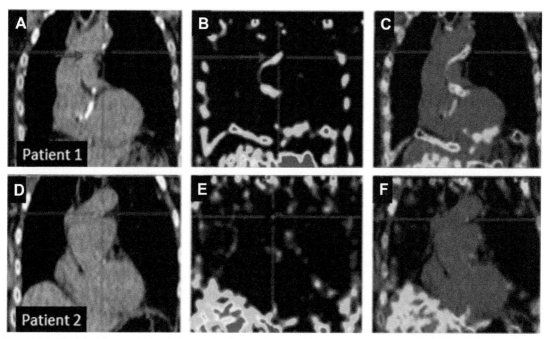

Fig. 1. 18F-Fluciclatide uptake in the aorta. Patient 1 (*top row*) demonstrates aortic calcification, as indicated by the *red arrow* in the CT scan (*A*). 18F-Fluciclatide uptake is highlighted by the *red arrow* in the Patlak slope parametric image (*B*). Patient 2 (*bottom row*) lacks aortic calcification in sagittal CT (*D*) and associated 18F-fluciclatide uptake (*E*). Fused CT and Patlak slope parametric images are seen for Patients 1 and 2 in *C* and *F*, respectively. (*Modified from* Jenkins WS, Vesey AT, Vickers A, Neale A, Moles C, Connell M, et al. In vivo alpha-V beta-3 integrin expression in human aortic atherosclerosis. Heart Br Card Soc 2019;105:1868–75. https://doi.org/10.1136/heartjnl-2019-315103; with permission.)

facilitating inflammation and plaque formation in atherosclerosis to examine the utility of ^{68}Ga-pentixafor, a ligand of the cysteine-X-cysteine chemokine receptor 4 (CXCR4), located on macrophages, in the imaging of atherosclerosis following acute myocardial infarction.[40] Using PET/CT, the authors found that there was significantly increased CXCR4 expression colocalized with CD68$^+$ cells, which are markers of inflammation, in atherosclerotic lesions. Hyafil and colleagues[41] also used the interaction between ^{68}Ga-pentixafor and CXCR4, to examine its efficacy in identifying the presence of plaques in the vasculature through PET/MR imaging. Using the right carotid artery and abdominal aorta of seven rabbits fed an atherogenic diet, the authors found that ^{68}Ga-pentixafor uptake was significantly increased in regions of atherosclerotic plaque development, and the uptake decreased on injection of AMD3100, a CXCR4 inhibitor. These data suggest that ^{68}Ga-pentixafor might be a specific radiolabel for inflammatory cells present in plaques and a potential candidate for PET/MR imaging of atherosclerosis. Another study from the same group used a different tracer, 2-(5-fluoro-pentyl)-2-methylmalonic acid ([^{18}F]ML-

10), a marker for apoptosis, to determine whether it could identify plaque formation in atherosclerotic rabbits.[42] Using autoradiography to localize the tracer and PET to obtain target-to-background ratios, the authors found that the tracer was an effective marker of plaques containing apoptotic cells. Meletta and coworkers[43] used ^{11}C-RS-016, a ligand for cannabinoid receptor type 2, which, like the CXCR4 receptor, is expressed on activated immune cells, such as macrophages, to determine if it could be used as an alternative to ^{18}F-FDG in PET. Using human carotid plaques and apolipoprotein E knockout mouse models of atherosclerosis, the authors observed the accumulation of ^{11}C-RS-016 in the plaques elicited in the mouse models through in vivo PET imaging, and they also acknowledged that the tracer accumulated in the human plaques using in vitro autoradiography. The authors did state, however, that the tracer did not distinguish between vulnerable and nonvulnerable atherosclerotic plaques in the mice models, which presents a limitation to investigate in the future. Another study from the same group used a mouse model of shear stress-induced atherosclerosis and various tracers, including ^{11}C-AM7 and ^{18}F-AC74, both of which target CD80, a marker of inflammation.[44] They found that although ^{18}F-FDG and ^{18}F-fluoro-D-mannose were significantly increased in areas of plaque formation, ^{18}F-AC74 did not accumulate in the plaques at all, and the target-to-background ratio observed with ^{11}C-AM7 uptake was low, which poses a challenge to detecting the earliest signs of atherosclerotic development. Tarkin and colleagues[45,46] used the somatostatin receptor ligand ^{68}Ga-DOTATATE to take advantage of the receptor's location on activated macrophages in the pathogenesis of atherosclerosis for imaging purposes. They determined, using PET, that not only is ^{68}Ga-DOTATATE an effective radiotracer for the identification of inflammation related to atherosclerosis, but it was also superior to ^{18}F-FDG in distinguishing between high- and low-risk coronary plaques. However, Malmberg and colleagues[47] compared ^{68}Ga-DOTATATE with ^{64}Cu-DOTATATE, also a somatostatin receptor ligand, in the evaluation of atherosclerotic risk in 60 patients with neuroendocrine tumors. They found that ^{64}Cu-DOTATATE uptake, but not ^{68}Ga-DOTATATE uptake, was significantly associated with cardiovascular risk, as demonstrated by Framingham risk score. Taken together, these contradictory findings demonstrate a continued need for further investigation into somatostatin receptor ligands as a reliable representation of atherosclerotic development.

Translocator protein (TSPO) ligands have been used in the evaluation of atherosclerosis, because they are specific in detecting the presence of monocytes and macrophages, which are inflammatory components in the plaque formation process.[48] Ammirati and coworkers[49] assessed the efficacy of ^{11}C-PK11195 in visualizing atherosclerotic lesions using PET and CT angiography in a cohort of nine patients with carotid plaques. Although the study was small, the authors determined that ^{11}C-PK11195 uptake in carotid plaques was inversely correlated with the concentration of an activated subset of monocytes expressing CD14[++]CD16[−]HLA-DR[+]; the authors use these results to conclude that certain subsets of monocytes may be preferentially recruited to areas of plaque development, although the authors acknowledge that other underlying mechanisms may be responsible for these findings. Hellberg and colleagues[50] used the next-generation TSPO ligand ^{18}F-flutriciclamide (^{18}F-GE-180), to evaluate the presence of plaques in mouse models of atherosclerosis. They showed that, although ^{18}F-GE-180 was uptaken into macrophages, which are indicative of plaque accumulation, the amount of tracer present in plaque-damaged areas was not significantly higher than the amount present in healthy vascular tissue. Thus, although TSPOs have been used to visualize atherosclerotic plaques through PET/CT, not all of them have been equally successful and their eligibility for imaging atherosclerosis is still lacking.

INFLAMMATORY DISORDERS OF THE HEART
Coronary Artery Disease/Acute Coronary Syndrome

Acute coronary syndrome represents a subcategory of coronary artery disease, characterized by the thickening of and the formation of plaques in the walls of the coronary arteries.[51] Although some coronary artery diseases are asymptomatic, the hallmark of acute coronary syndrome is unstable angina.[52,53] Because of the nature of these disorders, imaging techniques using radiotracers to assess inflammation and perfusion can be used.

Radiolabeled oxygen is a common tracer used in the detection of cardiovascular flow reserve. ^{15}O-H$_2$O PET is the gold standard for perfusion imaging, and Driessen and colleagues[54] performed ^{15}O-H$_2$O PET in 53 patients to evaluate the effects of coronary revascularization to restore blood flow to prevent coronary artery disease. They observed significant increases in fractional flow reserve and myocardial perfusion as a result of percutaneous coronary intervention, which demonstrates the success of percutaneous coronary intervention in restoring cardiac blood flow, and the ability of ^{15}O-H$_2$O to be used as a PET tracer to monitor these changes. Everaars and colleagues[55] also used ^{15}O-H$_2$O PET to investigate myocardial perfusion. The authors compared this technique with Doppler flow velocity and thermodilution to assess coronary flow reserve in 40 patients with suspected coronary artery disease. They observed a strong correlation between the coronary flow reserve measurements made by Doppler and ^{15}O-H$_2$O PET but noted that thermodilution was only mildly correlated to either technique, which suggests that ^{15}O-H$_2$O PET may be a comparable technique to Doppler in evaluating coronary flow reserve. Bom and coworkers[56] recently found that, in 648 patients with known or suspected coronary artery disease, individuals who experienced abnormal coronary flow reserve and hyperemic myocardial blood flow as measured by ^{15}O-H$_2$O PET were more likely to experience myocardial infarction or death during a median follow-up period of 6.9 years post measurements. This work demonstrates the importance of ^{15}O-H$_2$O PET in monitoring myocardial perfusion, stressing its importance as a prognostic factor in further pathologic developments.

Rubidium tracers are used in clinical work-up in the identification of coronary artery disease. von Scholten and colleagues used ^{82}Rb, a known radiotracer used for myocardial perfusion imaging to monitor changes in myocardial blood flow, in PET/CT scans of 60 patients with type 2 diabetes to evaluate coronary flow reserve.[57–59] They found that, although these individuals did not present with any known CVDs, ^{82}Rb PET/CT identified reduced coronary flow reserve and higher coronary artery calcium scores in normoalbuminuric patients compared with control subjects and in patients with albuminuria compared with control subjects. They also observed increased coronary artery calcium scores in patients with albuminuria compared with normoalbuminuric patients. This study highlights the potential of ^{82}Rb PET/CT in the early detection of cardiovascular dysfunction in patients where overt pathologic symptoms are not yet apparent.

Unlike atherosclerosis in general, there are limited studies using TSPO receptors in the assessment of coronary artery disease. Verweij and colleagues[60] used ^{18}F-DPA-714 PET/CT to target the TSPO receptor present in myeloid cells in bone marrow. They determined that, in patients with acute-phase postacute coronary syndrome, ^{18}F-DPA-714 uptake was increased, which reflects the participation of myeloid cells in the inflammatory response associated with this pathology. Further studies are warranted to elucidate the efficacy of TSPO receptors as PET markers of inflammation in coronary artery disease, and at the moment there is no evidence of such.

Sarcoidosis

Sarcoidosis is characterized by the formation of granulomas, composed of multinucleated giant cells and lymphocytes, throughout the body.[61,62] Although this disorder has variable presentations, a small percentage of patients develop cardiac manifestations, which most commonly presents with granuloma formation in the myocardium.[63] These complications can lead to various cardiac disorders, including heart block, conduction interference, arrhythmias, and heart failure.[64] Like atherosclerosis, cardiac sarcoidosis is characterized by inflammation, which makes it possible for the use of nonconventional radiotracers that target key players in these processes. Importantly, only about half of patients who are determined to have had the disease at autopsy were ever diagnosed with it during their lifetime, and early detection might spare patients from more severe systemic complications, which indicates a need to expand the current repertoire of diagnostic methods used to identify cardiac sarcoidosis.[65]

Weinberg and colleagues[66] performed ^{18}F-NaF and ^{18}F-FDG PET/CT scans on three patients with cardiac sarcoidosis to determine their detection of this pathology. They found that the ^{18}F-FDG uptake pattern observed was consistent with myocardial inflammation, which is a hallmark of the disease, but ^{18}F-NaF did not detect any uptake representative of sarcoidosis. Norikane and coworkers[67] used ^{18}F-fluorothymidine (^{18}F-FLT) in a case study of a patient with cardiac sarcoidosis, and they observed increased uptake in the left ventricle and in the lymph nodes, which decreased after the patient was treated with immunosuppressive therapy.

A later study by Norikane and colleagues[68] compared the use of ^{18}F-FDG and ^{18}F-FLT in PET/CT to detect cardiac sarcoidosis in 20 patients (**Fig. 2**). Although the uptake of ^{18}F-FLT in inflammatory lesions was lower than ^{18}F-FDG uptake, the authors determined that the sensitivity, specificity, and accuracy of the two radiotracers were comparable, and they acknowledged that ^{18}F-FLT may be easier for patients to tolerate, because it does not require the dietary changes necessary for successful ^{18}F-FDG administration. Gormsen and colleagues[69] also stressed the importance of minimal dietary changes for patients, in their case comparing ^{18}F-FDG and ^{68}Ga-DOTA-Nal-octreotide (^{68}Ga-DOTANOC), a somatostatin receptor ligand, in detecting suspected sarcoidosis in 19 patients. Although only three patients were eventually diagnosed with cardiac sarcoidosis, 11 of the 19 ^{18}F-FDG PET/CT scans were rated as inconclusive, compared with none of the ^{68}Ga-DOTA-d-Phe(1)-Tyr(3)-octreotide (^{68}Ga-DOTATOC) PET/CT scans, which also demonstrated higher diagnostic accuracy. In addition to examining aluminum fluoride-18-labeled 1,4,7-triazacyclononane-1,4,7-triacetic acid conjugated folate (^{18}F-FOL) uptake in inflamed myocardium, Jahandediah and colleagues[70] also identified increased uptake in cardiac sarcoidosis lesions, because of their expression of folate receptor beta. These studies indicate a potential for both gallium-based and ^{18}F-FLT tracers in the identification of sarcoidosis via PET, but a global PET-based investigatory approach should be taken in future studies because of the systemic nature of sarcoidosis.

Cardiomyopathy

One of the primary causes of heart failure is cardiomyopathy, a term that includes conditions that impede the heart's ability to function properly in either forceful pumping of blood or electrical conduction.[71] Animal models of cardiomyopathy

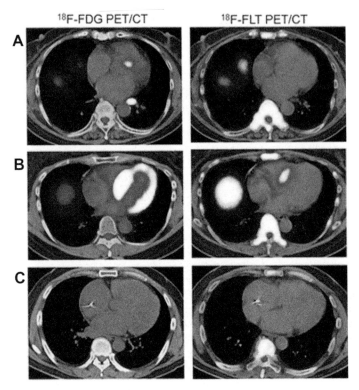

Fig. 2. (*A–C*) Fused PET/CT images demonstrating different cardiac uptake patterns of ^18F-FDG (*left*) and ^18F-FLT (*right*) in three patients with sarcoidosis. (*A*) Focal ^18F-FDG but no ^18F-FLT uptake in the basal anteroseptal myocardium. (*B*) Widespread ^18F-FDG but only focal ^18F-FLT uptake in the upper basal anteroseptal myocardium. (*C*) Neither ^18F-FDG nor ^18F-FLT uptake in the myocardium. (*From* Norikane T, Yamamoto Y, Maeda Y, Noma T, Dobashi H, Nishiyama Y. Comparative evaluation of 18F-FLT and 18F-FDG for detecting cardiac and extra-cardiac thoracic involvement in patients with newly diagnosed sarcoidosis. EJNMMI Res 2017;7:69. https://doi.org/10.1186/s13550-017-0321-0; with permission.)

have been used to investigate new nonconventional PET radiotracers. Houson and colleagues[72] used rats with isoproterenol-induced cardiomyopathy to assess the efficacy of ^18F-glucaric acid (^18F-FGA), an oxidized derivative of ^18F-FDG, in identifying myocardial injury. They determined that ^18F-FGA uptake was significantly increased in damaged rat hearts, whereas uptake was negligible in healthy hearts, which may qualify it as a candidate to be used in the assessment of myocardial injury. Sharma and colleagues[73] identified a compound referred to by this group as ^68Ga-Galmydar, as a promising radiotracer to be used in PET/CT for myocardial perfusion imaging, as tested in rat models. Savapackiam and colleagues[74] expanded on this study to investigate ^68Ga-Galmydar in identifying doxorubicin-associated cardiomyopathy in rat models (**Fig. 3**). They determined that this radiotracer could identify doxorubicin-induced cardiomyopathy in its early stages, which may indicate the use of this compound in improving existing diagnostic capabilities.

Heart Failure

Heart failure is caused by many different underlying diseases, but it is defined as the state of cardiovascular health when the heart is no longer able to supply adequate cardiac output to the rest of the body.[75] Although there have been few publications surrounding the use of non-^18F-FDG and non-^18F-NaF radiotracers in the study of heart failure, one recent study raised the possibility of the use of these compounds in PET/CT to assess cardiac performance. Byrne and colleagues[76] used ^82Rb as a tracer in PET/CT to compare myocardial perfusion between 27 control patients and 114 patients with nonischemic systolic heart failure, some of whom also presented with atrial fibrillation. Using this technique, the authors determined that patients with nonischemic systolic heart failure exhibited significantly lower myocardial perfusion than control subjects, particularly if they were experiencing atrial fibrillation at the time of the scan. This may suggest a role for ^82Rb in addition to ^15O-H$_2$O or other alternative radiotracers in the monitoring of cardiac perfusion in heart failure patients, which may be elucidated in studies that assess total-body perfusion in individuals with this condition.

INFECTIOUS DISEASES OF THE HEART

Viral infections can cause many cardiovascular complications, characterized most commonly by the location of the subsequent inflammation produced.[77] Myocarditis, or inflammation of the

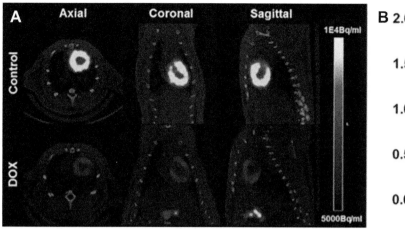
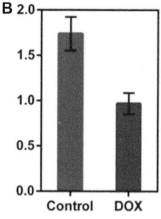

Fig. 3. Uptake of ^{68}Ga-Galmydar in the hearts of Sprague-Dawley rats. (*A*) Axial (*left*), coronal (*middle*), and sagittal (*right*) images of cardiac ^{68}Ga-Galmydar uptake in a control rat (*top row*) and in a rat treated with doxorubicin (DOX) for 5 days leading up to image acquisition to induce cardiotoxicity (*bottom row*). (*B*) Decreased ^{68}Ga-Galmydar uptake in DOX-treated rats. Images were obtained 60 minutes following tail-vein injection of the radiotracer. (*From* Sivapackiam J, Kabra S, Speidel S, Sharma M, Laforest R, Salter A, et al. 68Ga-Galmydar: A PET imaging tracer for noninvasive detection of Doxorubicin-induced cardiotoxicity. PLOS ONE 2019;14:e0215579. https://doi.org/10.1371/journal.pone.0215579; with permission.)

myocardium, has been one of the cardiac disorders most frequently investigated using non-^{18}F-FDG and non-^{18}F-NaF radiotracers.[78]

Kim and coworkers[79] used PET and a rat model of experimental autoimmune myocarditis to examine the diagnostic accuracy of two TSPO radiotracers, ^{18}F-fluoromethyl-PBR28 (an aryloxyanalide analogue) and ^{18}F-CB251 (an imidazopyridine). Comparing the heart-to-lung uptake ratios in healthy and diseased rats, the authors determined that, whereas ^{18}F-fluoromethyl-PBR28 did not exhibit a significant difference between heart and lung uptake, ^{18}F-CB251 did, which may indicate that an imidazopyridine-based compound may have promise in the detection of myocarditis. Jahandideh and coworkers[70] also used rats to evaluate myocardial damage, through an autoimmune myocarditis model induced by injected porcine cardiac myosin. To do this, they used ^{18}F-FOL as a tracer and found that the uptake of this tracer was significantly increased in damaged myocardium.[70] Maya and colleagues[80] used a similar rat model of experimental autoimmune myocarditis but used ^{11}C-methionine as a radiotracer instead of ^{18}F-FOL (**Fig. 4**). They found that ^{11}C-methionine uptake in inflammatory lesions were well correlated to ^{18}F-FDG uptake and histologic findings, which demonstrates the feasibility of this tracer in the detection of myocarditis. Lee and colleagues[81] used a tracer they referred to as ^{68}Ga-NOTA-MSA in a rat model of myocarditis to determine whether measuring the concentration of macrophages that

express mannose receptors could accurately reflect the myocarditis disease state. They found this tracer was, in fact, successful as a PET tracer in identifying myocarditis, even before signs of the disease could be identified in echocardiography.

Pericarditis is characterized by the inflammation of the fibrous pericardial sac, which sits outside of the epicardium.[82] There have been limited studies in the use of non-^{18}F-FDG and non-^{18}F-NaF radiotracers in the study of this pathology. Lapa and colleagues[83] evaluated the efficacy of somatostatin receptor-based PET/CT using a cohort of 12 patients exhibiting pericarditis/myocarditis or subacute myocardial infarction. Not only did somatostatin receptor–based PET/CT yield increased uptake in these patients, but the results were comparable with cardiac MR imaging. These results suggest the potential for more novel radiotracers to improve the existing imaging modalities available for cardiac disease monitoring.

Although ^{18}F-FDG has been used in several studies in the imaging of bacterial endocarditis, the inflammation of the inner lining of the heart and cardiac valves, there have been little to no data published regarding alternative tracers to visualize this pathology.[84–88] Panizzi and colleagues synthesized ^{64}Cu-DTPA-ProT, which has been shown to identify the presence of coagulase-positive *Staphylococcus aureus* endocarditis in mice by targeting staphylocoagulase.[89,90] Further studies should be conducted to

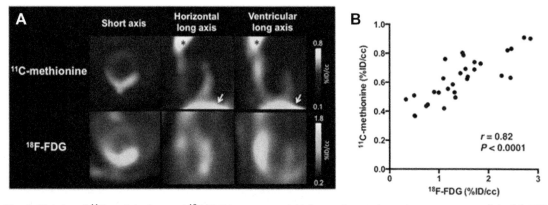

Fig. 4. Uptake of ^{11}C-methionine and ^{18}F-FDG in a rat model of experimental autoimmune myocarditis. (*A*) PET images of the short axis (*left*), horizontal long axis (*middle*), and ventricular long axis (*right*) of ^{11}C-methionine uptake (*top row*) and ^{18}F-FDG uptake (*bottom row*) of the myocardium. *Arrows* on the *top middle* and *right* panels are indicative of liver uptake of ^{11}C-methionine, whereas the *asterisks* in these panels are indicative of thymus uptake. (*B*) Significant correlation between ^{11}C-methionine and ^{18}F-FDG uptake in these regions, indicating a potential for ^{11}C-methionine as a cardiac tracer for experimental autoimmune myocarditis. (*From* Maya Y, Werner RA, Schütz C, Wakabayashi H, Samnick S, Lapa C, et al. 11C-Methionine PET of Myocardial Inflammation in a Rat Model of Experimental Autoimmune Myocarditis. J Nucl Med 2016;57:1985–90. https://doi.org/10.2967/jnumed.116.174045; with permission.)

expand on alternative radiotracers to be used in the detection of endocarditis caused by *S aureus* and by other bacterial species.

There have been limited studies conducted regarding parasitic infections of the heart in relation to non-^{18}F-FDG/^{18}F-NaF radiotracers, but the information that is available demonstrates potential utility of these tracers in total-body PET imaging. Chagas disease is a parasitic infection that classically damages the cardiovascular system, but also can cause damage to other regions of the body, leading to death through myocarditis, meningoencephalitis, or bronchopneumonia.[91] The causative organism *Trypanosoma cruzi* incites an initial inflammatory response, which may be followed by chronic infection.[92,93] Individuals with chronic infection may remain asymptomatic, or they may develop more severe complications, such as cardiomyopathy as a result of damage to β_1-adrenergic receptors or type 2 muscarinic acetylcholine receptors, both of which are found primarily at the heart.[94,95] Importantly, non-^{18}F-FDG and non-^{18}F-NaF radiotracers may have the capacity to identify evidence of parasitic disease, in addition to the various other endogenous pathologies that can occur. Moll-Bernardes and co-workers[96] conducted a case study with a 68-year-old man with Chagas disease, who had experienced ventricular tachycardia and ischemia as a result. They determined that ^{18}F-FDG and ^{68}Ga-DOTATOC demonstrated increased uptake in damaged areas of the heart, and they acknowledged that tracers, such as ^{68}Ga-DOTATOC,

may be advantageous over ^{18}F-FDG, because they do not accumulate in healthy myocardium on administration, which may be a potential improvement to the imaging of this disease in the future.

POTENTIAL FOR NON-^{18}F-FDG/^{18}F-NaF TRACERS IN CARDIOVASCULAR MEDICINE

This comprehensive review demonstrates that a great deal of progress has been made to assess CVD with non-^{18}F-FDG and non-^{18}F-NaF radiotracers. Unfortunately, except for myocardial perfusion tracers, there is limited evidence for the utility of other PET compounds in assessing various CVDs at the molecular and cellular levels. It is quite evident that ^{18}F-FDG and ^{18}F-NaF have been validated to a great extent as effective molecular and cellular probes for detecting and characterizing many disorders. Unfortunately, by conducting numerous research studies in this domain, effort and money have been spent with almost no clear return. These failures are mainly because of the lack of understanding of this technology and the true nature of the CVD processes, which together have led to the generation of misleading results. The limited spatial resolution of PET (8–10 mm), in association with substantial cardiopulmonary motions, are two pitfalls which, when combined, make it impossible to use this imaging technique to visualize plaques that are no more than a few hundred microns large in the coronary arteries and only slightly more sizable in the carotid arteries and aorta.[20] Therefore, ^{18}F-FDG and ^{18}F-NaF will remain the most valuable tracers for assessing CVD for the foreseeable future.

CLINICS CARE POINTS

- Cardiovascular disease was the leading cause of death globally in 2016, and it is projected to contribute significantly to increasing healthcare costs in the future.

- Non-FDG/NaF radiotracers have shown some utility in monitoring parameters such as myocardial perfusion, but evidence in other diseases is largely limited.

- FDG and NaF have demonstrated clear utility in the clinical evaluation of many cardiovascular pathologies and would thus be the optimal choices for the global evaluation of these diseases.

DISCLOSURE

The authors have nothing to disclose.

REFERENCES

1. Olvera Lopez E, Ballard BD, Jan A. Cardiovascular disease. StatPearls, Treasure Island (FL): StatPearls Publishing; 2020.
2. Benjamin EJ, Muntner P, Alonso A, et al. Heart disease and stroke statistics-2019 update: a report from the American Heart Association. Circulation 2019;139:e56–528.
3. Salerno M, Kramer CM. Advances in cardiovascular MRI for diagnostics: applications in coronary artery disease and cardiomyopathies. Expert Opin Med Diagn 2009;3:673–87.
4. Saeed M, Van TA, Krug R, et al. Cardiac MR imaging: current status and future direction. Cardiovasc Diagn Ther 2015;5:290–310.
5. Dave JK, Mc Donald ME, Mehrotra P, et al. Recent technological advancements in cardiac ultrasound imaging. Ultrasonics 2018;84:329–40.
6. Savino K, Ambrosio G. Handheld ultrasound and focused cardiovascular echography: use and information. Medicina (Mex) 2019;55:423.
7. Stokes MB, Roberts-Thomson R. The role of cardiac imaging in clinical practice. Aust Prescr 2017;40:151–5.
8. Krueger M, Cronin P, Sayyouh M, et al. Significant incidental cardiac disease on thoracic CT: what the general radiologist needs to know. Insights Imaging 2019;10:10.
9. Li Z, Gupte AA, Zhang A, et al. Pet imaging and its application in cardiovascular diseases. Methodist Debakey Cardiovasc J 2017;13:29–33.
10. Santos BS, Ferreira MJ. Positron emission tomography in ischemic heart disease. Rev Port Cardiol 2019;38:599–608.
11. Kazakauskaitė E, Žaliaduonytė-Pekšienė D, Rumbinaitė E, et al. Positron emission tomography in the diagnosis and management of coronary artery disease. Medicina (Mex) 2018;54:47.
12. Lameka K, Farwell MD, Ichise M. Positron emission tomography. Handb Clin Neurol 2016;135:209–27.
13. Vaidyanathan S, Patel CN, Scarsbrook AF, et al. FDG PET/CT in infection and inflammation: current and emerging clinical applications. Clin Radiol 2015;70:787–800.
14. Borja AJ, Hancin EC, Dreyfuss AD, et al. 18F-FDG-PET/CT in the quantification of photon radiation therapy-induced vasculitis. Am J Nucl Med Mol Imaging 2020;10:66–73.
15. Al-Zaghal A, Aras M, Borja AJ, et al. Detection of pulmonary artery atherosclerosis by FDG-PET/CT: a new observation. Am J Nucl Med Mol Imaging 2020;10:127.
16. Feng H, Wang X, Chen J, et al. Nuclear imaging of glucose metabolism: beyond 18F-FDG. Contrast Media Mol Imaging 2019. https://doi.org/10.1155/2019/7954854.
17. Gaudieri V, Zampella E, D'Antonio A, et al. 18F-sodium fluoride and vascular calcification: some like it hot. J Nucl Cardiol 2020. https://doi.org/10.1007/s12350-020-02125-0.
18. Raynor WY, Borja AJ, Rojulpote C, et al. 18F-sodium fluoride: an emerging tracer to assess active vascular microcalcification. J Nucl Cardiol 2020. https://doi.org/10.1007/s12350-020-02138-9.
19. Borja AJ, Rojulpote C, Hancin EC, et al. An update on the role of total-body PET imaging in the evaluation of atherosclerosis. PET Clin 2020;15:477–85.
20. Alavi A, Werner TJ, Høilund-Carlsen PF. What can be and what cannot be accomplished with PET to detect and characterize atherosclerotic plaques. Springer. J Nucl Cardiol 2018;25(6):2012–5.
21. Machado J, Hopes K, Little D, et al. P315improving the cardiac fasting protocol in 18F-FDG PET/CT imaging. Eur Heart J Cardiovasc Imaging 2019;20. https://doi.org/10.1093/ehjci/jez148.043.
22. Osborne MT, Hulten EA, Murthy VL, et al. Patient preparation for cardiac fluorine-18 fluorodeoxyglucose positron emission tomography imaging of inflammation. J Nucl Cardiol 2017;24:86–99.
23. Elman S, Yang K-C, Soine L. Impact of unfractionated heparin on cardiac sarcoidosis evaluation with cardiac PET: not worth the added effort and risk? J Nucl Med 2016;57:453.

24. Blomberg BA, Thomassen A, de Jong PA, et al. Impact of personal characteristics and technical factors on quantification of sodium 18F-fluoride uptake in human arteries: prospective evaluation of healthy subjects. J Nucl Med 2015;56:1534–40.
25. Pahwa R, Jialal I. Atherosclerosis. StatPearls, Treasure. Island (FL): StatPearls Publishing; 2019.
26. Rafieian-Kopaei M, Setorki M, Doudi M, et al. Atherosclerosis: process, indicators, risk factors and new hopes. Int J Prev Med 2014;5:927–46.
27. Bergheanu SC, Bodde MC, Jukema JW. Pathophysiology and treatment of atherosclerosis. Neth Heart J 2017;25:231–42.
28. Frink RJ. Inflammatory Atherosclerosis: Characteristics of the Injurious Agent. Sacramento (CA): Heart Research Foundation; 2002. Chapter 2, The Smooth Muscle Cell. The Pivot in Atherosclerosis. Available at: https://www.ncbi.nlm.nih.gov/books/NBK2018/
29. Hutcheson JD, Goettsch C, Bertazzo S, et al. Genesis and growth of extracellular-vesicle-derived microcalcification in atherosclerotic plaques. Nat Mater 2016;15:335–43.
30. Nakahara T, Narula J, Strauss HW. NaF uptake in unstable plaque: what does fluoride uptake mean? Eur J Nucl Med Mol Imaging 2018;45:2250–2.
31. Nakahara T, Dweck MR, Narula N, et al. Coronary artery calcification: from mechanism to molecular imaging. JACC Cardiovasc Imaging 2017;10:582–93.
32. Zhu Y, Xian X, Wang Z, et al. Research progress on the relationship between atherosclerosis and inflammation. Biomolecules 2018;8:80.
33. Finney AC, Stokes KY, Pattillo CB, et al. Integrin signaling in atherosclerosis. Cell Mol Life Sci 2017;74:2263–82.
34. Rosas E, Sobenin I, Orekhov A, et al. Importance of receptor-targeted systems in the battle against atherosclerosis. Curr Pharm Des 2013;19:5897–903.
35. Jenkins WS, Vesey AT, Vickers A, et al. In vivo alpha-V beta-3 integrin expression in human aortic atherosclerosis. Heart 2019;105:1868–75.
36. Guibbal F, Meneyrol V, Ait-Arsa I, et al. Synthesis and automated labeling of [18F]Darapladib, a Lp-PLA2 ligand, as potential PET imaging tool of atherosclerosis. ACS Med Chem Lett 2019;10:743–8.
37. Senders ML, Que X, Cho YS, et al. PET/MR imaging of malondialdehyde-acetaldehyde epitopes with a human antibody detects clinically relevant atherothrombosis. J Am Coll Cardiol 2018;71:321–35.
38. Li X, Bauer W, Israel I, et al. Targeting P-selectin by gallium-68-labeled fucoidan positron emission tomography for noninvasive characterization of vulnerable plaques: correlation with in vivo 17.6T MRI. Arterioscler Thromb Vasc Biol 2014;34:1661–7.
39. Derlin T, Sedding DG, Dutzmann J, et al. Imaging of chemokine receptor CXCR4 expression in culprit and nonculprit coronary atherosclerotic plaque using motion-corrected [68Ga]pentixafor PET/CT. Eur J Nucl Med Mol Imaging 2018;45:1934–44.
40. Martins-Green M, Petreaca M, Wang L. Chemokines and their receptors are key players in the orchestra that regulates wound healing. Adv Wound Care 2013;2:327–47.
41. Hyafil F, Pelisek J, Laitinen I, et al. Imaging the cytokine receptor CXCR4 in atherosclerotic plaques with the radiotracer 68Ga-Pentixafor for PET. J Nucl Med 2017;58:499–506.
42. Hyafil F, Tran-Dinh A, Burg S, et al. Detection of apoptotic cells in a rabbit model with atherosclerosis-like lesions using the positron emission tomography radiotracer [18F]ML-10. Mol Imaging 2015;14:433–42.
43. Meletta R, Slavik R, Mu L, et al. Cannabinoid receptor type 2 (CB2) as one of the candidate genes in human carotid plaque imaging: evaluation of the novel radiotracer [11C]RS-016 targeting CB2 in atherosclerosis. Nucl Med Biol 2017;47:31–43.
44. Meletta R, Steier L, Borel N, et al. CD80 Is upregulated in a mouse model with shear stress-induced atherosclerosis and allows for evaluating CD80-targeting PET tracers. Mol Imaging Biol 2017;19:90–9.
45. Tarkin JM, Joshi FR, Evans NR, et al. Detection of atherosclerotic inflammation by 68Ga-DOTATATE PET compared to [18F]FDG PET imaging. J Am Coll Cardiol 2017;69:1774–91.
46. Tarkin, J. M. (2017). Atherosclerotic inflammation imaging using somatostatin receptor-2 positron emission tomography (Doctoral thesis).https://doi.org/10.17863/CAM.15485
47. Malmberg C, Ripa RS, Johnbeck CB, et al. 64Cu-DOTATATE for noninvasive assessment of atherosclerosis in large arteries and its correlation with risk factors: head-to-head comparison with 68Ga-DOTATOC in 60 patients. J Nucl Med 2015;56:1895–900.
48. Evans NR, Tarkin JM, Chowdhury MM, et al. PET imaging of atherosclerotic disease: advancing plaque assessment from anatomy to pathophysiology. Curr Atheroscler Rep 2016;18:30.
49. Ammirati E, Moroni F, Magnoni M, et al. Carotid artery plaque uptake of 11C-PK11195 inversely correlates with circulating monocytes and classical CD14++CD16− monocytes expressing HLA-DR. Int J Cardiol Heart Vasc 2018;21:32–5.
50. Hellberg S, Liljenbäck H, Eskola O, et al. Positron emission tomography imaging of macrophages in atherosclerosis with 18F-GE-180, a radiotracer for translocator protein (TSPO). Contrast Media Mol Imaging 2018;2018:9186902.
51. Sanchis-Gomar F, Perez-Quilis C, Leischik R, et al. Epidemiology of coronary heart disease and acute coronary syndrome. Ann Transl Med 2016;4:256.
52. Singh A, Museedi AS, Grossman SA. Acute coronary syndrome. StatPearls, Treasure Island (FL): StatPearls Publishing; 2020.

53. Regmi M, Siccardi MA. Coronary artery disease prevention. StatPearls, Treasure Island (FL): StatPearls Publishing; 2020.

54. Driessen RS, Danad I, Stuijfzand WJ, et al. Impact of revascularization on absolute myocardial blood flow as assessed by serial [15O]H2O positron emission tomography imaging: a comparison with fractional flow reserve. Circ Cardiovasc Imaging 2018;11:e007417.

55. Everaars H, de Waard GA, Driessen RS, et al. Doppler flow velocity and thermodilution to assess coronary flow reserve: a head-to-head comparison with [15O]H2O PET. JACC Cardiovasc Interv 2018; 11:2044–54.

56. Bom MJ, van Diemen PA, Driessen RS, et al. Prognostic value of [15O]H2O positron emission tomography-derived global and regional myocardial perfusion. Eur Heart J Cardiovasc Imaging 2020;21:777–86.

57. Chatal J-F, Rouzet F, Haddad F, et al. Story of rubidium-82 and advantages for myocardial perfusion PET imaging. Front Med (Lausanne) 2015;2:65.

58. Klein R, Ocneanu A, Renaud JM, et al. Consistent tracer administration profile improves test-retest repeatability of myocardial blood flow quantification with 82Rb dynamic PET imaging. J Nucl Cardiol 2018;25:929–41.

59. von Scholten BJ, Hasbak P, Christensen TE, et al. Cardiac (82)Rb PET/CT for fast and non-invasive assessment of microvascular function and structure in asymptomatic patients with type 2 diabetes. Diabetologia 2016;59:371–8.

60. Verweij SL, Stiekema LCA, Delewi R, et al. Prolonged hematopoietic and myeloid cellular response in patients after an acute coronary syndrome measured with 18F-DPA-714 PET/CT. Eur J Nucl Med Mol Imaging 2018;45:1956–63.

61. Broos CE, van Nimwegen M, Hoogsteden HC, et al. Granuloma formation in pulmonary sarcoidosis. Front Immunol 2013;4:437.

62. Ipek E, Demirelli S, Ermis E, et al. Sarcoidosis and the heart: a review of the literature. Intractable Rare Dis Res 2015;4:170–80.

63. Doughan AR, Williams BR. Cardiac sarcoidosis. Heart 2006;92:282–8.

64. Sedaghat-Hamedani F, Kayvanpour E, Hamed S, et al. The chameleon of cardiology: cardiac sarcoidosis before and after heart transplantation. ESC Heart Fail 2019;7:692–6.

65. Sekhri V, Sanal S, DeLorenzo LJ, et al. Cardiac sarcoidosis: a comprehensive review. Arch Med Sci 2011;7:546–54.

66. Weinberg RL, Morgenstern R, DeLuca A, et al. F-18 sodium fluoride PET/CT does not effectively image myocardial inflammation due to suspected cardiac sarcoidosis. J Nucl Cardiol 2017;24:2015–8.

67. Norikane T, Yamamoto Y, Maeda Y, et al. 18F-FLT PET imaging in a patient with sarcoidosis with cardiac involvement. Clin Nucl Med 2015;40:433–4.

68. Norikane T, Yamamoto Y, Maeda Y, et al. Comparative evaluation of 18F-FLT and 18F-FDG for detecting cardiac and extra-cardiac thoracic involvement in patients with newly diagnosed sarcoidosis. EJNMMI Res 2017;7:69.

69. Gormsen LC, Haraldsen A, Kramer S, et al. A dual tracer 68Ga-DOTANOC PET/CT and 18F-FDG PET/CT pilot study for detection of cardiac sarcoidosis. EJNMMI Res 2016;6:52.

70. Jahandideh A, Uotila S, Stahle M, et al. Folate receptor β targeted PET imaging of macrophages in autoimmune myocarditis. J Nucl Med 2020. https://doi.org/10.2967/jnumed.119.241356.

71. Wexler R, Elton T, Pleister A, et al. Cardiomyopathy: an overview. Am Fam Physician 2009;79:778–84.

72. Houson HA, Nkepang GN, Hedrick AF, et al. Imaging of isoproterenol-induced myocardial injury with 18F labeled fluoroglucaric acid in a rat model. Nucl Med Biol 2018;59:9–15.

73. Sharma V, Sivapackiam J, Harpstrite SE, et al. A generator-produced gallium-68 radiopharmaceutical for PET imaging of myocardial perfusion. PLoS One 2014;9:e109361.

74. Sivapackiam J, Kabra S, Speidel S, et al. 68Ga-Galmydar: a PET imaging tracer for noninvasive detection of doxorubicin-induced cardiotoxicity. PLoS One 2019;14:e0215579.

75. Zimmer A, Bagchi AK, Vinayak K, et al. Innate immune response in the pathogenesis of heart failure in survivors of myocardial infarction. Am J Physiol Heart Circ Physiol 2018;316:H435–45.

76. Byrne C, Hasbak P, Kjær A, et al. Myocardial perfusion during atrial fibrillation in patients with non-ischaemic systolic heart failure: a cross-sectional study using Rubidium-82 positron emission tomography/computed tomography. Eur Heart J Cardiovasc Imaging 2019;20:233–40.

77. Fong IW. New perspectives of infections in cardiovascular disease. Curr Cardiol Rev 2009;5:87–104.

78. Cooper LT. Myocarditis. N Engl J Med 2009;360: 1526–38.

79. Kim GR, Paeng JC, Jung JH, et al. Assessment of TSPO in a rat experimental autoimmune myocarditis model: a comparison study between [18F]Fluoromethyl-PBR28 and [18F]CB251. Int J Mol Sci 2018;19:276.

80. Maya Y, Werner RA, Schütz C, et al. 11C-Methionine PET of myocardial inflammation in a rat model of experimental autoimmune myocarditis. J Nucl Med 2016;57:1985–90.

81. Lee S-P, Im H-J, Kang S, et al. Noninvasive imaging of myocardial inflammation in myocarditis using 68Ga-tagged mannosylated human serum albumin positron emission tomography. Theranostics 2017; 7:413–24.

82. Dababneh E, Siddique MS. Pericarditis. StatPearls, Treasure Island (FL): StatPearls Publishing; 2020.

83. Lapa C, Reiter T, Li X, et al. Imaging of myocardial inflammation with somatostatin receptor based PET/CT: a comparison to cardiac MRI. Int J Cardiol 2015;194:44–9.

84. Kouijzer IJE, Vos FJ, Janssen MJR, et al. The value of 18F-FDG PET/CT in diagnosing infectious endocarditis. Eur J Nucl Med Mol Imaging 2013;40:1102–7.

85. Yan J, Zhang C, Niu Y, et al. The role of 18F-FDG PET/CT in infectious endocarditis: a systematic review and meta-analysis. Int J Clin Pharmacol Ther 2016;54:337–42.

86. Kestler M, Muñoz P, Rodríguez-Créixems M, et al. Role of (18)F-FDG PET in patients with infectious endocarditis. J Nucl Med 2014;55:1093–8.

87. Jiménez-Ballvé A, Pérez-Castejón MJ, Delgado-Bolton RC, et al. Assessment of the diagnostic accuracy of 18F-FDG PET/CT in prosthetic infective endocarditis and cardiac implantable electronic device infection: comparison of different interpretation criteria. Eur J Nucl Med Mol Imaging 2016;43:2401–12.

88. McDonald JR. Acute infective endocarditis. Infect Dis Clin North Am 2009;23:643–64.

89. Shan L. 64Cu-Diethylenetriamine pentaacetic acid-NH-CO-CH2-S-CH2-Phe-Pro-Arg-CH2-prothrombin. Mol. Imaging contrast agent database MICAD. Bethesda (MD): National Center for Biotechnology Information (US); 2004.

90. Panizzi P, Nahrendorf M, Figueiredo J-L, et al. In vivo detection of Staphylococcus aureus endocarditis by targeting pathogen-specific prothrombin activation. Nat Med 2011;17:1142–6.

91. Teixeira ARL, Nitz N, Guimaro MC, et al. Chagas disease. Postgrad Med J 2006;82:788–98.

92. Lidani KCF, Andrade FA, Bavia L, et al. Chagas disease: from discovery to a worldwide health problem. Front Public Health 2019;7:166.

93. Nguyen T, Waseem M. Chagas disease (American Trypanosomiasis). StatPearls, Treasure Island (FL): StatPearls Publishing; 2020.

94. De Bona E, Lidani KCF, Bavia L, et al. Autoimmunity in chronic Chagas disease: a road of multiple pathways to cardiomyopathy? Front Immunol 2018;9:1842.

95. Gordan R, Gwathmey JK, Xie L-H. Autonomic and endocrine control of cardiovascular function. World J Cardiol 2015;7:204–14.

96. Moll-Bernardes RJ, de Oliveira RS, de Brito ASX, et al. Can PET/CT be useful in predicting ventricular arrhythmias in Chagas disease? J Nucl Cardiol 2020. https://doi.org/10.1007/s12350-019-02014-1.

Radionuclide Imaging of Cardiac Amyloidosis

Vladimir Joseph, MD[a], Howard M. Julien, MD, MPH[a], Paco E. Bravo, MD[a,b,c],*

KEYWORDS

- Cardiac amyloidosis • SPECT • PET • Molecular imaging

KEY POINTS

- Bone scintigraphy has high diagnostic accuracy for evaluating individuals with suspected transthyretin cardiac amyloidosis but poor performance for detecting light chain cardiac amyloidosis.
- It is likely that cross-sectional imaging with single-photon emission computed tomography (SPECT) or SPECT/computed tomography eventually will replace planar imaging during bone scintigraphy.
- Amyloid-specific probes, such as florbetapir and florbetaben, remain investigational; however, they appear to be sensitive and specific biomarkers to detect both light chain and transthyretin cardiac amyloidosis.

INTRODUCTION

Amyloidosis is a systemic infiltrative disease characterized by the pathologic deposition of abnormally folded proteins known as amyloid fibrils.[1] These proteins circulate in the plasma, deposit diffusely in tissue extracellularly, and eventually aggregate into an amyloid plaque. This extracellular deposition and aggregation is known to result in vital organ dysfunction.[1] Amyloid deposition occurs in the myocardial interstitium and intramyocardial vessels, subsequently leading to diastolic and systolic dysfunction, perfusion defects, conduction abnormalities, and arrhythmias.[2] Virtually any organ system can be affected, but the prognosis of the disease largely is due to the extent of cardiac involvement, because this is the leading cause of morbidity and mortality in systemic amyloidosis.[3]

Although several amyloid fibrils can infiltrate the heart, immunoglobulin light chain (AL) and transthyretin (ATTR) unquestionably are the most common amyloid fibril types affecting the myocardium and are the focus of this revision.

PATHOBIOLOGY AND PROGNOSIS

ATTR is a plasma protein produced by the liver that primarily is involved with the systemic transport of thyroxine (T4) and retinol (vitamin A1).[4] Genetic mutations and aging can cause ATTR to disassemble into fibrils that eventually form amyloid plaques[5] and eventually manifest in 2 distinct forms: mutant ATTR called familial amyloid cardiomyopathy, also known as familial amyloidotic polyneuropathy, which arises from an autosomal dominant genetic disorder that results in the misfolding of ATTR protein due to a mutated or variant ATTR gene, and a nonhereditary form or wild-type ATTR, which is a nongenetic, sporadic, disease caused by misaggregation of wild-type ATTR [6–8] Cardiac involvement can be variable in hereditary ATTR amyloidosis (rare in TTR-Val30Met and approximately 90% in TTR-Thr60Ala mutation)

Funding Source: Supported in part by the Institute for Translational Medicine and Therapeutics (ITMAT:Philadelphia, PA, USA) Transdisciplinary Program in Translational Medicine and Therapeutics.
a Division of Cardiovascular Medicine, Department of Medicine, Perelman School of Medicine, University of Pennsylvania, Philadelphia, PA, USA; b Division of Nuclear Medicine and Clinical Molecular Imaging, Department of Radiology, Perelman School of Medicine, University of Pennsylvania, Philadelphia, PA, USA; c Division of Cardiothoracic Imaging, Department of Radiology, Perelman School of Medicine, University of Pennsylvania, Philadelphia, PA, USA
* Corresponding author. Hospital of the University of Pennsylvania, 3400 Civic Center Boulevard, 11-154 South Pavilion, Philadelphia, PA 19104.
E-mail address: paco.bravo@pennmedicine.upenn.edu

and is seen in almost all patients with wild-type ATTR.

Immunoglobulin AL amyloidosis, on the other hand, is a monoclonal plasma cell proliferative disorder caused by extracellular deposition of AL fibrils in various tissues and organs, with predominant involvement of the heart (60%–75%), and kidney (50%–60%) and less commonly the liver (15%), peripheral/autonomic nervous system (10%), and gastrointestinal tract (5%–10%), causing disease by progressively damaging the structure and function of the affected tissue.[6,8,9]

From a pathophysiology viewpoint, the structural and molecular mechanisms underlying amyloid-mediated cardiac damage are elucidated only partially. Structurally, cardiac amyloid infiltration leads to a significant increment in left ventricular (LV) mass, with preferential involvement for the basal and mid-LV segments, a process that appears to be the result of diffuse expansion of the extracellular matrix from amyloid deposition.[10] Importantly, LV mass is associated strongly with reduced myocardial strain on echocardiography, a sensitive parameter of cardiac function that has been found to be an independent predictor of survival in amyloidosis.[11] Therefore, a mechanical and/or passive restrictive effect from amyloid infiltration has been proposed as a cause of cardiac dysfunction in both ATTR and AL. More recent experimental and clinical observations, however, also support a more direct cytotoxic-mediated role of the AL fibrils in the heart.[12–14] Cardiac amyloid deposition typically is much more substantial in the ATTR than in the AL type, but serum markers of myocardial tissue damage, such as N-terminal fragment of the probrain natriuretic peptide and troponin, generally are higher in AL.[15] This dissonance is postulated to be correlated to the more rapidly depositing and toxic effect of AL amyloid in comparison to the ATTR type,[16] which also may help explain the differences in outcomes. In the presence of heart failure symptoms, cardiac ATTR amyloidosis portends a more favorable prognosis than cardiac AL amyloidosis with median survival typically 3 years to 5 years from diagnosis as opposed to AL disease median survival of less than 1 year.[16] Consequently, discerning between the subtypes is critical as prognostication and treatment options differ significantly between the etiologies.[6,17]

DIAGNOSIS

The gold standard of diagnosis remains endomyocardial biopsy with Congo red staining resulting in apple-green birefringence of amyloid deposits under polarized light, followed either by mass spectroscopy or immunohistochemical staining, which is required for typing of the amyloid fibril.[18] Endomyocardial biopsy, however, is not widely available and carries procedural risks making it less than ideal for routine screening. As a result, multimodality imaging has emerged as the strategy of choice for evaluation and management of individuals with suspected amyloid heart disease, which typically includes a combination of structural and tissue characterization techniques, including echocardiography, contrast-enhanced cardiac magnetic resonance (CMR), and radionuclide imaging modalities, such as single-photon emission computed tomography (SPECT) and PET.

In this respect, radionuclide imaging has gained great clinical relevance in recent years to the point that has become the standard of care for the noninvasive diagnosis of ATTR cardiomyopathy. On the other hand, accurate detection of AL remains challenging. With the advent of more-specific amyloid probes, however, the noninvasive diagnosis of AL seems more feasible than before.

According to their molecular mechanism of binding, radiopharmaceuticals can be divided into non–amyloid-specific and amyloid-specific agents (Table 1). In general, the former tracers are more specific for ATTR, whereas, the latter seem to bind more avidly to AL.

NON–AMYLOID-SPECIFIC RADIOTRACERS (BONE SCINTIGRAPHY)

Bone-seeking radiopharmaceuticals (bone scintigraphy), including technetium 99m (99mTc) 3,3-diphosphono-1,2-propanodicarboxylic acid (DPD), 99mTc hydroxymethylene diphosphonate (HMDP), 99mTc methylene diphosphonate (MDP), and 99mTc pyrophosphate (PYP) have been tested successfully and become key markers in the detection of amyloidosis in general and ATTR in particular. They became clinically relevant after they were found to accumulate within extraosseous tissue, including the heart, incidentally during whole-body planar imaging for noncardiac indications (Fig. 1). Subsequent studies have shown the preferential selectivity of these tracers for ATTR.

From a procedural perspective, bone scintigraphy imaging has been historically performed using planar images acquired between 1 hour and 3 hours after the radiotracer administration. The advent of SPECT and SPECT/CT (Fig. 2), however, has let to questioning the actual utility of planar imaging because it is not infrequent to encounter significant blood pool activity in the cardiac region, particularly at 1 hour, that might be confused

Table 1
Summary of most important radiopharmaceutical for evaluation of individuals with suspected cardiac amyloidosis

Targeted Nuclear Imaging Probes for Cardiac Amyloidosis					
Category	Molecular Targets	Modality	Uptake Time	Amyloid–Subtype Affinity	Cardiac Amyloid Uptake
Non–amyloid-specific binding *Bone-seeking radionuclides*					
99mTc-PYP	Microcalcifications	Planar/SPECT	60–90 min	ATTR >> AL	Positive
99mTc-DPD	Microcalcifications	Planar/SPECT	180 min	ATTR >> AL	Positive
99mTc-HMDP	Microcalcifications	Planar/SPECT	180 min	ATTR >> AL	Positive
Amyloid-specific binding *Thioflavin T derivatives*					
11C-PIB	β-Amyloid plaque	PET	4–30 min	AL > ATTR	Positive
18F-florbetaben	β-Amyloid plaque	PET	4–30 min	AL > ATTR	Positive
18F-flutemetamol	β-Amyloid plaque	PET	20 min	AL > ATTR	Positive
Stilbene derivatives					
18F-florbetapir	β-Amyloid plaque	PET	4–30 min	AL > ATTR	Positive

with LV wall activity without cross-sectional imaging with SPECT or SPECT/CT (**Fig. 3**). Consequently, it is highly conceivable that SPECT or SPECT/CT eventually will replace planar imaging in the foreseeable future.

From a molecular basis, the exact mechanism of uptake in amyloidosis is not understood completely, although the current consensus is that it appears to be related to the level of microcalcifications present in amyloid deposits.[19] For example, Stats and Stone[19] investigated calcium staining and macrophage expression in cardiac tissue of patients with ATTR and AL amyloidosis. They found significantly greater extent of microcalcifications in cases of ATTR compared with AL, whereas macrophage expression was significantly lower in ATTR than AL,[19] indicating that the increased level of microcalcifications, and not macrophage expression, may explain the enhanced affinity of bone-seeking probes for ATTR over AL amyloidosis, as described later.

Technetium Tc 99m Pyrophosphate

99mTc-PYP is an ATTR-specific single-photon emitter tracer that readily identifies ATTR cardiac amyloidosis.[20] In a single-center, blinded, prospective cohort study, 45 subjects (12 AL, 16 wild-type ATTR, and 17 mutant ATTR) underwent 99mTc-PYP scintigraphy cardiac imaging and were scored based on cardiac retention of the tracer; subjects with ATTR cardiac amyloid had a significantly higher cardiac retention scores: visual and quantitative (heart–to–contralateral uptake ratio). A heart–to–contralateral lung ratio of greater than 1.5 correlated to 97% sensitivity and 100% specificity for identifying ATTR cardiac amyloidosis.[21]

Technetium Tc 99m 3,3-Diphosphono-1,2-Propanodicarboxylicacid

99mTc–DPD is another single-photon radiotracer with high affinity for ATTR. Peruguni and colleagues,[22] studied 35 subjects (15 ATTR, 10 AL, and 10 controls) and found that tracer retention of 99mTc-DPD was significantly higher in ATTR subjects than in AL and control patients. Control and AL subjects showed no uptake of 99mTc-DPD and ATTR subjects showed increased uptake with 100% sensitivity.[22]

Technetium Tc 99m Hydroxymethylene Diphosphonate

99mTc–HMDP scintigraphy is available outside of the United States and has performed at least as well as 99mTc-DPD or 99mTc-PYP scintigraphy in differentiating ATTR from AL.[23] In a retrospective Italian study of 65 patients (26 with AL and 39 with ATTR [16 mutant ATTR, 23 wild-type ATTR])

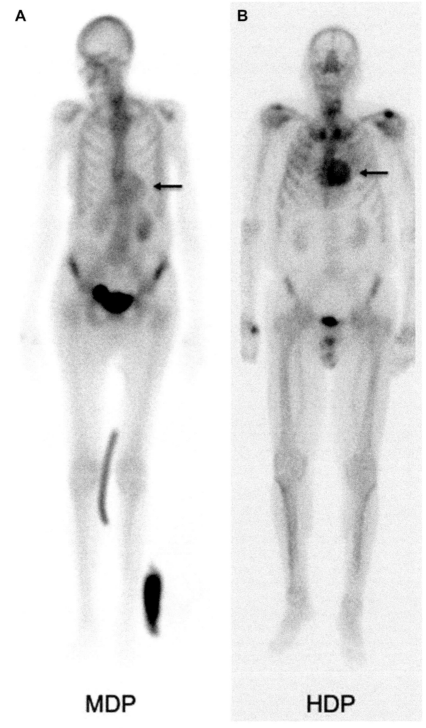

Fig. 1. Incidental myocardial uptake (*arrows*) of 99mTc–MDP (*A*) and 99mTc–hydroxydiphosphonate (HDP) (*B*) in 2 elderly male patients undergoing bone scintigraphy for bone metastasis evaluation. Notice that cardiac uptake would be considered grade II (similar to adjacent rib uptake) in patient in (*A*), and grade III (significantly greater than ribs) for patient in (*B*). Both patients had history of explained heart failure.

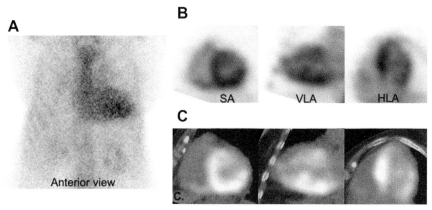

Fig. 2. Planar chest (*A*), and cardiac SPECT (*B*), and SPECT/CT fused (*C*) images acquired 1 hour after 99mTc–PYP IV administration on a 75-year-old woman with heart failure symptoms. Images show intense myocardial uptake, significantly greater than blood pool, and nearby rib activity. Overall, imaging findings are strongly suggestive of cardiac TTR amyloidosis. HLA, horizontal long axis; SA, short axis; VLA, vertical long axis.

underwent 99mTc-HMDP scintigraphy; of the 26 AL patients, only 2 showed a visual heart uptake score of grade 1 whereas 24 showed no uptake. All ATTR patients showed 99mTc-HMDP uptake. This correlated to a positive 99mTc-HMDP scintigraphy with 100% sensitivity and 96% specificity for ATTR cardiac amyloidosis identification.[24]

The strongest evidence of the true diagnostic accuracy of bone scintigraphy in cardiac amyloidosis, however, was elucidated by Gillmore and collaborators[25] in a large multicenter study that included 1217 patients with suspected cardiac amyloidosis who were imaged with either 99mTc–DPD, 99mTc–PYP, or 99mTc–MDP. Of them, 31% underwent endomyocardial biopsy, whereas the remaining only underwent extracardiac biopsies. Overall, 43% and 10% of patients

eventually were identified as having confirmed cardiac ATTR and AL amyloidosis, respectively. Remarkably, bone scintigraphy had greater than 99% sensitivity and 86% specificity for detecting ATTR, with false-positive results occurring mostly from uptake (typically mild) in patients with AL amyloidosis. The sensitivity of bone scintigraphy, however, decreased to 90% whereas the specificity increased to 97% when only moderate (grade 2) or intense (grade 3) myocardial tracer uptake was considered abnormal for ATTR. This indicates that most false-positive scans for ATTR typically exhibit mild (grade 1) radiotracer activity in the heart. Additionally, the combined findings of grade 2 or grade 3 myocardial radiotracer uptake on bone scintigraphy in the absence of a monoclonal protein in serum or urine had a specificity and

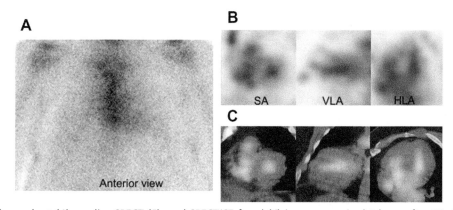

Fig. 3. Planar chest (*A*), cardiac SPECT (*B*), and SPECT/CT fused (*C*) images acquired 1 hour after 99mTc–PYP IV administration on a 54-year-old man with clinical suspicion for hereditary TTR amyloidosis. Planar images suggest mild uptake in the cardiac region. SPECT and SPECT/CT images confirm, however, that myocardial uptake is localized to the blood pool and not the LV wall. Thus, findings are not consistent with ATTR infiltration. HLA, horizontal long axis; SA, short axis; VLA, vertical long axis.

positive predictive value for cardiac ATTR amyloidosis of 100%.

In summary, if carefully performed, bone scintigraphy has an extremely high accuracy for establishing the diagnosis of cardiac ATTR amyloidosis but poor sensitivity and specificity to detect cardiac AL amyloidosis.[25]

AMYLOID-SPECIFIC PROBES

Over the past 15 years, there have been tremendous efforts in the development of novel probes for the detection of amyloid deposition. All these probes share a common structure and are quite specific for amyloid imaging. The next section reviews the most relevant ones related to cardiac imaging.

Thioflavin T and Stilbene Derivatives

Thioflavin T is a benzothiazole stain that exhibits enhanced fluorescence upon binding to amyloid fibrils and, hence, is used routinely in clinical practice as a potent fluorescent marker of amyloid deposits in tissue, both in vitro and ex vivo.[26–29] The radiopharmaceuticals, ^{11}C-Pittsburgh compound B (PiB),[30] ^{18}F-flutemetamol, and ^{18}F-florbetaben,[31] are benzothiazoles whereas ^{18}F-florbetapir[32] is a stilbene derivative with a very similar structure. These radiotracers selectively bind to β-amyloid plaques and originally were designed as an aid to establish the clinical diagnosis of Alzheimer disease.

C-11 Pittsburgh Compound B

C11-PIB is a PET tracer that has been shown to identify both AL and ATTR cardiac amyloid. In a study that included 5 patients with ATTR, 5 with AL, and 5 healthy volunteers, Antoni and colleagues[33] observed that myocardial retention index (RI) of 11C-PIB was significantly higher in both types of amyloidosis patients when compared with healthy controls (0.054 min^{-1}– 0.025 min^{-1}). A comparison between ATTR and AL myocardial uptake, however, was not performed. With its short half-life of 20 minutes, the use of 11C-PIB is limited to PET centers with an on-site cyclotron and currently it is not Food and Drug Administration approved for the diagnosis of cardiac amyloidosis.

18F-Florbetapir

18F-florbetapir is a stilbene-derived PET tracer with long half-life (109 min) as well as high affinity and specificity for amyloid β.[34] Dorbala and colleagues[35] explored the use of 18F-florbetapir in evaluating cardiac amyloidosis and found that florbetaben PET/CT not only is able to detect cardiac amyloidosis but also may be able to potentially differentiate between the subtypes (**Fig. 4**). In a prospective case-control pilot study of 14 subjects, 9 subjects with known cardiac amyloidosis and 5 control subjects without amyloidosis who underwent 18F-florbetapir PET/CT, myocardial RI/target-to-background ratio (TBR) of 18F-florbetapir was significantly higher in the amyloid subjects than in the control subjects (median RI was 0.043 min^{-1}–0.023 min^{-1}). In addition, myocardial retention was significantly higher in the AL patients rather than the ATTR patients despite a significantly lower myocardial mass noted in the AL subjects. Suggesting greater affinity of 18F-florbetapir for AL cardiac amyloid and may reflect amyloid disease activity.[35]

18F-Florbetaben

F18-florbetaben is another PET tracer with diagnostic ability for cardiac amyloid (**Fig. 5**). In a prospective 14-patient pilot study (5 with AL, 5 with

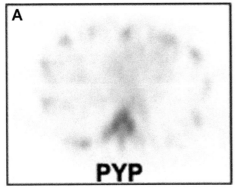
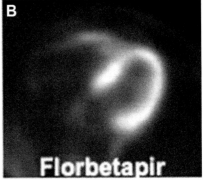

Fig. 4. Differences in myocardial uptake between 99mTc–PYP (*A*) and ^{18}F-florbetapir (*B*) in a patient with heart failure due to AL amyloidosis. Please notice the diffuse intense myocardial uptake of florbetapir in contrast to the lack of PYP binding in the same patient. (Image courtesy of Sharmila Dorbala, MD from Brigham and Women's Hospital.)

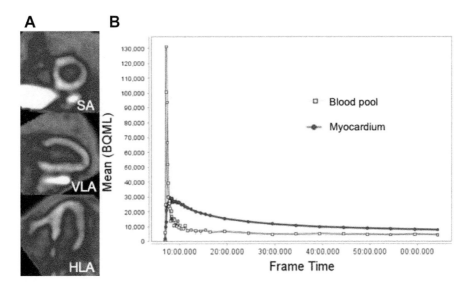

Fig. 5. Abnormally increased myocardial 18F florbetaben uptake in an individual with heart failure due to AL amyloidosis involvement. Cardiac static (summed 10–60 minutes) images (*A*) and time activity curves of blood pool and myocardial activity on dynamic images (0–60 minutes) (*B*). HLA, horizontal long axis; SA, short axis; VLA, vertical long axis.

ATTR, and 4 controls with hypertensive heart disease) who underwent PET/CT utilizing 18F-florbetaben–target-to-background SUV ratio and myocardial 18F-forbetaben retention were measured and were significantly higher in amyloid patients than in hypertensive controls. A median myocardial 18F-florbetaben RI was 0.043 min^{-1} in AL patients, 0.035 min^{-1} in ATTR patients, and 0.010 min^{-1} in hypertensive controls,[31] again showing the higher binding avidity of these probes for AL.

18F-Flutemetamol

18F-flutemetamol is another PET tracer that has demonstrated the ability to diagnose cardiac amyloid. In a retrospective study of 12 patients (3 control subjects without cardiac amyloidosis and 9 subjects with known cardiac amyloidosis) who underwent 18F-flutemetamol PET/CT, cardiac uptake of 18F-flutemetamol was noted in all patients with cardiac amyloidosis except 1, and none was noted in the control arm. The TBR was significantly higher in amyloidosis patients than in control subjects: 1.46 versus 1.06 (*P* = .033). There was only 1 AL patient in the cardiac amyloid arm and that patient had a higher TBR than ATTR patients: TBR 3.0 versus TBR median 1.44.[36]

CLINICAL APPLICATIONS AND FUTURE DIRECTIONS

In the United States, only bone scintigraphy with or without SPECT/CT currently is approved for imaging cardiac amyloidosis, whereas the more-specific PET probes, such as florbetapir and florbetaben, remain investigational, at least for cardiac imaging. Patients evaluated for cardiac amyloidosis typically present with heart failure symptoms, and the current recommendations emphasize the importance of simultaneously screening or excluding the possibility of underlying AL by checking free AL and serum and/or urine immunofixation. In the absence of a monoclonal protein, a grade 2/3 positive myocardial bone scan has a positive predictive value greater than 99% for ATTR and now is considered a definitive diagnosis, obviating cardiac biopsy. The next step, in those positive cases, is genetic testing to distinguish between hereditary versus wild-type ATTR. On the other hand, a negative bone scan requires additional work-up, including biochemical testing to rule out AL, as discussed previously, and/or hopefully in the future the use of any of the available amyloid-specific PET probes, as illustrated in **Fig. 4**.

Additional areas of future investigation will include the use of quantitative radionuclide imaging techniques to assess treatment response in both AL and ATTR amyloidosis[10] as well as the accuracy of these methods for early detection.[37]

In summary, PET and SPECT technologies have revolutionized our ability to diagnose cardiac amyloidosis, thus allowing early detection, differentiation of amyloid types, and potentially tracking disease progression in the future.

CLINICS CARE POINTS

- A negative myocardial bone scan with single-photon probes has sensitivity and negative predictive value close to 100% to exclude the possibility of cardiac ATTR amyloidosis.

- Similarly, myocardial radiotracer uptake on bone scintigraphy in the absence of a monoclonal protein in serum or urine has a specificity and positive predictive value for cardiac ATTR amyloidosis close to 100%.

- Bone scintigraphy is not helpful to detect AL cardiac amyloidosis.

ACKNOWLEDGMENTS

The authors would like to thank Sharmila Dorbala, MD, from Brigham and Women's Hospital for facilitating some illustrations.

DISCLOSURE

The authors report no conflicts.

REFERENCES

1. Lachmann HJ, Hawkins PN. Systemic amyloidosis. Curr Opin Pharmacol 2006;6:214–20.
2. Falk RH. Diagnosis and management of the cardiac amyloidoses. Circulation 2005;112:2047–60.
3. Merlini G, Seldin DC, Gertz MA. Amyloidosis: pathogenesis and new therapeutic options. J Clin Oncol 2011;29:1924–33.
4. Hamilton JA, Benson MD. Transthyretin: a review from a structural perspective. Cell Mol Life Sci 2001;58:1491–521.
5. Kelly JW. Mechanisms of amyloidogenesis. Nat Struct Biol 2000;7:824–6.
6. Martinez-Naharro A, Hawkins PN, Fontana M. Cardiac amyloidosis. Clin Med (Lond) 2018;18:s30–5.
7. Witteles RM, Bokhari S, Damy T, et al. Screening for transthyretin amyloid cardiomyopathy in everyday practice. JACC Heart Failure 2019;7:709–16.
8. Ruberg FL, Berk JL. Transthyretin (ttr) cardiac amyloidosis. Circulation 2012;126:1286–300.
9. Muchtar E, Gertz MA, Kumar SK, et al. Improved outcomes for newly diagnosed al amyloidosis between 2000 and 2014: cracking the glass ceiling of early death. Blood 2017;129:2111–9.
10. Bravo PE, Fujikura K, Kijewski MF, et al. Relative apical sparing of myocardial longitudinal strain is explained by regional differences in total amyloid mass rather than the proportion of amyloid deposits. JACC Cardiovasc Imaging 2019;12(7 Pt 1):1165–73.
11. Buss SJ, Emami M, Mereles D, et al. Longitudinal left ventricular function for prediction of survival in systemic light-chain amyloidosis: incremental value compared with clinical and biochemical markers. J Am Coll Cardiol 2012;60:1067–76.
12. Liao R, Jain M, Teller P, et al. Infusion of light chains from patients with cardiac amyloidosis causes diastolic dysfunction in isolated mouse hearts. Circulation 2001;104:1594–7.
13. Mishra S, Guan J, Plovie E, et al. Human amyloidogenic light chain proteins result in cardiac dysfunction, cell death, and early mortality in zebrafish. Am J Physiol Heart Circ Physiol 2013;305:H95–103.
14. Palladini G, Lavatelli F, Russo P, et al. Circulating amyloidogenic free light chains and serum n-terminal natriuretic peptide type b decrease simultaneously in association with improvement of survival in al. Blood 2006;107:3854–8.
15. Suhr OB, Anan I, Backman C, et al. Do troponin and b-natriuretic peptide detect cardiomyopathy in transthyretin amyloidosis? J Intern Med 2008;263:294–301.
16. Rapezzi C, Merlini G, Quarta CC, et al. Systemic cardiac amyloidoses: disease profiles and clinical courses of the 3 main types. Circulation 2009;120:1203–12.
17. Fontana M, Chung R, Hawkins PN, et al. Cardiovascular magnetic resonance for amyloidosis. Heart Fail Rev 2015;20:133–44.
18. Vrana JA, Gamez JD, Madden BJ, et al. Classification of amyloidosis by laser microdissection and mass spectrometry-based proteomic analysis in clinical biopsy specimens. Blood 2009;114:4957–9.
19. Stats MA, Stone JR. Varying levels of small microcalcifications and macrophages in attr and al cardiac amyloidosis: implications for utilizing nuclear medicine studies to subtype amyloidosis. Cardiovasc Pathol 2016;25:413–7.
20. Hongo M, Hirayama J, Fujii T, et al. Early identification of amyloid heart disease by technetium-99m-pyrophosphate scintigraphy: a study with familial amyloid polyneuropathy. Am Heart J 1987;113:654–62.
21. Bokhari S, Castano A, Pozniakoff T, et al. 99m)tc-pyrophosphate scintigraphy for differentiating light-chain cardiac amyloidosis from the transthyretin-related familial and senile cardiac amyloidoses. Circ Cardiovasc Imaging 2013;6:195–201.
22. Perugini E, Guidalotti PL, Salvi F, et al. Noninvasive etiologic diagnosis of cardiac amyloidosis using 99mtc-3,3-diphosphono-1,2-propanodicarboxylic acid scintigraphy. J Am Coll Cardiol 2005;46:1076–84.
23. Galat A, Rosso J, Guellich A, et al. Usefulness of (99m)tc-hmdp scintigraphy for the etiologic

diagnosis and prognosis of cardiac amyloidosis. Amyloid 2015;22:210–20.

24. Cappelli F, Gallini C, Di Mario C, et al. Accuracy of 99mtc-hydroxymethylene diphosphonate scintigraphy for diagnosis of transthyretin cardiac amyloidosis. J Nucl Cardiol 2019;26:497–504.

25. Gillmore JD, Maurer MS, Falk RH, et al. Nonbiopsy diagnosis of cardiac transthyretin amyloidosis. Circulation 2016;133:2404–12.

26. Hobbs JR, Morgan AD. Fluorescence microscopy with thioflavine-t in the diagnosis of amyloid. J Pathol Bacteriol 1963;86:437–42.

27. Klunk WE, Wang Y, Huang GF, et al. Uncharged thioflavin-t derivatives bind to amyloid-beta protein with high affinity and readily enter the brain. Life Sci 2001;69:1471–84.

28. Biancalana M, Koide S. Molecular mechanism of thioflavin-t binding to amyloid fibrils. Biochim Biophys Acta 2010;1804:1405–12.

29. Khurana R, Coleman C, Ionescu-Zanetti C, et al. Mechanism of thioflavin t binding to amyloid fibrils. J Struct Biol 2005;151:229–38.

30. Klunk WE, Engler H, Nordberg A, et al. Imaging brain amyloid in alzheimer's disease with pittsburgh compound-b. Ann Neurol 2004;55:306–19.

31. Law WP, Wang WY, Moore PT, et al. Cardiac amyloid imaging with 18f-florbetaben pet: a pilot study. J Nucl Med 2016;57:1733–9.

32. Clark CM, Schneider JA, Bedell BJ, et al. Use of florbetapir-pet for imaging beta-amyloid pathology. JAMA 2011;305:275–83.

33. Antoni G, Lubberink M, Estrada S, et al. In vivo visualization of amyloid deposits in the heart with 11c-pib and pet. J Nucl Med 2013;54:213–20.

34. Park MA, Padera RF, Belanger A, et al. 18f-florbetapir binds specifically to myocardial light chain and transthyretin amyloid deposits: autoradiography study. Circ Cardiovasc Imaging 2015;8. 10.1161/CIRCIMAGING.114.002954 e002954.

35. Dorbala S, Vangala D, Semer J, et al. Imaging cardiac amyloidosis: a pilot study using (1)(8)f-florbetapir positron emission tomography. Eur J Nucl Med Mol Imaging 2014;41:1652–62.

36. Dietemann S, Nkoulou R. Amyloid pet imaging in cardiac amyloidosis: a pilot study using (18)f-flutemetamol positron emission tomography. Ann Nucl Med 2019;33:624–8.

37. Cuddy SAM, Bravo PE, Falk RH, et al. Improved quantification of cardiac amyloid burden in systemic light chain amyloidosis: redefining early disease? JACC Cardiovasc Imaging 2020;13:1325–36.

Novel Musculoskeletal and Orthopedic Applications of ¹⁸F-Sodium Fluoride PET

William Y. Raynor, BS[a,b], Austin J. Borja, BA[a,c], Emily C. Hancin, MS, BA[a,d], Thomas J. Werner, MSc[a], Abass Alavi, MD, MD (Hon), PhD (Hon), DSc (Hon)[a], Mona-Elisabeth Revheim, MD, PhD, MHA[a,e,f],*

KEYWORDS

- Fracture • Osteoarthritis • Ankylosing spondylitis • Temporomandibular disorder • Arthroplasty
- Infection • Osteoporosis • Osteosarcoma

KEY POINTS

- ¹⁸F-sodium fluoride (NaF) PET can detect causes of bone pain and traumatic injuries that cannot be successfully visualized by other modalities such as radiography, bone scintigraphy, computed tomography, and magnetic resonance. Thus, NaF-PET may contribute to the assessment of occult fractures, child abuse, and stress-related injuries.
- NaF-PET is an excellent modality to assess osteoarthritis, ankylosing spondylitis, and temporomandibular joint dysfunction. More studies are needed to determine its potential role in inflammatory arthropathies such as rheumatoid arthritis and psoriatic arthritis.
- Complications of orthopedic surgery such as hardware loosening and infection are readily visualized by NaF-PET. Heterotopic ossification after surgery is another possible imaging target that requires further exploration.
- Metabolic bone diseases such as osteoporosis and Paget disease can be evaluated over time with NaF-PET to determine effects of pharmacologic interventions such as bisphosphonates and teriparatide.
- NaF-PET may have a role in assessing primary bone tumors such as osteosarcoma, helping to determine response to treatment and guiding patient management decisions.

INTRODUCTION

The bone-seeking properties of ¹⁸F-sodium fluoride (NaF) were first described in 1962 by Blau and colleagues,[1] who used this positron-emitting radiotracer in skeletal scintigraphy. Both high uptake by bone and rapid plasma clearance of NaF were determined to be advantages in imaging skeletal metabolism.[2] The mechanism of NaF uptake relies on the exchange of OH^- for $^{18}F^-$, converting hydroxyapatite on the surface of the bone matrix to fluorapatite.[2,3] One hour after NaF is administered intravenously, only 10% remains in the plasma compartment because of a first-pass

Conflict of interest: The authors have declared no conflicts of interest.

[a] Department of Radiology, Hospital of the University of Pennsylvania, 3400 Spruce Street, Philadelphia, PA 19104, USA; [b] Drexel University College of Medicine, 2900 West Queen Lane, Philadelphia, PA 19129, USA; [c] Perelman School of Medicine at the University of Pennsylvania, 3400 Civic Center Boulevard, Philadelphia, PA 19104, USA; [d] Lewis Katz School of Medicine at Temple University, 3500 North Broad Street, Philadelphia, PA 19140, USA; [e] Division of Radiology and Nuclear Medicine, Oslo University Hospital, Sognsvannsveien 20, Oslo 0372, Norway; [f] Institute of Clinical Medicine, Faculty of Medicine, University of Oslo, Problemveien 7, Oslo 0315, Norway

* Corresponding author. Division of Radiology and Nuclear Medicine, Oslo University Hospital, Sognsvannsveien 20, Oslo 0372, Norway.

E-mail address: monar@ous-hf.no

PET Clin 16 (2021) 295–311
https://doi.org/10.1016/j.cpet.2020.12.006

extraction rate of 100%, allowing excellent contrast resolution.[4]

However, the use of NaF was largely abandoned after the introduction of phosphate-based tracers labeled with [99m]Tc.[4] The first of these was ^{99m}Tc-polyphosphate, which was described in 1971,[5] followed by ^{99m}Tc-methylene diphosphonate in 1975.[6] Compared with NaF, bone scintigraphy (BS) with ^{99m}Tc-labeled agents had the advantage of a longer half-life (6.0 hours vs 110 minutes) and photons with lower energy (140-keV vs 511-keV), allowing easier detection by conventional gamma cameras.[4,7–9] Over the next 4 decades, developments in PET scanners allowed the detection of high-energy photons, resulting in the widespread adoption of many ^{18}F-based tracers.[3,4] As PET imaging with 2-deoxy-2-[^{18}F]fluoro-D-glucose (FDG) continues to expand, increased efficiency in the production and delivery of ^{18}F-labeled tracers has resulted in greater NaF availability.[9] Several properties of NaF, such as lower protein binding and higher plasma clearance, justify its superiority to ^{99m}Tc-labeled tracers.[10] In addition, the increased spatial resolution of PET compared with gamma cameras presents a significant advantage.[7] Consequently, the promise of high-resolution skeletal imaging has sparked a growing interest in assessing musculoskeletal disorders by NaF-PET.

Quantitative PET parameters used to measure new bone formation include bone plasma clearance expressed as K_i and bone uptake expressed as a standardized uptake value (SUV).[11] Calculation of plasma clearance is based on rate constants that describe the movement of NaF between plasma, bone extracellular fluid, and bone mineral compartments. To obtain these data, the Hawkins method represents the standard protocol, requiring 60-minute dynamic imaging and arterial or venous sampling and only allowing the assessment of a single skeletal site at a time.[12] More recently, simplified methods of estimating K_i have been developed, such as that proposed by Siddique and colleagues,[13] which nonetheless requires 4 venous blood samples taken at 10-minute intervals starting 30 minutes after tracer administration. Alternatively, NaF uptake can be measured throughout the skeleton with a single static scan and no need for blood sampling. SUV represents the detected activity concentration in an area, normalized to the administered activity and the patient's body weight or lean body mass.[11]

A major focus of NaF-PET imaging has been the assessment of skeletal metastases from prostate and breast cancer.[10] Although NaF-PET represents a sensitive method of detecting osteoblastic

changes, other PET tracers are available that are more appropriate in this domain. Because bone metastases start with seeding of the red marrow by malignant cells, PET imaging with FDG, ^{18}F-fluciclovine (FACBC), radiolabeled choline, or prostate-specific membrane antigen ligands constitutes a more direct approach and has the advantage of detecting intramedullary lesions that have not resulted in reactive bone remodeling.[14,15] By contrast, indirect evidence of metastasis provided by bone imaging modalities is not appropriate for detecting cancer cell activity, unless malignant cells themselves express osteoblastic activity, as in osteosarcoma.[16] Rather, NaF-PET, combined with computed tomography (CT) or magnetic resonance (MR) for anatomic correlation, has a promising role in the imaging of benign musculoskeletal disorders that cause direct changes in osteoblastic activity. This article discusses the novel applications and utility of NaF in the assessment of musculoskeletal trauma, arthropathies, back pain, orthopedic complications, metabolic bone disease, and other osseous and soft tissue disorders.

MUSCULOSKELETAL TRAUMA

The first-line imaging modality to assess for traumatic fracture is conventional radiography, and CT can be used to detect and characterize occult and complex fractures with high sensitivity.[17] Recent investigations have suggested the superiority of NaF-PET/CT to conventional modalities in the detection of pathologic fractures, fatigue fractures, and occult fractures.[18–22] Jeon and colleagues[23] retrospectively analyzed NaF-PET/CT images obtained a median of 290 days after ankle injury in a study that included 95 patients with fracture, 12 with Achilles tendon rupture, 12 with ligament injury, and 2 with complex regional pain syndrome. All patients with fractures were found to have NaF-avid lesions, and only 8 in the nonfracture group had negative NaF-PET/CT findings. Further, various PET parameters, including maximum SUV (SUVmax), mean SUV (SUVmean), metabolic target volume (MTV), and total lesion activity (TLA = SUVmean × MTV) were all inversely correlated with ankle range of motion. The feasibility of imaging stress fractures with NaF-PET/MR was investigated in 20 patients with foot pain by Crönlein and colleagues.[24] Despite negative findings on radiography, 4 stress fractures and 7 stress reactions involving the foot and ankle were identified by PET/MR. A comparative study between PET/CT and PET/MR by the same group found that both hybrid modalities identified the same 42 lesions across 22 subjects with foot pain of unclear cause.[25] They reported that NaF uptake expressed as SUVmax and SUVmean was highly correlated between PET/CT and PET/MR. Although PET/CT was noted as being superior for the diagnosis of osteoarthritis, the ability to assess bone marrow resulted in PET/MR being favored in the diagnosis of stress fractures and bone marrow edema. Spriet and colleagues[26] reported a study of 9 racehorses, in which NaF-PET/CT imaging was performed on 16 forelimbs and 4 hindlimbs. The investigators found that NaF-PET/CT detected lesions that were not present on BS, CT, or MR, and they concluded that early detection of stress injuries by PET could play a role in preventing catastrophic fractures in horseracing.

Indications for NaF-PET/CT in children and young adults have primarily been for benign disorders.[27] The bones of the thorax and extremities have been observed to have increased NaF avidity in cases of fracture and stress injury.[21] As with BS, NaF uptake may be present at the pubic synchondrosis as part of normal development.[28,29] One application of NaF-PET/CT that has been proposed is in the evaluation of child abuse. In a study of 22 pediatric patients with suspicion of having been abused, Drubach and colleagues[21] found that although high-detail skeletal survey detected 156 fractures, imaging with NaF-PET detected 200 fractures (**Fig. 1**). The investigators calculated the sensitivities of NaF-PET and skeletal survey by comparing baseline imaging studies with follow-up skeletal survey imaging performed 10 to 24 days later. The results suggested that NaF-PET was superior to baseline skeletal survey in detecting fractures involving bones of the thorax, such as the ribs, sternum, scapulae, and clavicles, with a sensitivity of 92%. The sensitivity of NaF-PET in detecting posterior rib fractures was determined to be 93%. At the same time, NaF-PET was found to be inferior in the detection of classic metaphyseal fractures, with a sensitivity of 67%, whereas skeletal survey had a sensitivity of 80%. Overall for all lesions, NaF-PET was found to have a sensitivity of 85%, whereas skeletal survey had a sensitivity of 72%, and the investigators concluded that, in addition to initial radiographic evaluation to assess for metaphyseal fractures, further imaging with NaF-PET may warrant consideration in order to uncover injuries that would otherwise not be evident until follow-up imaging.

In general, the preliminary investigations into the assessment of traumatic injury by NaF-PET/CT and NaF-PET/MR show great promise. To gain a better understanding of how this technology can best be used in a variety of clinical scenarios, larger prospective trials are urgently needed.

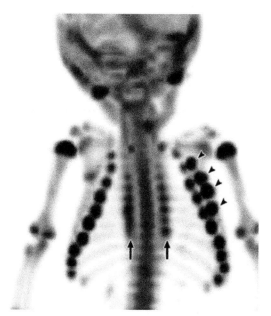

Fig. 1. Maximum intensity projection NaF-PET in a 2-month-old boy. Multiple posterior rib fractures (*arrows*) and left lateral anterior rib fractures (*arrowheads*) are visualized bilaterally. (*From* Drubach LA, Johnston PR, Newton AW, Perez-Rossello JM, Grant FD, Kleinman PK. Skeletal trauma in child abuse: detection with 18F-NaF PET. Radiology. 2010;255(1):173-181; with permission.)

ARTHROPATHIES

NaF has shown success in visualizing changes associated with joint degeneration such as in osteoarthritis (OA) and temporomandibular disorder (TMD).[30–39] Both FDG and NaF activities at the knee were assessed in 97 subjects in a study by Al-Zaghal and colleagues,[40] who found uptake of both tracers was correlated with body mass index. Studies from the same group have similarly found associations between body mass index and NaF uptake at the sacroiliac and hip joints, which are often involved in OA.[41,42] A retrospective study in 34 subjects by Khaw and colleagues[30] showed increased NaF uptake measured at the joints of the elbows, hands, knees, and feet with higher subject body weight, which is a major factor in degenerative joint disease. The interaction between cartilage and bone at the knee in patients with early signs of OA has been successfully imaged by NaF-PET/MR, and an association between NaF activity and pain was described in cases without morphologic abnormalities.[35] This finding suggests that NaF activity can explain underlying pathophysiology before changes are evident on conventional modalities, a notion that is supported by a study that found, in 172 NaF-avid lesions associated with knee pain or injury, that 63 appeared normal on MR.[34] In addition to the potential for early diagnosis, the predictive power of NaF-PET was shown in a study of 57 hip joints by Kobayashi and colleagues,[36] who showed that SUVmax predicted pain worsening and minimum joint space narrowing. Regarding the assessment of TMD, NaF-PET/CT seems feasible in diagnosis and determining the response to treatment.[32,38]

Conventional BS is commonly used in joint diseases such as rheumatoid arthritis (RA), ankylosing spondylitis (AS), and psoriatic arthritis (PsA). In a meta-analysis of 25 studies, the sensitivity of BS in detecting AS in 361 patients was 51.8%, with a sensitivity of 49.4% for detecting sacroiliitis in 255 patients.[43] In contrast, the higher sensitivity of MR has resulted in its replacement of BS as the first-line modality for spondyloarthropathies at some institutions.[4] A major limitation of MR is the limited field of view obtained by whole-body MR, which often does not include distal extremities. As investigators continue to assess its validity, NaF-PET/CT may represent a useful modality in assessing various inflammatory joint diseases.

Although visualization of inflammation with FDG is suitable for imaging RA and PsA,[44–50] several studies have reported the utility of NaF in imaging AS.[51–60] Son and colleagues[54] examined 49 patients with AS and 19 patients without AS, all of whom had inflammatory low back pain for at least 3 months. Enthesopathy, syndesmophytes, and sacroiliitis were identified on NaF-PET/CT. Overall, NaF-PET/CT was found to have a sensitivity of 79.6% and a specificity of 84.2% in the diagnosis of AS. A study by Strobel and colleagues[61] used NaF-PET/CT to evaluate sacroiliitis in 15 patients with AS and 13 patients with mechanical back pain. By calculating the ratio of NaF uptake in the sacroiliac joint to the uptake in the sacrum, the investigators used a cutoff of 1.3 as indicating sacroiliitis. Using this method, the sensitivity of NaF-PET/CT in sacroiliitis was found to be 80% with a specificity of 77%. To compare modalities in AS, whole-body MR and NaF-PET/CT were used to image 10 patients with AS.[62] At the sacroiliac joint, NaF uptake was found to correlate with bone marrow edema on MR, and there was a modest correlation at the spine. The investigators explained that the correlation was weaker than expected, possibly because of NaF-PET/CT portraying bone remodeling that occurs independently from inflammation. In a study of 12 patients with AS imaged by NaF-PET/MR, Park and colleagues[56] found that baseline NaF uptake was independently associated with syndesmophyte formation on radiography at 2-year follow-up. These findings may indicate utility for NaF-PET

combined with both CT and MR in the evaluation of AS and a need for further investigation into this field of study.

Using NaF-PET/CT to assess the effects of treatment regimens, Bruijnen and colleagues[63] studied 12 patients with active AS receiving anti–tumor necrosis factor therapy (**Fig. 2**). Imaging was performed at baseline and 12 weeks after initiation of treatment. In patients who responded to treatment after 24 weeks, NaF uptake was found to decrease at the costovertebral and sacroiliac joints after 12 weeks, whereas no significant changes were observed in nonresponders. Although NaF uptake at 12 weeks correlated with clinical evaluation at 24 weeks, clinical evaluation at 12 weeks did not correlate with later clinical evaluation. This finding suggests that NaF-PET/CT can predict eventual treatment efficacy, even when PET findings contradict early clinical evidence. Other studies examining patients with AS treated with anti–tumor necrosis factor therapy have found success in predicting treatment response from NaF uptake measured from baseline NaF-PET/CT images.[52,53]

A limited number of studies have examined NaF activity at the joints in RA and PsA. In a preclinical trial using mice with glucose-6-phosphate isomerase–induced arthritis, NaF-PET/CT was found to correlate with the degree of bone destruction.[64] Another trial using a murine model found that anti–tumor necrosis factor therapy resulted in increased NaF activity at growth plates and was associated with increased osteoblasts, osteoid formation, and trabecular bone mass.[65] Watanabe and colleagues[66] assessed the hands of 12 patients with RA by FDG-PET/CT and NaF-PET/CT to compare the utility of the 2 tracers. SUVmax of both tracers as measured in the joints were found to correlate with one another. The NaF-PET parameter calculated by summing SUVmax from the metacarpophalangeal joints, proximal interphalangeal joints, and regions of the wrists was associated with the disease activity score in 28 joints, the modified health assessment questionnaire (mHAQ), radiographic progression, and the presence of erosions. Jonnakuti and colleagues[67] reported that NaF uptake in the knees of patients with RA was associated with Kellgren-Lawrence grading, suggesting that NaF-PET/CT can track bone changes associated with RA over time. Tan and colleagues[68] imaged 234 distal interphalangeal joints from 10 patients with PsA, 10 patients with OA, and 10 healthy controls. Compared with that of OA, NaF uptake in PsA involved the distal phalanges more diffusely, with increased uptake at the tufts, periosteum, and entheses. As imaging with NaF-PET is applied to

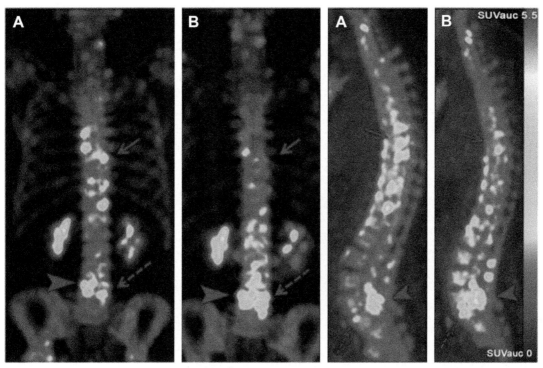

Fig. 2. Baseline (*A*) and 12-week follow-up (*B*) NaF-PET images of an patient with AS starting anti–tumor necrosis factor therapy. Although NaF activity in some AS lesions decreased (*solid arrows*), activity in other lesions increased (*dashed arrows*). Uptake at the facet joints was considered to be a result of osteoarthritis (*arrowheads*). (*From* Bruijnen STG, Verweij NJF, van Duivenvoorde LM, et al. Bone formation in ankylosing spondylitis during anti-tumour necrosis factor therapy imaged by 18F-fluoride positron emission tomography. Rheumatology (Oxford). 2018;57(4):631-638; with permission.)

new areas, it is imperative that, in addition to OA and AS, its potential role to portray bone involvement in other arthropathies is considered and investigated on a large scale.

BACK PAIN

Analogous to previous studies that used BS and single-photon emission CT (SPECT),[69–74] NaF-PET/CT has been used to assess benign causes of back pain.[75–77] Athletes are particularly at risk of injuries resulting from repetitive hyperextension (**Fig. 3**).[78] A common cause of low back pain in young athletes is spondylolysis, defined as a defect or stress fracture involving the pars interarticularis that commonly affects the lumbar spine. Pars fractures show increased bone turnover until the bone is finished healing.[77,79] Grant and colleagues[9] report that, in their experience, correlation with CT confirms pars fracture in about half of cases with abnormal NaF uptake, with the other half likely representing patients with pars stress without spondylolysis. The investigators also reported that, generally, normal NaF uptake corresponds to normal anatomy of the pars

interarticularis on CT, except in cases of long-standing spondylolysis where bone turnover is at baseline.

Not only does NaF-PET/CT facilitate the diagnosis of pars stress but it can also help diagnose other potential causes of back pain, such as facet arthropathy.[80–82] The observation that NaF uptake at the cervical, thoracic, and lumbar spine is associated with increased body weight in healthy individuals suggests that NaF-PET/CT can detect early changes in the spine related to degeneration.[83] In 42 adult patients with back pain and no history of spine surgery, NaF-PET/CT scans identified the cause of pain in 37 (88%) of the patients.[82] Furthermore, NaF activity at lumbar facet joints has been found to correlate with both MR findings and clinical disability.[80] Mabray and colleagues[81] observed that, in 30 adult patients who underwent imaging by NaF-PET/CT, uptake of NaF was only weakly correlated with CT Pathria grade of facet osteoarthropathy. Thereby, the investigators reasoned that the assessment of bone turnover with NaF provided new information that can be used to supplement structural data provided by CT.

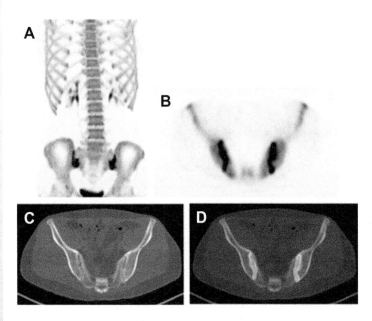

Fig. 3. NaF-PET maximum intensity projection (*A*), transaxial (*B*), and fused PET/CT (*D*) images in an 18-year-old female dancer with extension-based low back pain show significant activity at the sacroiliac joints, whereas minimal abnormality is apparent on CT (*C*). (*From* Grant FD. 18F-fluoride PET and PET/CT in children and young adults. PET Clin. 2014;9(3):287-297; with permission.)

Although many causes of back pain are related to muscular injuries or abnormalities associated with intervertebral discs, osseous involvement is common. Therefore, NaF-PET should be considered as the imaging modality of choice in these cases even when malignancy is not suspected. In a study of 15 adolescent patients with back pain, Ovadia and colleagues[77] found that NaF-PET/CT revealed positive findings in 10 patients, which included spondylolysis, frank fracture, osteoid osteoma, osteitis pubis, sacroiliitis, and disc herniation. Pseudoarthrosis associated with lumbosacral transitional vertebrae is another cause of back pain that can be evaluated by NaF-PET/CT.[27] Lim and colleagues[76] identified back pain caused by vertebral body ring apophyseal injury and stress or injury at the spinous process, pars interarticularis, pedicle, sacroiliac joint, and transitional vertebra-sacral articulation. Usmani and colleagues[84] reported the case of a 34-year-old woman with severe low back pain, whose L5 vertebra contained a hemisacralized left transverse process. The transverse-sacral articulation showed NaF avidity, consistent with Bertolotti syndrome. A study in 55 patients with lumbosacral transitional vertebrae by the same investigators showed a strong correlation between NaF uptake and the presence of symptoms.[85] These early studies and case reports show the significant utility of NaF-PET in the evaluation of musculoskeletal back pain, warranting further investigation into the potential role PET may play in the diagnosis, management, and follow-up of this serious cause of disability.

ORTHOPEDIC COMPLICATIONS

Faced with an aging population, the prevalence of OA is increasing, and joint replacement surgery is becoming more common.[86,87] Postsurgical complications include instability, infection, fracture, and loosening, and the ability to discriminate between infection and aseptic loosening has important implications for patient management.[88–91] The first-line modality after hip or knee arthroplasty is radiography, which can show subsequent fractures and dislocations. Although the high sensitivity of 3-phase BS can be used to rule out postsurgical loosening and infection,[92] the addition of anatomic information in SPECT/CT can improve the otherwise low specificity.[93] Scintigraphy with gallium-67 (Ga67) and indium-111 (111In)–labeled white blood cells represent other methods of increasing the specificity of 3-phase BS.[94–96]

Several studies have indicated that NaF-PET has utility in assessing complications related to hip arthroplasty.[97–119] Increased NaF activity can indicate stem loosening in patients experiencing pain but with equivocal radiograph findings.[99] To determine the efficacy of denosumab in preventing periprosthetic bone loss, which contributes to loosening, Nyström and colleagues[100] quantified bone turnover with NaF-PET. They noted that, in patients treated with denosumab, the increase in uptake after surgery was not as great as the increase in the patients receiving placebo. Even higher uptake in septic loosening is observed compared with aseptic loosening. By visually assessing the proportion of the bone-implant interface that showed NaF avidity, Kobayashi and colleagues[109] diagnosed infection in 65 hip prostheses by NaF-PET/CT with a sensitivity of 95% and a specificity of 98%. In a comparative study between NaF-PET/CT and FDG-PET/CT, 42 patients with painful hip prostheses suspected of loosening underwent imaging before revision arthroplasty to determine whether or not infection was present.[102] The sensitivity and specificity of NaF-PET/CT were 75% and 96%, respectively, whereas the sensitivity and specificity of FDG-PET/CT were 94% and 92%, respectively. Although imaging with NaF resulted in higher specificity, the investigators argued that the overall diagnostic performance with FDG was more suitable for routine clinical practice. As an analog to 3-phase BS, multiphase NaF-PET has been proposed to assess for infection. In a demonstration of early-phase imaging in a patient with cellulitis, Li and colleagues[120] suggested that NaF-PET images acquired 2 minutes after tracer administration can be used to visualize increased regional blood flow at infected areas. Although future investigations may assess the feasibility of this method in a larger number of patients, there is currently limited evidence regarding early-phase NaF-PET in infection. Choe and colleagues[108] found that, by using NaF-PET to identify active lesions in total hip arthroplasty patients, they achieved a higher accuracy of tissue sampling in the diagnosis of periprosthetic infection. Besides hip arthroplasty, NaF-PET has been used to image knee, ankle, and shoulder arthroplasties.[121–125] A study that included 24 hip and 13 knee prostheses found that NaF-PET/CT had a sensitivity of 95% and a specificity of 87% in diagnosing periprosthetic loosening (**Fig. 4**).[123] The viability and fusion of femoral allografts in 7 patients who underwent reverse total shoulder arthroplasty was assessed by NaF-PET/CT, which showed a similar amount of uptake in the allografts as in reference vertebrae.[121]

Spinal orthopedics is another area that may benefit from NaF-PET, which may have a role in predicting healing and identifying complications such as nonunion, pseudarthrosis, infection, and hardware loosening.[126–131] In pediatrics, Grant[27] reported utility in determining the cause of pain in children who underwent spinal fusion surgery for scoliosis. Fischer and colleagues[132] studied 20 patients who underwent cervical or lumbar intercorporal fusion and found that increased NaF activity could be visualized in cervical cages for up to 8 years after intervention and up to 10 years in lumbar cages (**Fig. 5**). The investigators suggested that this may represent unsuccessful

fusion, which could be a result of stress or micro-instability. In a comparison between NaF-PET/CT, plain radiography, and CT, fusion was assessed in 8 patients after en bloc spondylectomy.[133] Although radiographs and CT showed successful fusion in all patients, NaF-PET/CT findings indicated nonunion in each case, showing a large discrepancy in findings between these modalities.

Although more studies are needed, other orthopedic applications of NaF-PET include assessing the effects of Taylor Spatial Frame treatment,[134] as well as determining the progression of graft incorporation after anterior cruciate ligament reconstruction.[135] NaF activity can also be informative for surgical planning. In patients with hip fractures, decreased NaF activity was predictive of future need for joint replacement surgery.[136] In a study of patients with osteonecrosis, 9 out of 17 hips had NaF avidity in the absence of findings on BS, SPECT, and MR, which shows the importance of this modality.[137] Patients with posttraumatic and postsurgical chronic osteomyelitis after unsuccessful surgical intervention were imaged by both FDG-PET/CT and NaF-PET/CT in a study by Christersson and colleagues.[138] In all 8 patients assessed, PET determined the culprit sequestrum, and, in 4 patients, an additional sequestrum with no clinical signs was identified. Follow-up revealed no clinical indications of recurrence and negative PET findings in all patients. Because both the disorder and the treatment often directly affect bone activity in orthopedics, it is logical that imaging with NaF-PET has a large role to play in managing patients before and after surgical procedures. Preliminary studies in this area are very promising, and future studies should focus on surgical planning as well as using NaF-PET to investigate the healing process or associated complications after treatment, which could be overlooked by conventional modalities.

METABOLIC BONE DISEASES

Osteoporosis is a systemic disease of bone, in which reduced bone mass results in greater fragility and risk of fracture. Because osteoporosis mostly occurs in elderly men and postmenopausal women, its prevalence is expected to increase with current demographic trends.[139] Osteoporotic fractures often involve the vertebrae, hip, distal forearm, or shoulder.[140] To assess for osteoporosis, bone mineral density (BMD) determined by dual x-ray absorptiometry (DXA) and expressed as a T score is the current standard of care. Representing the number of standard deviations from average BMD in a young healthy population, a T score between −1.0 and −2.5 is diagnostic for

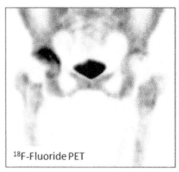
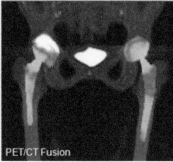
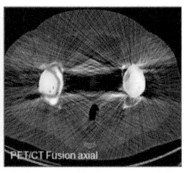

¹⁸F-Fluoride PET   PET/CT Fusion   PET/CT Fusion axial

Fig. 4. NaF-PET and PET/CT images of a 72-year-old woman who underwent total hip arthroplasty 12 years earlier. High NaF uptake involving the right acetabular component suggests loosening. No loosening is suspected in the right femoral component or in either components of the left arthroplasty. (*From* Koob S, Gaertner FC, Jansen TR, et al. Diagnosis of peri-prosthetic loosening of total hip and knee arthroplasty using (18)F-Fluoride PET/CT. Oncotarget. 2019;10(22):2203-2211; with permission.)

osteopenia, whereas a T score less than −2.5 is considered osteoporosis.[139] However, some investigators have questioned the accuracy of DXA-derived BMD,[141–143] and 1 study found that most women with hip fracture had T scores more than −2.5, showing the low sensitivity of this technique.[144] Rather than BMD, bone turnover can be used to evaluate patients for osteoporosis. However, established methods face certain limitations.[145] Bone turnover markers can be used to evaluate overall metabolic activity but suffer from low sensitivity and cannot assess individual skeletal sites. Alternatively, transiliac biopsy after double labeling with tetracycline is invasive and limited to 1 area of the skeleton.

Bone imaging with functional modalities such as PET is a sensitive method that can overcome the limitations associated with other bone turnover assessments.[146,147] A study by Piert and colleagues[148] used NaF-PET to assess bone turnover at the vertebrae of healthy pigs and compared their findings with histomorphometric data derived from iliac crest biopsies. The influx rate and volume flux of NaF were found to correlate with the mineral apposition rate, and the investigators concluded that NaF-PET may represent a noninvasive method of following metabolic bone diseases over time, decreasing the need for invasive bone biopsies. NaF-PET has had success in detecting both postmenopausal and glucocorticoid-induced osteoporosis.[149–153] A study of 71 male and 68 female subjects observed a decrease in NaF uptake at the femoral neck with age, correlating with BMD from CT.[154] In patients diagnosed with osteoporosis by DXA, NaF activity at the lumbar spine is significantly lower than in healthy persons and in patients with osteopenia.[151–153] Bone formation at other skeletal sites

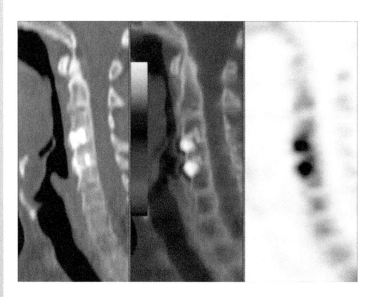

Fig. 5. Low-dose CT (*left*), fused NaF-PET/CT (*middle*), and NaF-PET (*right*) images of a 52-year-old male patient who underwent 2 adjacent intercorporal fusions (C3/4, C4/5). At 79 months postoperatively, both cervical cages still show increased NaF activity. (*From* Fischer DR, Zweifel K, Treyer V, et al. Assessment of successful incorporation of cages after cervical or lumbar intercorporal fusion with [(18)F]fluoride positron-emission tomography/computed tomography. Eur Spine J. 2011;20(4):640-648; with permission.)

as determined by NaF-PET include the pelvis, tibia, parietal bone, humerus, and sternum.[155,156]

The effects of antiresorptive therapy with bisphosphonates result in a rapid decrease in osteoclast activity, followed by a gradual decrease in osteoblast metabolism. Several studies have observed this expected decrease in bone formation after treatment with risedronate and alendronate.[151,157–159] Uchida and colleagues[151] observed a significant decrease in SUV at the lumbar spine after 3 months of treatment with alendronate, whereas no significant changes in serum bone-specific alkaline phosphate were observed until 6 months, and DXA did not show a significant change until 12 months. In 11 postmenopausal women treated with alendronate and 9 treated with risedronate, Frost and colleagues[160] found that NaF activity remained suppressed in the spine in both groups 12 months after discontinuation of therapy. However, after 12 months of discontinuation in the alendronate group, an increase in NaF uptake at the hip and femoral shaft was seen.

In contrast, teriparatide therapy causes increased activity in both osteoblasts and osteoclasts. As expected, increased bone turnover at the spine, femoral shaft, and pelvis portrayed by NaF-PET was described in a study of 18 postmenopausal women after 6 months of teriparatide therapy.[161] A study by the same group saw significantly greater NaF clearance at the hip, femoral neck, lumbar spine, and pelvis in patients after 12 weeks of taking teriparatide, whereas no changes were observed in a control group taking calcium and vitamin D only.[156]

Paget disease, characterized by increased osteoclast activity followed by increased osteoblast activity, and renal osteodystrophy, in which chronic kidney disease results in abnormally low or high bone turnover, are other disorders that may benefit from NaF-PET assessment.[162–167] NaF activity is higher in pagetic bones and has been found to decrease after 1 month of treatment with bisphosphonates, followed by a further decrease after 6 months.[166] Despite normal biomarkers, increased NaF activity was observed in most patients. In 11 patients with renal osteodystrophy, Messa and colleagues[167] determined that clearance of NaF could differentiate between high bone turnover in secondary hyperparathyroidism and low-turnover bone disease. Further, NaF clearance correlated with serum alkaline phosphatase and parathyroid hormone levels as well as with histomorphometric data. After parathyroidectomy and medical therapy in 2 patients, NaF clearance was found to decrease by approximately 30% to 40%. These studies imply that NaF-PET is much more sensitive than the existing

approaches for assessing the involvement of bones throughout the body in a variety of metabolic disorders. Although the implementation of routine PET imaging may present challenges in terms of cost and radiation exposure, NaF-PET could play a key role in therapy development, in which sensitive tests are needed to evaluate early biological effects in vivo.

OTHER OSSEOUS AND SOFT TISSUE DISORDERS

Aside from the aforementioned major applications of NaF-PET in bone and joint disorders, an array of other potential areas of investigation have been suggested by preliminary observations. Osteonecrosis, including medication-related osteonecrosis of the jaw, seems to be a promising area in need of further study,[168–172] in addition to assessment of fibrous dysplasia.[173,174] Increased NaF uptake in the otic capsule in patients with otosclerosis compared with healthy controls suggests a potential role in diagnosis.[175] With regard to benign primary bone tumors, both osteoid osteoma and osteoblastoma are known to show NaF avidity.[77,176–178] Similarly, malignancies such as osteosarcoma and Ewing sarcoma can be identified with this modality.[179–182] Case reports show the successful identification of osteosarcoma metastases by NaF-PET in the lungs, in the right ventricle of the heart, and in the abdominal and paraspinal muscles.[183–185] Further, by detecting greater osteosarcoma disease extent than was apparent on structural imaging, NaF-PET contributed to the decision in 1 case of changing from curative intent to palliative intent.[186]

Regarding disorders arising from nonosseous structures, NaF activity has been observed in Langerhans cell histiocytosis, in which focal uptake was observed throughout the skeleton.[187] Significant uptake has also been shown in a case of vertebral body hemangioma.[10] Other neoplasms reported to show NaF activity include neurofibroma,[188] meningioma,[189] uterine leiomyoma,[190,191] ovarian cancer,[192] bladder cancer,[193] glioblastoma,[194] and medullary thyroid carcinoma.[195] Certain normal tissues, such as breast tissue, have moderate NaF activity at baseline,[196] which can even be appreciated in drug-induced gynecomastia in men.[197] NaF-PET can also show physiologic calcification of intracranial structures,[198,199] as well as heterotopic ossification after surgery.[200] In addition, NaF uptake has been reported in the gastrointestinal wall caused by hypercalcemia[201] and as a sequela of Japanese schistosomiasis.[202] Although the significance of these findings is still unclear, an important extraosseous indication for NaF-PET is in the evaluation of vascular microcalcification, with the possibility of NaF surpassing FDG as the PET tracer of choice in assessing atherosclerotic activity.[203,204]

SUMMARY

The rise of NaF-PET and its combination with CT and MR present new opportunities to assess benign musculoskeletal disorders with a greater sensitivity compared with conventional approaches. In particular, conditions affecting the skeleton and joints stand to benefit greatly from PET findings that would otherwise be missed on conventional radiographs, BS, CT, or MR. As a result, previously undetermined causes of bone pain may be elucidated, and sites of occult traumatic injury could be discovered, findings that have important implications for patient care. In addition to its diagnostic role, NaF-PET can be used to evaluate pharmacologic and surgical interventions designed to treat osseous structures. Orthopedic surgeons in particular are faced with managing complications that can be better characterized by NaF-PET than with other modalities. Moreover, drugs such as teriparatide and bisphosphonates cause direct changes in NaF activity before the effects are evident by any other means. As clinicians continue to gain a better understanding of this modality, its future role in other bone and soft tissue disorders is still undetermined, and large-scale prospective studies are warranted to investigate its utility.

CLINICS CARE POINTS

- Although NaF-PET/CT can be used to detect bone metastases, PET tracers that portray tumor activity such as FDG or radiolabeled PSMA ligands are more appropriate in this setting.
- Many benign musculoskeletal conditions can be detected by NaF-PET, which can play a role in diagnosis and monitoring.
- NaF-PET and its hybrid modalities can assist in orthopedic planning as well as in evaluation for postsurgical complications such as infection.
- PET quantification allows precise evaluation of metabolic bone diseases. NaF uptake reflects bone turnover, pathologic changes in which are present years before changes in bone mineral density.

DISCLOSURE

The authors have nothing to disclose.

REFERENCES

1. Blau M, Nagler W, Bender MA. Fluorine-18: a new isotope for bone scanning. J Nucl Med 1962;3: 332–4.
2. Blau M, Ganatra R, Bender MA. 18 F-fluoride for bone imaging. Semin Nucl Med 1972;2(1):31–7.
3. Raynor W, Houshmand S, Gholami S, et al. Evolving role of molecular imaging with (18)F-sodium fluoride PET as a biomarker for calcium metabolism. Curr Osteoporos Rep 2016;14(4):115–25.
4. Beheshti M. (18)F-Sodium Fluoride PET/CT and PET/MR imaging of bone and joint disorders. PET Clin 2018;13(4):477–90.
5. Subramanian G, McAfee JG. A new complex of 99mTc for skeletal imaging. Radiology 1971;99(1): 192–6.
6. Subramanian G, McAfee JG, Blair RJ, et al. Technetium-99m-methylene diphosphonate–a superior agent for skeletal imaging: comparison with other technetium complexes. J Nucl Med 1975;16(8): 744–55.
7. Blake GM, Fogelman I. Bone radionuclide imaging, quantitation and bone densitometry. In: McCready R, Gnanasegaran G, Bomanji JB, editors. A history of radionuclide studies in the UK: 50th Anniversary of the British Nuclear Medicine Society; Springer. Cham (CH): 2016. p. 111–20.
8. Williams LE. Anniversary paper: nuclear medicine: fifty years and still counting. Med Phys 2008;35(7): 3020–9.
9. Grant FD, Fahey FH, Packard AB, et al. Skeletal PET with 18F-fluoride: applying new technology to an old tracer. J Nucl Med 2008;49(1):68–78.
10. Bastawrous S, Bhargava P, Behnia F, et al. Newer PET application with an old tracer: role of 18F-NaF skeletal PET/CT in oncologic practice. Radiographics 2014;34(5):1295–316.
11. Austin AG, Raynor WY, Reilly CC, et al. Evolving role of MR imaging and PET in assessing osteoporosis. PET Clin 2019;14(1):31–41.
12. Blake GM, Puri T, Siddique M, et al. Site specific measurements of bone formation using [(18)F] sodium fluoride PET/CT. Quant Imaging Med Surg 2018;8(1):47–59.
13. Siddique M, Blake GM, Frost ML, et al. Estimation of regional bone metabolism from whole-body 18F-fluoride PET static images. Eur J Nucl Med Mol Imaging 2012;39(2):337–43.
14. Walker SM, Lim I, Lindenberg L, et al. Positron emission tomography (PET) radiotracers for prostate cancer imaging. Abdom Radiol (N Y) 2020; 45(7):2165–75.

15. Aydin A, Yu JQ, Zhuang H, et al. Detection of bone marrow metastases by FDG-PET and missed by bone scintigraphy in widespread melanoma. Clin Nucl Med 2005;30(9):606–7.

16. Raynor WY, Al-Zaghal A, Zadeh MZ, et al. Metastatic seeding attacks bone marrow, not bone: rectifying ongoing misconceptions. PET Clin 2019; 14(1):135–44.

17. Jarraya M, Hayashi D, Roemer FW, et al. Radiographically occult and subtle fractures: a pictorial review. Radiol Res Pract 2013;2013:370169.

18. Usmani S, Marafi F, Al Kandari F, et al. Adductor insertion avulsion syndrome with stress fracture in morbidly obese patient diagnosed on (18)f-sodium fluoride positron emission tomography-computed tomography. Indian J Nucl Med 2019;34(3):256–7.

19. Seifert P, Konig V, Hofmann GO, et al. Devitalized bone in a multi-fragment femoral shaft fracture detected by (18)F-NaF PET-CT. Nuklearmedizin 2016; 55(5):N52–3.

20. Dua SG, Purandare NC, Shah S, et al. F-18 fluoride PET/CT in the detection of radiation-induced pelvic insufficiency fractures. Clin Nucl Med 2011;36(10): e146–9.

21. Drubach LA, Johnston PR, Newton AW, et al. Skeletal trauma in child abuse: detection with 18F-NaF PET. Radiology 2010;255(1):173–81.

22. Hsu WK, Feeley BT, Krenek L, et al. The use of 18F-fluoride and 18F-FDG PET scans to assess fracture healing in a rat femur model. Eur J Nucl Med Mol Imaging 2007;34(8):1291–301.

23. Jeon TJ, Kim S, Park J, et al. Use of (18)F-sodium fluoride bone PET for disability evaluation in ankle trauma: a pilot study. BMC Med Imaging 2018; 18(1):34.

24. Cronlein M, Rauscher I, Beer AJ, et al. Visualization of stress fractures of the foot using PET-MRI: a feasibility study. Eur J Med Res 2015;20:99.

25. Rauscher I, Beer AJ, Schaeffeler C, et al. Evaluation of 18F-fluoride PET/MR and PET/CT in patients with foot pain of unclear cause. J Nucl Med 2015; 56(3):430–5.

26. Spriet M, Espinosa-Mur P, Cissell DD, et al. (18) F-sodium fluoride positron emission tomography of the racing Thoroughbred fetlock: validation and comparison with other imaging modalities in nine horses. Equine Vet J 2019;51(3):375–83.

27. Grant FD. (1)(8)fluoride PET and PET/CT in children and young adults. PET Clin 2014;9(3):287–97.

28. Hardoff R, Gips S. Ischiopubic synchondrosis. Normal finding, increased pubic uptake on bone scintigraphy. Clin Nucl Med 1992;17(2):139.

29. Cawley KA, Dvorak AD, Wilmot MD. Normal anatomic variant: scintigraphy of the ischiopubic synchondrosis. J Nucl Med 1983;24(1):14–6.

30. Khaw TH, Raynor WY, Borja AJ, et al. Assessing the effects of body weight on subchondral bone formation with quantitative (18)F-sodium fluoride PET. Ann Nucl Med 2020;34(8):559–64.

31. Tibrewala R, Bahroos E, Mehrabian H, et al. [(18) F]-Sodium fluoride PET/MR imaging for bone-cartilage interactions in hip osteoarthritis: a feasibility study. J Orthop Res 2019;37(12):2671–80.

32. Suh MS, Park SH, Kim YK, et al. (18)F-NaF PET/CT for the evaluation of temporomandibular joint disorder. Clin Radiol 2018;73(4):414.e7-13.

33. Al-Zaghal A, Raynor W, Khosravi M, et al. Applications of PET imaging in the evaluation of musculoskeletal diseases among the geriatric population. Semin Nucl Med 2018;48(6):525–34.

34. Kogan F, Fan AP, McWalter EJ, et al. PET/MRI of metabolic activity in osteoarthritis: a feasibility study. J Magn Reson Imaging 2017;45(6):1736–45.

35. Savic D, Pedoia V, Seo Y, et al. Imaging bone-cartilage interactions in osteoarthritis using [(18) F]-NaF PET-MRI. Mol Imaging 2016;15:1–12.

36. Kobayashi N, Inaba Y, Yukizawa Y, et al. Use of 18F-fluoride positron emission tomography as a predictor of the hip osteoarthritis progression. Mod Rheumatol 2015;25(6):925–30.

37. Hirata Y, Inaba Y, Kobayashi N, et al. Correlation between mechanical stress by finite element analysis and 18F-fluoride PET uptake in hip osteoarthritis patients. J Orthop Res 2015;33(1):78–83.

38. Lee JW, Lee SM, Kim SJ, et al. Clinical utility of fluoride-18 positron emission tomography/CT in temporomandibular disorder with osteoarthritis: comparisons with 99mTc-MDP bone scan. Dentomaxillofac Radiol 2013;42(2):29292350.

39. Temmerman OP, Raijmakers PG, Kloet R, et al. In vivo measurements of blood flow and bone metabolism in osteoarthritis. Rheumatol Int 2013; 33(4):959–63.

40. Al-Zaghal A, Yellanki DP, Ayubcha C, et al. CT-based tissue segmentation to assess knee joint inflammation and reactive bone formation assessed by (18)F-FDG and (18)F-NaF PET/CT: effects of age and BMI. Hell J Nucl Med 2018; 21(2):102–7.

41. Al-Zaghal A, Yellanki DP, Kothekar E, et al. Sacroiliac joint asymmetry regarding inflammation and bone turnover: assessment by FDG and NaF PET/CT. Asia Ocean J Nucl Med Biol 2019;7(2):108–14.

42. Yellanki DP, Kothekar E, Al-Zaghal A, et al. Efficacy of (18)F-FDG and (18)F-NaF PET/CT imaging: a novel semi-quantitative assessment of the effects of age and obesity on hip joint inflammation and bone degeneration. Hell J Nucl Med 2018;21(3): 181–5.

43. Song IH, Carrasco-Fernandez J, Rudwaleit M, et al. The diagnostic value of scintigraphy in assessing sacroiliitis in ankylosing spondylitis: a systematic literature research. Ann Rheum Dis 2008;67(11): 1535–40.

44. Hotta M, Minamimoto R, Kaneko H, et al. Fluoro-deoxyglucose PET/CT of arthritis in rheumatic diseases: a pictorial review. Radiographics 2020; 40(1):223–40.

45. Raynor WY, Jonnakuti VS, Zirakchian Zadeh M, et al. Comparison of methods of quantifying global synovial metabolic activity with FDG-PET/CT in rheumatoid arthritis. Int J Rheum Dis 2019;22(12): 2191–8.

46. Fosse P, Kaiser MJ, Namur G, et al. (18)F- FDG PET/CT joint assessment of early therapeutic response in rheumatoid arthritis patients treated with rituximab. Eur J Hybrid Imaging 2018;2(1):6.

47. Bhattarai A, Nakajima T, Sapkota S, et al. Diagnostic value of 18F-fluorodeoxyglucose uptake parameters to differentiate rheumatoid arthritis from other types of arthritis. Medicine (Baltimore) 2017; 96(25):e7130.

48. Chaudhari AJ, Ferrero A, Godinez F, et al. High-resolution (18)F-FDG PET/CT for assessing disease activity in rheumatoid and psoriatic arthritis: findings of a prospective pilot study. Br J Radiol 2016;89(1063):20160138.

49. Mountz JM, Alavi A, Mountz JD. Emerging optical and nuclear medicine imaging methods in rheumatoid arthritis. Nat Rev Rheumatol 2012;8(12): 719–28.

50. Yun M, Kim W, Adam LE, et al. F-18 FDG uptake in a patient with psoriatic arthritis: imaging correlation with patient symptoms. Clin Nucl Med 2001;26(8): 692–3.

51. Hancin EC, Borja AJ, Nikpanah M, et al. PET/MR imaging in musculoskeletal precision imaging - third wave after X-ray and MR. PET Clin 2020; 15(4):521–34.

52. Lee SJ, Kim JY, Choi YY, et al. Predictive value of semi-quantitative index from F-18-fluoride PET/CT for treatment response in patients with ankylosing spondylitis. Eur J Radiol 2020;129:109048.

53. Kim K, Son SM, Goh TS, et al. Prediction of response to tumor necrosis value-alpha blocker is suggested by (18)F-NaF SUVmax but not by quantitative pharmacokinetic analysis in patients with ankylosing spondylitis. AJR Am J Roentgenol 2020;214(6):1352–8.

54. Son SM, Kim K, Pak K, et al. Evaluation of the diagnostic performance of (18)F-NaF positron emission tomography/computed tomography in patients with suspected ankylosing spondylitis according to the Assessment of SpondyloArthritis International Society criteria. Spine J 2020;20(9):1471–9.

55. Sawicki LM, Lutje S, Baraliakos X, et al. Dual-phase hybrid (18) F-Fluoride Positron emission tomography/MRI in ankylosing spondylitis: investigating the link between MRI bone changes, regional hyperaemia and increased osteoblastic activity. J Med Imaging Radiat Oncol 2018;62(3):313–9.

56. Park EK, Pak K, Park JH, et al. Baseline increased 18F-fluoride uptake lesions at vertebral corners on positron emission tomography predict new syndesmophyte development in ankylosing spondylitis: a 2-year longitudinal study. Rheumatol Int 2017; 37(5):765–73.

57. Idolazzi L, Salgarello M, Gatti D, et al. 18F-fluoride PET/CT for detection of axial involvement in ankylosing spondylitis: correlation with disease activity. Ann Nucl Med 2016;30(6):430–4.

58. Buchbender C, Ostendorf B, Ruhlmann V, et al. Hybrid 18F-labeled Fluoride Positron Emission Tomography/Magnetic Resonance (MR) imaging of the sacroiliac joints and the spine in patients with axial spondyloarthritis: a pilot study exploring the link of MR bone pathologies and increased osteoblastic activity. J Rheumatol 2015;42(9): 1631–7.

59. Lee SG, Kim IJ, Kim KY, et al. Assessment of bone synthetic activity in inflammatory lesions and syndesmophytes in patients with ankylosing spondylitis: the potential role of 18F-fluoride positron emission tomography-magnetic resonance imaging. Clin Exp Rheumatol 2015;33(1):90–7.

60. Bruijnen ST, van der Weijden MA, Klein JP, et al. Bone formation rather than inflammation reflects ankylosing spondylitis activity on PET-CT: a pilot study. Arthritis Res Ther 2012;14(2):R71.

61. Strobel K, Fischer DR, Tamborrini G, et al. 18F-fluoride PET/CT for detection of sacroiliitis in ankylosing spondylitis. Eur J Nucl Med Mol Imaging 2010;37(9):1760–5.

62. Fischer DR, Pfirrmann CW, Zubler V, et al. High bone turnover assessed by 18F-fluoride PET/CT in the spine and sacroiliac joints of patients with ankylosing spondylitis: comparison with inflammatory lesions detected by whole body MRI. EJNMMI Res 2012;2(1):38.

63. Bruijnen STG, Verweij NJF, van Duivenvoorde LM, et al. Bone formation in ankylosing spondylitis during anti-tumour necrosis factor therapy imaged by 18F-fluoride positron emission tomography. Rheumatology (Oxford) 2018;57(4):631–8.

64. Irmler IM, Gebhardt P, Hoffmann B, et al. 18 F-Fluoride positron emission tomography/computed tomography for noninvasive in vivo quantification of pathophysiological bone metabolism in experimental murine arthritis. Arthritis Res Ther 2014; 16(4):R155.

65. Hayer S, Zeilinger M, Weiss V, et al. Multimodal [(18) F]FDG PET/CT is a direct readout for inflammatory bone repair: a longitudinal study in TNFalpha transgenic mice. J Bone Miner Res 2019; 34(9):1632–45.

66. Watanabe T, Takase-Minegishi K, Ihata A, et al. 18) F-FDG and (18)F-NaF PET/CT demonstrate coupling of inflammation and accelerated bone

turnover in rheumatoid arthritis. Mod Rheumatol 2016;26(2):180–7.

67. Jonnakuti VS, Raynor WY, Taratuta E, et al. A novel method to assess subchondral bone formation using [18F]NaF-PET in the evaluation of knee degeneration. Nucl Med Commun 2018;39(5):451–6.

68. Tan AL, Tanner SF, Waller ML, et al. High-resolution [18F]fluoride positron emission tomography of the distal interphalangeal joint in psoriatic arthritis–a bone-enthesis-nail complex. Rheumatology (Oxford) 2013;52(5):898–904.

69. Strobel K, Burger C, Seifert B, et al. Characterization of focal bone lesions in the axial skeleton: performance of planar bone scintigraphy compared with SPECT and SPECT fused with CT. AJR Am J Roentgenol 2007;188(5):W467–74.

70. Takemitsu M, El Rassi G, Woratanarat P, et al. Low back pain in pediatric athletes with unilateral tracer uptake at the pars interarticularis on single photon emission computed tomography. Spine (Phila Pa 1976) 2006;31(8):909–14.

71. Reinartz P, Schaffeldt J, Sabri O, et al. Benign versus malignant osseous lesions in the lumbar vertebrae: differentiation by means of bone SPET. Eur J Nucl Med 2000;27(6):721–6.

72. De Maeseneer M, Lenchik L, Everaert H, et al. Evaluation of lower back pain with bone scintigraphy and SPECT. Radiographics 1999;19(4):901–12 [discussion: 912–4].

73. Bellah RD, Summerville DA, Treves ST, et al. Low-back pain in adolescent athletes: detection of stress injury to the pars interarticularis with SPECT. Radiology 1991;180(2):509–12.

74. Collier BD, Johnson RP, Carrera GF, et al. Painful spondylolysis or spondylolisthesis studied by radiography and single-photon emission computed tomography. Radiology 1985;154(1):207–11.

75. Drubach LA, Connolly SA, Palmer EL 3rd. Skeletal scintigraphy with 18F-NaF PET for the evaluation of bone pain in children. AJR Am J Roentgenol 2011; 197(3):713–9.

76. Lim R, Fahey FH, Drubach LA, et al. Early experience with fluorine-18 sodium fluoride bone PET in young patients with back pain. J Pediatr Orthop 2007;27(3):277–82.

77. Ovadia D, Metser U, Lievshitz G, et al. Back pain in adolescents: assessment with integrated 18F-fluoride positron-emission tomography-computed tomography. J Pediatr Orthop 2007;27(1):90–3.

78. Goetzinger S, Courtney S, Yee K, et al. Spondylolysis in young athletes: an overview emphasizing nonoperative management. J Sports Med 2020; 2020:9235958.

79. Zukotynski K, Curtis C, Grant FD, et al. The value of SPECT in the detection of stress injury to the pars interarticularis in patients with low back pain. J Orthop Surg Res 2010;5:13.

80. Jenkins NW, Talbott JF, Shah V, et al. [(18)F]-Sodium fluoride PET MR-based localization and quantification of bone turnover as a biomarker for facet joint-induced disability. AJNR Am J Neuroradiol 2017;38(10):2028–31.

81. Mabray MC, Brus-Ramer M, Behr SC, et al. (18)F-Sodium Fluoride PET-CT hybrid imaging of the lumbar facet joints: tracer uptake and degree of correlation to CT-graded arthropathy. World J Nucl Med 2016;15(2):85–90.

82. Gamie S, El-Maghraby T. The role of PET/CT in evaluation of Facet and Disc abnormalities in patients with low back pain using (18)F-Fluoride. Nucl Med Rev Cent East Eur 2008;11(1):17–21.

83. Ayubcha C, Zirakchian Zadeh M, Stochkendahl MJ, et al. Quantitative evaluation of normal spinal osseous metabolism with 18F-NaF PET/CT. Nucl Med Commun 2018;39(10):945–50.

84. Usmani S, Ahmed N, Marafi F, et al. Bertolotti syndrome demonstrated on 18F-NaF PET/CT. Clin Nucl Med 2017;42(6):480–2.

85. Usmani S, Ahmed N, Marafi F, et al. 18)F-sodium fluoride bone PET-CT in symptomatic lumbosacral transitional vertebra. Clin Radiol 2020;75(8):643. e1-10.

86. Koh YG, Jung KH, Hong HT, et al. Optimal design of patient-specific total knee arthroplasty for improvement in wear performance. J Clin Med 2019;8(11):2023.

87. Tzatzairis T, Fiska A, Ververidis A, et al. Minimally invasive versus conventional approaches in total knee replacement/arthroplasty: a review of the literature. J Orthop 2018;15(2):459–66.

88. Markes AR, Cheung E, Ma CB. Failed reverse shoulder arthroplasty and recommendations for revision. Curr Rev Musculoskelet Med 2020;13(1): 1–10.

89. Kwak JM, Koh KH, Jeon IH. Total elbow arthroplasty: clinical outcomes, complications, and revision surgery. Clin Orthop Surg 2019;11(4):369–79.

90. Chalmers PN, Boileau P, Romeo AA, et al. Revision reverse shoulder arthroplasty. J Am Acad Orthop Surg 2019;27(12):426–36.

91. Deshmukh S, Omar IM. Imaging of hip arthroplasties: normal findings and hardware complications. Semin Musculoskelet Radiol 2019;23(2):162–76.

92. Niccoli G, Mercurio D, Cortese F. Bone scan in painful knee arthroplasty: obsolete or actual examination? Acta Biomed 2017;88(2S):68–77.

93. Van den Wyngaert T, Paycha F, Strobel K, et al. SPECT/CT in postoperative painful hip arthroplasty. Semin Nucl Med 2018;48(5):425–38.

94. Thelu-Vanysacker M, Frederic P, Charles-Edouard T, et al. SPECT/CT in postoperative shoulder pain. Semin Nucl Med 2018;48(5):469–82.

95. Palestro CJ, Love C. Role of nuclear medicine for diagnosing infection of recently implanted lower

extremity arthroplasties. Semin Nucl Med 2017; 47(6):630–8.

96. Yue B, Tang T. The use of nuclear imaging for the diagnosis of periprosthetic infection after knee and hip arthroplasties. Nucl Med Commun 2015; 36(4):305–11.

97. Ullmark G, Sorensen J, Nilsson O, et al. Bone mineralisation adjacent to cemented and uncemented acetabular cups: analysis by [18F]-fluoride-PET in a randomised clinical trial. Hip Int 2020;30(6): 745–51.

98. Tezuka T, Kobayashi N, Hyonmin C, et al. Influence of hydroxyapatite coating for the prevention of bone mineral density loss and bone metabolism after total hip arthroplasty: assessment using (18)F-fluoride positron emission tomography and dual-energy X-ray absorptiometry by randomized controlled trial. Biomed Res Int 2020;2020:4154290.

99. Ullmark G. Occult hip prosthetic loosening diagnosed by [18F] Fluoride-PET/CT. Arthroplast Today 2020;6(3):548–51.

100. Nyström A, Kiritopoulos D, Ullmark G, et al. Denosumab prevents early periprosthetic bone loss after uncemented total hip arthroplasty: results from a randomized placebo-controlled clinical trial. J Bone Miner Res 2020;35(2):239–47.

101. Ullmark G, Sorensen J, Maripuu E, et al. Fingerprint pattern of bone mineralisation on cemented and uncemented femoral stems: analysis by [18F]-fluoride-PET in a randomised clinical trial. Hip Int 2019;29(6):609–17.

102. Kumar R, Kumar R, Kumar V, et al. Potential clinical implication of (18) F-FDG PET/CT in diagnosis of periprosthetic infection and its comparison with (18) F-Fluoride PET/CT. J Med Imaging Radiat Oncol 2016;60(3):315–22.

103. Kumar R, Kumar R, Kumar V, et al. Comparative analysis of dual-phase 18F-fluoride PET/CT and three phase bone scintigraphy in the evaluation of septic (or painful) hip prostheses: a prospective study. J Orthop Sci 2016;21(2):205–10.

104. Bernstein P, Beuthien-Baumann B, Kotzerke J, et al. Periacetabular bone metabolism following hip revision surgery. PET-based evaluation of allograft osteointegration. Nuklearmedizin 2014;53(4): 147–54.

105. Ullmark G, Nilsson O, Maripuu E, et al. Analysis of bone mineralization on uncemented femoral stems by [18F]-fluoride-PET: a randomized clinical study of 16 hips in 8 patients. Acta Orthop 2013;84(2): 138–44.

106. Ullmark G, Sorensen J, Nilsson O. Analysis of bone formation on porous and calcium phosphate-coated acetabular cups: a randomised clinical [18F]fluoride PET study. Hip Int 2012;22(2):172–8.

107. Ullmark G, Sundgren K, Milbrink J, et al. Metabolic development of necrotic bone in the femoral head

following resurfacing arthroplasty. A clinical [18F] fluoride-PET study in 11 asymptomatic hips. Acta Orthop 2012;83(1):22–5.

108. Choe H, Inaba Y, Kobayashi N, et al. Use of 18F-fluoride PET to determine the appropriate tissue sampling region for improved sensitivity of tissue examinations in cases of suspected periprosthetic infection after total hip arthroplasty. Acta Orthop 2011;82(4):427–32.

109. Kobayashi N, Inaba Y, Choe H, et al. Use of F-18 fluoride PET to differentiate septic from aseptic loosening in total hip arthroplasty patients. Clin Nucl Med 2011;36(11):e156–61.

110. Ullmark G, Sundgren K, Milbrink J, et al. Femoral head viability following resurfacing arthroplasty. A clinical positron emission tomography study. Hip Int 2011;21(1):66–70.

111. Kuo J, Foster C, Shelton D. Particle disease on fluoride-18 (NaF) PET/CT imaging. J Radiol Case Rep 2011;5(5):24–30.

112. Zoccali C, Teori G, Salducca N. The role of FDG-PET in distinguishing between septic and aseptic loosening in hip prosthesis: a review of literature. Int Orthop 2009;33(1):1–5.

113. Ullmark G, Sorensen J, Nilsson O. Bone healing of severe acetabular defects after revision arthroplasty. Acta Orthop 2009;80(2):179–83.

114. Ullmark G, Sundgren K, Milbrink J, et al. Osteonecrosis following resurfacing arthroplasty. Acta Orthop 2009;80(6):670–4.

115. Temmerman OP, Raijmakers PG, Heyligers IC, et al. Bone metabolism after total hip revision surgery with impacted grafting: evaluation using H2 15O and [18F]fluoride PET; a pilot study. Mol Imaging Biol 2008;10(5):288–93.

116. Ullmark G, Sorensen J, Langstrom B, et al. Bone regeneration 6 years after impaction bone grafting: a PET analysis. Acta Orthop 2007;78(2):201–5.

117. Forrest N, Welch A, Murray AD, et al. Femoral head viability after Birmingham resurfacing hip arthroplasty: assessment with use of [18F] fluoride positron emission tomography. J Bone Joint Surg Am 2006;88(Suppl 3):84–9.

118. Sorensen J, Ullmark G, Langstrom B, et al. Rapid bone and blood flow formation in impacted morselized allografts: positron emission tomography (PET) studies on allografts in 5 femoral component revisions of total hip arthroplasty. Acta Orthop Scand 2003;74(6):633–43.

119. Piert M, Winter E, Becker GA, et al. Allogenic bone graft viability after hip revision arthroplasty assessed by dynamic [18F]fluoride ion positron emission tomography. Eur J Nucl Med 1999;26(6): 615–24.

120. Li Y, Schiepers C, Lake R, et al. Clinical utility of (18)F-fluoride PET/CT in benign and malignant bone diseases. Bone 2012;50(1):128–39.

121. Hochreiter J, Mattiassich G, Hitzl W, et al. Quantitative in vivo assessment of bone allograft viability using (18)F-fluoride PET/CT after glenoid augmentation in reverse shoulder arthroplasty: a pilot study. Eur J Orthop Surg Traumatol 2019;29(7):1399–404.

122. Dyke JP, Garfinkel JH, Volpert L, et al. Imaging of bone perfusion and metabolism in subjects Undergoing total ankle arthroplasty using (18)F-fluoride positron emission tomography. Foot Ankle Int 2019;40(12):1351–7.

123. Koob S, Gaertner FC, Jansen TR, et al. Diagnosis of peri-prosthetic loosening of total hip and knee arthroplasty using (18)F-Fluoride PET/CT. Oncotarget 2019;10(22):2203–11.

124. Son HJ, Jeong YJ, Yoon HJ, et al. Visual pattern and serial quantitation of (18)F-Sodium Fluoride PET/CT in asymptomatic patients after hip and knee arthroplasty. Nucl Med Mol Imaging 2016; 50(4):308–21.

125. Sterner T, Pink R, Freudenberg L, et al. The role of [18F]fluoride positron emission tomography in the early detection of aseptic loosening of total knee arthroplasty. Int J Surg 2007;5(2):99–104.

126. Constantinescu CM, Jacobsen MK, Gerke O, et al. Fusion and healing prediction in posterolateral spinal fusion using (18)F-Sodium Fluoride-PET/CT. Diagnostics (Basel) 2020;10(4):226.

127. Pouldar D, Bakshian S, Matthews R, et al. Utility of 18F sodium fluoride PET/CT imaging in the evaluation of postoperative pain following surgical spine fusion. Musculoskelet Surg 2017;101(2): 159–66.

128. Seifen T, Rodrigues M, Rettenbacher L, et al. The value of (18)F-fluoride PET/CT in the assessment of screw loosening in patients after intervertebral fusion stabilization. Eur J Nucl Med Mol Imaging 2015;42(2):272–7.

129. Peters M, Willems P, Weijers R, et al. Pseudarthrosis after lumbar spinal fusion: the role of (1)(8)F-fluoride PET/CT. Eur J Nucl Med Mol Imaging 2015;42(12):1891–8.

130. Peters MJ, Wierts R, Jutten EM, et al. Evaluation of a short dynamic 18F-fluoride PET/CT scanning method to assess bone metabolic activity in spinal orthopedics. Ann Nucl Med 2015;29(9):799–809.

131. Quon A, Dodd R, Iagaru A, et al. Initial investigation of (1)(8)F-NaF PET/CT for identification of vertebral sites amenable to surgical revision after spinal fusion surgery. Eur J Nucl Med Mol Imaging 2012;39(11):1737–44.

132. Fischer DR, Zweifel K, Treyer V, et al. Assessment of successful incorporation of cages after cervical or lumbar intercorporal fusion with [(18)F]fluoride positron-emission tomography/computed tomography. Eur Spine J 2011;20(4):640–8.

133. Pumberger M, Prasad V, Druschel C, et al. Quantitative in vivo fusion assessment by (18)F-fluoride PET/CT following en bloc spondylectomy. Eur Spine J 2016;25(3):836–42.

134. Sanchez-Crespo A, Christiansson F, Thur CK, et al. Predictive value of [(18)F]-fluoride PET for monitoring bone remodeling in patients with orthopedic conditions treated with a Taylor spatial frame. Eur J Nucl Med Mol Imaging 2017;44(3):441–8.

135. Sorensen J, Michaelsson K, Strand H, et al. Long-standing increased bone turnover at the fixation points after anterior cruciate ligament reconstruction: a positron emission tomography (PET) study of 8 patients. Acta Orthop 2006;77(6):921–5.

136. Schiepers C, Broos P, Miserez M, et al. Measurement of skeletal flow with positron emission tomography and 18F-fluoride in femoral head osteonecrosis. Arch Orthop Trauma Surg 1998; 118(3):131–5.

137. Dasa V, Adbel-Nabi H, Anders MJ, et al. F-18 fluoride positron emission tomography of the hip for osteonecrosis. Clin Orthop Relat Res 2008;466(5): 1081–6.

138. Christersson A, Larsson S, Sorensen J. Presurgical localization of infected avascular bone segments in chronic complicated posttraumatic osteomyelitis in the lower extremity using dual-tracer PET/CT. EJNMMI Res 2018;8(1):65.

139. Akkawi I, Zmerly H. Osteoporosis: current concepts. Joints 2018;6(2):122–7.

140. Sozen T, Ozisik L, Basaran NC. An overview and management of osteoporosis. Eur J Rheumatol 2017;4(1):46–56.

141. Pennington Z, Ehresman J, Lubelski D, et al. Assessing underlying bone quality in spine surgery patients: a narrative review of dual-energy X-ray absorptiometry (DXA) and alternatives. Spine J 2020. https://doi.org/10.1016/j.spinee.2020.08.020.

142. Albano D, Agnollitto PM, Petrini M, et al. Operator-Related Errors and Pitfalls in Dual Energy X-ray absorptiometry: how to recognize and avoid them. Acad Radiol 2020. https://doi.org/10.1016/j.acra.2020.07.028.

143. Choksi P, Jepsen KJ, Clines GA. The challenges of diagnosing osteoporosis and the limitations of currently available tools. Clin Diabetes Endocrinol 2018;4:12.

144. Kinoshita H, Tamaki T, Hashimoto T, et al. Factors influencing lumbar spine bone mineral density assessment by dual-energy X-ray absorptiometry: comparison with lumbar spinal radiogram. J Orthop Sci 1998;3(1):3–9.

145. Frost ML, Blake GM, Fogelman I. (18)F-Fluoride PET in osteoporosis. PET Clin 2010;5(3):259–74.

146. Zhang V, Koa B, Borja AJ, et al. Diagnosis and monitoring of osteoporosis with total-body (18)F-sodium fluoride-PET/CT. PET Clin 2020;15(4):487–96.

147. Reilly CC, Raynor WY, Hong AL, et al. Diagnosis and monitoring of osteoporosis with (18)F-Sodium

Fluoride PET: an unavoidable path for the foreseeable future. Semin Nucl Med 2018;48(6):535–40.

148. Piert M, Zittel TT, Becker GA, et al. Assessment of porcine bone metabolism by dynamic. J Nucl Med 2001;42(7):1091–100.

149. Jassel IS, Siddique M, Frost ML, et al. The influence of CT and dual-energy X-ray absorptiometry (DXA) bone density on quantitative [(18)F] sodium fluoride PET. Quant Imaging Med Surg 2019;9(2):201–9.

150. Frost ML, Blake GM, Park-Holohan SJ, et al. Long-term precision of 18F-fluoride PET skeletal kinetic studies in the assessment of bone metabolism. J Nucl Med 2008;49(5):700–7.

151. Uchida K, Nakajima H, Miyazaki T, et al. Effects of alendronate on bone metabolism in glucocorticoid-induced osteoporosis measured by 18F-fluoride PET: a prospective study. J Nucl Med 2009;50(11):1808–14.

152. Frost ML, Fogelman I, Blake GM, et al. Dissociation between global markers of bone formation and direct measurement of spinal bone formation in osteoporosis. J Bone Miner Res 2004;19(11):1797–804.

153. Berding G, Kirchhoff TD, Burchert W, et al. [18F] fluoride PET indicates reduced bone formation in severe glucocorticoid-induced osteoporosis. Nuklearmedizin 1998;37(2):76–9.

154. Rhodes S, Batzdorf A, Sorci O, et al. Assessment of femoral neck bone metabolism using (18)F-sodium fluoride PET/CT imaging. Bone 2020;136:115351.

155. Win AZ, Aparici CM. Normal SUV values measured from NaF18- PET/CT bone scan studies. PLoS One 2014;9(9):e108429.

156. Frost ML, Moore AE, Siddique M, et al. (1)(8)F-fluoride PET as a noninvasive imaging biomarker for determining treatment efficacy of bone active agents at the hip: a prospective, randomized, controlled clinical study. J Bone Miner Res 2013;28(6):1337–47.

157. Frost ML, Blake GM, Cook GJ, et al. Differences in regional bone perfusion and turnover between lumbar spine and distal humerus: (18)F-fluoride PET study of treatment-naive and treated postmenopausal women. Bone 2009;45(5):942–8.

158. Frost ML, Cook GJ, Blake GM, et al. The relationship between regional bone turnover measured using 18F-fluoride positron emission tomography and changes in BMD is equivalent to that seen for biochemical markers of bone turnover. J Clin Densitom 2007;10(1):46–54.

159. Frost ML, Cook GJ, Blake GM, et al. A prospective study of risedronate on regional bone metabolism and blood flow at the lumbar spine measured by 18F-fluoride positron emission tomography. J Bone Miner Res 2003;18(12):2215–22.

160. Frost ML, Siddique M, Blake GM, et al. Regional bone metabolism at the lumbar spine and hip following discontinuation of alendronate and risedronate treatment in postmenopausal women. Osteoporos Int 2012;23(8):2107–16.

161. Frost ML, Siddique M, Blake GM, et al. Differential effects of teriparatide on regional bone formation using (18)F-fluoride positron emission tomography. J Bone Miner Res 2011;26(5):1002–11.

162. Aaltonen L, Koivuviita N, Seppanen M, et al. Correlation between (18)F-Sodium Fluoride positron emission tomography and bone histomorphometry in dialysis patients. Bone 2020;134:115267.

163. Cucchi F, Simonsen L, Abild-Nielsen AG, et al. 18F-Sodium fluoride PET/CT in paget disease. Clin Nucl Med 2017;42(7):553–4.

164. Derlin T, Weiberg D, Sohns JM. Multitracer molecular imaging of paget disease targeting bone remodeling, fatty acid metabolism, and PSMA expression on PET/CT. Clin Nucl Med 2016;41(12):991–2.

165. Frost ML, Compston JE, Goldsmith D, et al. (18)F-fluoride positron emission tomography measurements of regional bone formation in hemodialysis patients with suspected adynamic bone disease. Calcif Tissue Int 2013;93(5):436–47.

166. Installe J, Nzeusseu A, Bol A, et al. (18)F-fluoride PET for monitoring therapeutic response in Paget's disease of bone. J Nucl Med 2005;46(10):1650–8.

167. Messa C, Goodman WG, Hoh CK, et al. Bone metabolic activity measured with positron emission tomography and [18F]fluoride ion in renal osteodystrophy: correlation with bone histomorphometry. J Clin Endocrinol Metab 1993;77(4):949–55.

168. Kim Y, Lee HY, Yoon HJ, et al. Utility of 18F-fluorodeoxy glucose and 18F-sodium fluoride positron emission tomography/computed tomography in the diagnosis of medication-related osteonecrosis of the jaw: a preclinical study in a rat model. J Craniomaxillofac Surg 2016;44(4):357–63.

169. Kubota S, Inaba Y, Kobayashi N, et al. Prediction of femoral head collapse in osteonecrosis using 18F-fluoride positron emission tomography. Nucl Med Commun 2015;36(6):596–603.

170. Guggenberger R, Fischer DR, Metzler P, et al. Bisphosphonate-induced osteonecrosis of the jaw: comparison of disease extent on contrast-enhanced MR imaging, [18F] fluoride PET/CT, and conebeam CT imaging. AJNR Am J Neuroradiol 2013;34(6):1242–7.

171. Gayana S, Bhattacharya A, Kashyap R, et al. (18)F-fluoride PET/CT in avascular necrosis of the femoral head. Clin Nucl Med 2013;38(6):e265–6.

172. Aratake M, Yoshifumi T, Takahashi A, et al. Evaluation of lesion in a spontaneous osteonecrosis of the knee using 18F-fluoride positron emission tomography. Knee Surg Sports Traumatol Arthrosc 2009;17(1):53–9.

173. van der Bruggen W, Hagelstein-Rotman M, de Geus-Oei LF, et al. Quantifying skeletal burden in fibrous dysplasia using sodium fluoride PET/CT. Eur J Nucl Med Mol Imaging 2020;47(6):1527–37.

174. Lee H, Lee KS, Lee WW. 18F-NaF PET/CT findings in fibrous dysplasia. Clin Nucl Med 2015;40(11):912–4.

175. Waterval JJ, Vallinga M, Brans B, et al. 18F-fluoride PET/CT scan for quantification of bone metabolism in the inner ear in patients with otosclerosis–a pilot study. Clin Nucl Med 2013;38(9):677–85.

176. Bhure U, Roos JE, Strobel K. Osteoid osteoma: multimodality imaging with focus on hybrid imaging. Eur J Nucl Med Mol Imaging 2019;46(4):1019–36.

177. Seniaray N, Jain A. Osteoid osteoma mimicking inflammatory synovitis. Indian J Nucl Med 2017; 32(3):194–7.

178. Batouli A, Gholamrezanezhad A, Petrov D, et al. Management of primary osseous spinal tumors with PET. PET Clin 2019;14(1):91–101.

179. Broadhead ML, Lokmic Z, Tan ML, et al. Applying advanced imaging techniques to a murine model of orthotopic osteosarcoma. Front Surg 2015;2:36.

180. Campanile C, Arlt MJ, Kramer SD, et al. Characterization of different osteosarcoma phenotypes by PET imaging in preclinical animal models. J Nucl Med 2013;54(8):1362–8.

181. Franzius C, Hotfilder M, Poremba C, et al. Successful high-resolution animal positron emission tomography of human Ewing tumours and their metastases in a murine xenograft model. Eur J Nucl Med Mol Imaging 2006;33(12):1432–41.

182. Brenner W, Bohuslavizki KH, Eary JF. PET imaging of osteosarcoma. J Nucl Med 2003;44(6):930–42.

183. Usmani S, Marafi F, Rasheed R, et al. Unsuspected metastases to muscles in osteosarcoma detected on 18F-Sodium Fluoride PET-CT. Clin Nucl Med 2018;43(9):e343–5.

184. Chou YH, Ko KY, Cheng MF, et al. 18F-NaF PET/CT images of cardiac metastasis from osteosarcoma. Clin Nucl Med 2016;41(9):708–9.

185. Tse N, Hoh C, Hawkins R, et al. Positron emission tomography diagnosis of pulmonary metastases in osteogenic sarcoma. Am J Clin Oncol 1994; 17(1):22–5.

186. Brunkhorst T, Boerner AR, Bergh S, et al. Pretherapeutic assessment of tumour metabolism using a dual tracer PET technique. Eur J Nucl Med Mol Imaging 2002;29(10):1416.

187. Caoduro C, Ungureanu CM, Rudenko B, et al. 18F-fluoride PET/CT aspect of an unusual case of Erdheim-Chester disease with histologic features of Langerhans cell histiocytosis. Clin Nucl Med 2013;38(7):541–2.

188. Liu H, Chen Y, Yang L, et al. 18F-NaF uptake in retroperitoneal neurofibroma and uterine leiomyoma calcifications. Clin Nucl Med 2019;44(12): 991–2.

189. Woodhead GJ, Avery RJ, Kuo PH. Atlas of extraosseous findings detected by 18F-NaF PET/CT bone scan. Clin Nucl Med 2017;42(12):930–8.

190. Kothekar E, Raynor WY, Werner TJ, et al. 18F-NaF uptake in calcified uterine leiomyoma. Clin Nucl Med 2019;44(11):e620–1.

191. Al-Zaghal A, Werner TJ, Hoilund-Carlsen PF, et al. The detection of uterine leiomyoma (fibroid) calcifications on 18F-NaF PET/CT. Clin Nucl Med 2018; 43(8):e287–8.

192. Zhu Y, Chen Y, Huang Z, et al. Unsuspected metastatic ovarian cancer revealed by 18F-NaF PET/CT performed to evaluate lower-back pain. Clin Nucl Med 2017;42(2):154–6.

193. Shao F, Zou Y, Cai L, et al. Unexpected detection of urinary bladder cancer on dual phase 18F-NaF PET/CT in a patient with back pain. Clin Nucl Med 2016;41(11):902–4.

194. Ishimura M, Yamamoto Y, Mitamura K, et al. A case of glioblastoma with calcified region imaged with 18F-NaF PET/CT. Clin Nucl Med 2018;43(10):764–5.

195. Duarte PS, Marin JFG, De Carvalho JWA, et al. Brain metastasis of medullary thyroid carcinoma without macroscopic calcification detected first on 68Ga-dotatate and then on 18F-fluoride PET/CT. Clin Nucl Med 2018;43(8):623–4.

196. Sarikaya I, Sharma P, Sarikaya A. F-18 fluoride uptake in primary breast cancer. Ann Nucl Med 2018; 32(10):678–86.

197. Kothekar E, Raynor WY, Al-Zaghal A, et al. Incidental 18F-NaF uptake in drug-induced gynecomastia. Clin Nucl Med 2019;44(4):e303–4.

198. Usmani S, Marafi F, Al Kandari F, et al. Normal Variant 18F-sodium fluoride uptake in the falx cerebri ossification. Clin Nucl Med 2019;44(10):804–5.

199. Al-Zaghal A, Mehdizadeh Seraj S, Werner TJ, et al. Assessment of physiological intracranial calcification in healthy adults using (18)F-NaF PET/CT. J Nucl Med 2018. https://doi.org/10.2967/jnumed. 118.213678.

200. Seraj SM, Al-Zaghal A, Ostergaard B, et al. Identification of heterotopic ossification using 18F-NaF PET/CT. Clin Nucl Med 2019;44(4):319–20.

201. Shao F, Zhang S, Qi C, et al. Diffuse increased sodium fluoride gastric activity in a patient with hypercalcemia. Clin Nucl Med 2017;42(9):711–3.

202. Zhang W, Chen L, Wan Q, et al. 18F-NaF PET/CT finding in a patient with abdominal discomfort after schistosomiasis. Clin Nucl Med 2018;43(3):183–5.

203. Raynor WY, Borja AJ, Rojulpote C, et al. (18)F-sodium fluoride: an emerging tracer to assess active vascular microcalcification. J Nucl Cardiol 2020. https://doi.org/10.1007/s12350-020-02138-9.

204. Hoilund-Carlsen PF, Sturek M, Alavi A, et al. Atherosclerosis imaging with (18)F-sodium fluoride PET: state-of-the-art review. Eur J Nucl Med Mol Imaging 2020;47(6):1538–51.

Moving?

Make sure your subscription moves with you!

To notify us of your new address, find your **Clinics Account Number** (located on your mailing label above your name), and contact customer service at:

Email: journalscustomerservice-usa@elsevier.com

800-654-2452 (subscribers in the U.S. & Canada)
314-447-8871 (subscribers outside of the U.S. & Canada)

Fax number: 314-447-8029

Elsevier Health Sciences Division
Subscription Customer Service
3251 Riverport Lane
Maryland Heights, MO 63043

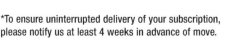

*To ensure uninterrupted delivery of your subscription, please notify us at least 4 weeks in advance of move.

ELSEVIER